Basic Gastro-enterology

Basic Gastro-enterology

including Diseases of the Liver

J. M. Naish M.D., F.R.C.P.
Consultant Physician, Frenchay Hospital, Bristol
Lecturer in Medicine, University of Bristol

and

Alan E. Read M.D., F.R.C.P.
Professor of Medicine, University of Bristol

with Chapters by

L. R. Celestin F.R.C.S.
Consultant Gastro-enterological Surgeon, Frenchay Hospital, Bristol
and
K. T. Evans F.R.C.P., F.F.R.
Professor of Radiodiagnosis, Welsh National School of Medicine, Cardiff

SECOND EDITION

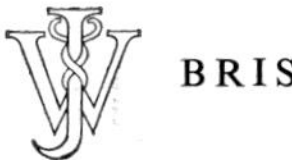 BRISTOL: JOHN WRIGHT & SONS LTD

First edition 1965
Second edition 1974

ISBN 0 7236 0346 4

Printed in Great Britain by John Wright & Sons Ltd., at The Stonebridge Press, Bristol

PREFACE

THE PRACTICE of gastro-enterology as a speciality has become much more widespread in Europe since the first edition of this book appeared. Within this speciality the frontiers of knowledge are steadily being driven outwards by teams of clinicians and scientists who concentrate on one aspect of the fundamental problems yet unsolved. The speciality is ever more popular with the young physician and scientist, and the tendency for some surgeons and radiologists to make gastro-enterology their special field of interest is also increasing. International working groups and subspeciality organizations are proliferating.

Against this background of accelerating advance we have attempted to rewrite and recast this volume, which we hope will remain, as before, an introduction to the fundamentals of the subject. Sadly, we pay tribute to the late Mr. T. J. Butler whose contributions to the first edition were so important. His successor in the hospital field, Mr. L. R. Celestin, has joined us in the production of this edition, and he has been able to use the same framework for the surgical chapters as T. J. Butler thought appropriate. The authors would like to record their gratitude to Dr. John Morris for his helpful criticism of the manuscript.

J. M. N.
A. E. R.

CONTENTS

Chapter 1

The Nervous System
and the Gastro-intestinal Tract

THIS COMPLEX subject must be introduced early, because to understand specific diseases and organ afflictions it is vital not only to appreciate the way in which the emotions may react upon those organs, but also to comprehend the importance of the functional derangements to which the alimentary tube is prone. Each organic disease must always be differentiated from the functional disturbance which mimics it, and each patient, whether his affliction is mainly structural or mainly functional, must be treated as a whole. Many patients with an organic disease actually suffer from the functional disturbances triggered by the organic disease.

Since patients do not die from them, the understanding of functional disorders is inhibited by the absence of pathological material. Knowledge is gained, not only from the experience of sufferers, but from animal experiments, the relevance of which may readily be doubted. The physiologist usually designs his experiments with organs which purposely have been detached from their normal regulatory device, the emotions. Experiments on human volunteers, or on patients whose organs have been exposed at operation, often throw light on the disorders (as distinct from the diseases) of the gut, but it must be confessed that knowledge is derived mainly from clinical experience. For these reasons the subject is one which appeals more to the practising doctor than to the student. The latter, working amongst the unrepresentative patient population of a hospital, is often unaware of the magnitude of the problem and the gaps in our knowledge, but later when his responsibilities are wide he will thirst to know more. This, therefore, must be a short introduction to a very big problem.

AETIOLOGY

To a large extent everyone is subject to nervous disorders of the gut. Few students can have escaped pre-examination nausea, few athletes pre-race diarrhoea. If the stimulus to gut disorder, whether it be fear, rage, or sexual excitement, is easily recognized by the sufferer, he will accept it. But if the emotional cause of his discomforts is not obvious to him, and if it continues, then he will feel ill.

This is the simplest concept, but behind environmental stress lies the constitution. Some people are born with such delicately tuned autonomic systems that 'the agitations of the soul communicate themselves directly to the body'. Alvarez (1956) tells the story of a man who dearly loved to play poker, but so intense were his reactions that when he drew a full house his face flushed and he often vomited. Another patient had diarrhoea not only after food but at the sight or sound of food. When walking in the town he had to cross the street to avoid restaurants, smells from which would provoke urgent defaecation. Yet another story concerns a girl who, when a proposal of marriage was made to her in a restaurant, promptly vomited. Her would-be husband was so upset by this that he did not dare to mention the subject again for a year!

Given, then, a finely adjusted nervous system and some physical or nervous stress, unpleasant symptoms rapidly assume the character of an illness. If, in addition, the patient becomes worried over the meaning of the symptoms, perhaps fearing cancer, the condition will become intractable. Alternatively, the patient quite subconsciously may find in the symptoms and consequent invalidism a way of escape from an intolerable emotional situation, and then again chronicity ensues.

There is certain experimental evidence which illustrates the workings of emotion on the gut. In animals under local anaesthesia, gut movements can be seen to be influenced by a variety of external stimuli, but section of the autonomic nerve supply abolishes these effects. In humans observed under the X-ray screen the pyloric valve mechanism is inhibited by fear and the stomach will not empty. Changes of mucosal colour and motility in response to emotion have been observed in the colon and stomach. Anxiety has been shown to produce strong non-propulsive contractions of the colon and constipation. Anxiety will make the mouth dry and the breath offensive.

It is easier to understand some of the mechanisms whereby disorders such as nausea, vomiting, abdominal cramps, diarrhoea, and constipation are caused than it is to understand how stress may cause a peptic ulcer to bleed or colitis to 'flare'. Aetiological concepts of psychosomatic disease are nebulous and rudimentary.

CLINICAL PICTURE
(Fig. 1)

Some of the gastro-intestinal manifestations of the neuroses can be summarized as follows:

1. *Anxiety State*
   Due to:
   a. Simple anxiety over a situation
   b. Neurotic or excessive anxiety
   c. Nosophobia (fear of certain diseases)
   SYMPTOMS IN GASTRO-INTESTINAL TRACT
   Dry mouth and foul breath
   Intestinal colic and rumbling

Nausea and heartburn
Discomfort after food
Spastic constipation or diarrhoea

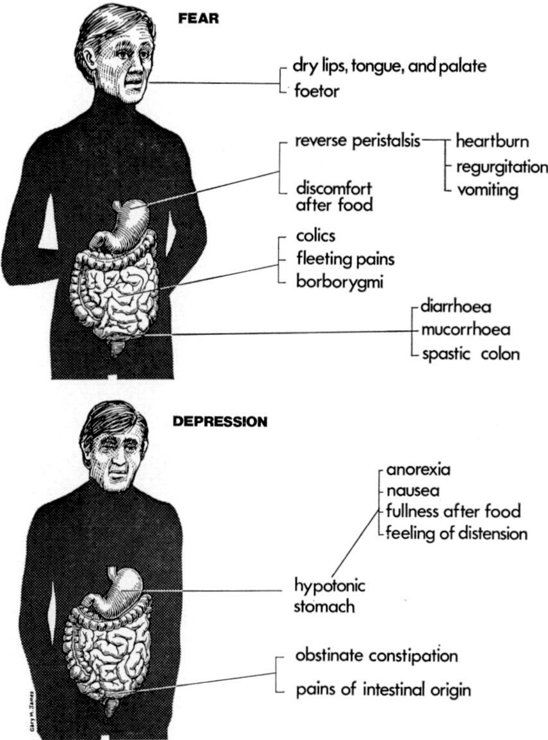

Fig. 1. Gastro-intestinal symptoms due to fear and depression.

2. *Depression*
   Due to:
   a. Undermining physical disease
   b. Emotional stress
   c. Endogenous
   SYMPTOMS IN GASTRO-INTESTINAL TRACT
   Loss of appetite and weight
   Nausea and food discomfort
   Constipation
   Conviction that serious organic disease is present

3. *Obsessional States*
   SYMPTOMS
   Bad breath and dirty tongue
   Food fads and dietary invalidism

Abdominal bloating and alleged distension with constipation
Diarrhoea which prevents social activities
Fixed conviction about poisoning, 'germs', etc.

In addition to the manifestations of fear, anxiety, depression, and obsession, there are a number of other reasons for gastro-intestinal distress which are not caused by structural disease. They can be grouped as follows:

A. *Constitutional Inadequacy*

There are patients who continually develop symptoms as a result of minor stresses and disappointments. They have an 'over-awareness' of their autonomic processes. Usually they are more comfortable when leading a quiet and restricted life. There is a continually changing pattern of symptoms, amongst which feelings of distension, disorders of appetite, and dietary fads are prominent.

B. *Habit Errors*

Food bolting and *aerophagy* cause belching and feelings of distension in the epigastrium. *Over-purgation* may cause cramps, rumblings, nausea, and heartburn. *Smoking* may cause strong segmentation movements of the colon with reflex nausea, distension, and heartburn. Eating in noisy or worrying surroundings may cause the same group of symptoms.

C. *Self Injury*

Patients often try to manipulate their relatives, friends, or employers by utilizing the functional virtuosity of the gastro-intestinal tract. Self-induced vomiting causes alarm to the onlookers but rarely causes harm to the patient. The vomitus is not severe or copious and the patient's good general condition is in contrast with the emotional aura which surrounds the act of vomiting or its colourful description. *Anorexia nervosa* is a more serious condition mainly occurring in girls soon after the menarche. They are often rebelling against morally dominant mothers, and they reject the female role. This leads them to a horror of growing round and plump, and they therefore starve themselves to maintain their juvenility. They develop a horror of food, especially carbohydrates. Pituitary function declines as a result of the starvation and they cease to menstruate. Death may occur as a result of intercurrent infection such as gastro-enteritis, but the prognosis is not so serious as it was in the past. Seventy per cent get better within three years, and progress is hastened if they can be removed from the anxiety-laden atmosphere of their own home. However, it is often difficult to find those who are capable of taking responsibility for such difficult young women, and as the condition is essentially one in which the patient is trying to manipulate or punish her parents, they usually tend to return home to do so. In adult cases, vomiting rather than anorexia is the dominant feature.

Other manipulative disorders include the patients who go from hospital to hospital with simulated 'acute abdominal' symptoms in the hope of being operated upon. Others may eat glass, paper, or dirt (pica). Others again may develop rectal irritability and mucus diarrhoea whenever they have to go out or meet people. Thus they can retreat from responsibilities.

D. *Spasmodic Disorders*

Under this heading are included diseases which are essentially functional but which are not necessarily related to neurosis. Often there is a genetic predisposition, and organic changes may result from disordered motility patterns if they continue long enough. The best example of such a disease is the *irritable colon syndrome*, which is often linked to irritability and reflex disorders of other parts of the gastro-intestinal tract. Some patients with this condition may ultimately develop a hypertrophy of the circular muscle of the sigmoid colon, and possibly diverticular disease (*Chapter 20*). Similar types of neuromuscular disorders are encountered in the oesophagus, and here also diverticula may develop in time (*Chapter 3*). It must be remembered that irritability and disordered muscular activity of one part of the gut often set up reflex disturbances in another part. A good example of this is the heartburn due to oesophageal contractions which often accompanies irritable colon symptoms.

DIAGNOSIS

The experienced gastro-enterologist may often suspect, after the patient's opening remarks, that his symptoms are due to a functional disturbance. From then on he will modify his interview technique, no longer relying on the straight answer to a question. The reason for this change of tactic is that the emotionally disturbed patient is often unable to give a coherent account of his symptoms; thus attempts to pressure him will only give a false picture in the mind of the physician and will effectively cut him off from the patient's inward fears which are the root cause of his abdominal distress. Interviews of such patients should be leisurely and permissive, with the physician relaxed as the patient talks. If he 'dries up', his last few words should be repeated with interest and curiosity; 'you were saying?' is a useful phrase. It must be remembered that the diagnostic interview is often the first step in therapy, and for this reason it must proceed gently and skilfully. Gradually a pattern will emerge which will suggest one or other of the groups of conditions mentioned earlier.

There are two important guiding principles to be followed in the process of diagnosis.

First, we should not make a firm diagnosis of a purely functional disorder until organic disease has been excluded.

Secondly, we should not diagnose a condition as functional simply because we think that we have excluded organic disease. The diagnosis of a functional disorder must be firmly based on positive evidence which points to emotional involvement. For instance, we should look for:

1. A cause for anxiety or depression.
2. An insecure background with a history of nervous inadequacy.

3. A pattern of symptoms which suggests exaggeration or inhibition of normal function.

4. Symptoms too widespread to be accounted for by a structural disease. Lastly, though organic disease may exist, symptoms may be entirely due to functional disorders.

The first general principle raises a difficult question—how far to carry the process of investigation to exclude organic disease. In some cases it may be unnecessary to do more than a thorough physical examination, in other cases simple screening tests such as a haemoglobin estimation, E.S.R., and faecal occult blood-tests may be required. In all cases of dyspepsia with an element of nosophobia it is best to have a barium meal done. The whole question must be decided on the index of clinical suspicion. Thus, if the diagnosis appears clear and positive, no investigations are necessary, but if the four criteria of a functional disorder are not present and if the trend of clinical suspicion is towards organic disease, then a very meticulous and thorough investigation may be demanded. It should not be forgotten, however, that repeated investigations in the milieu of a large hospital are damaging to the frightened or neurotic patient, who needs, above all, confident diagnosis and firm management, with as few investigations as possible.

MANAGEMENT AND TREATMENT

The interview is from the first moment therapeutic so the physician must strive towards empathy throughout.

Correct diagnosis means that the doctor will already know much about the patient's background and personality, and from this knowledge will come his plan of treatment.

First, he must be prepared to spot the depressed patient. Although often agitated, these people are ill and may require the skilled guidance of a psychiatrist, who has at his command treatments ranging from benzodiazopines for the mildest cases, through imipramine, amitryptylline, and mono-amine oxidase inhibitors to electroconvulsive therapy and modified leucotomy. This is the one group of patients that should usually be referred to the psychiatrist. Most patients with emotionally induced functional disorders are best managed by the physician who first makes the diagnosis.

Where anxiety is the main feature, the aim is to uncover the real source of trouble in the patient's life, rather than to bewilder him with too many detailed questions about the localization and timing of his symptoms. It is thus often wise to ask the patient quite early in the interview to give his opinion as to the cause of his own trouble. He can be asked if he believes he has an ulcer or a growth; some will reply yes, and so uncover rather superficial fears; others will reply honestly that they do not think so, in which case the way will be open for the physician to explain the mechanisms by which functional misbehaviour of the gut can cause pain and distress, and later to probe further into the real source of the patient's unhappiness.

Steps in treatment are:

1. Careful explanation of body mechanisms so that the cause of the pain or discomfort can be understood by the patient as being due to misbehaviour rather than to disease of his gut.

2. The illustration of the effect of emotion on the gastro-intestinal tract by simple experiences which the patient can recall such as tightening of the throat from emotion; salivation when hungry; bowel action when frightened; anorexia when frightened.

3. Firm reassurance on the absence of structural disease.

4. The dispelling of false notions, such as that the trouble is due to food poisoning, a 'germ in the system', or an ulcer or growth.

5. The uncovering of suppressed or ill-understood fears, which are then related in the patient's mind to his own symptoms.

6. Choosing a remedy which will give the patient some relief from the main symptoms, for example antispasmodics for cramps and spastic colon symptoms; barbiturates for anxious people; salicylates or ergotamine for migraine equivalents; codeine phosphate for nervous diarrhoea.

See them again after an interval.

Seek to build up confidence in your ability to help them, so that tensions are relaxed. Once improvement is noted and admitted, further progress will be made automatically as the patient loses his irrational fears and tensions.

In the case of the constitutionally inadequate, the 'explaining away' and alleviation of one set of symptoms is often followed by the development of new ones. At moments when it seems to the physician that all his effort is wasted, it is well to recall that these patients, by 'offering' their symptoms, are in fact offering themselves. Withdrawal of support is no answer, and though the doctor may despair of his patient, the patient is much more deeply grateful to, and dependent on, the doctor than he realizes. The burden must be accepted and the time given.

Diet

Worried or depressed patients often cannot eat normal food without discomfort. Consequently they may become 'faddy' and attribute their troubles to certain foods. This may lead to self-conditioning so that in time a certain food will always make them feel worse. In advising about diet, the doctor's job is gently to dispel misconceptions, yet it would be foolish for him to advise steak and chips twice a day for a depressed patient with a poor appetite. One solution is to advise an elimination type of diet, starting with foodstuffs least likely to cause hypersensitive reactions, and then gradually to build on this. This is a method beloved of 'food allergists'. Though allergic reactions to certain foodstuffs (e.g., mushrooms, shellfish, eggs, milk) certainly do occur, unpleasant symptoms after specific foods may well be due to emotional self-conditioning.

'Harmless foods' include lamb, chicken, potatoes, rice, macaroni, semolina, arrowroot, honey, jelly, baked bread slices, and fruit juices. It is perfectly possible to construct a diet adequate in calories, vitamins, and minerals from these. As treatment and reassurance proceed the diet can be built up, leaving the addition of items containing cooked fat and coarse vegetables to the last.

PROGNOSIS

Prognosis varies as much as the symptoms. Simple anxiety and nosophobia can be cured most easily. Depressive illnesses are often intractable. Constitutionally inadequate people will always be with us.

As Alvarez says, there are people in life, and there are many of them, whom you will have to help as long as they live. The obsessionals, the food faddists, and the 'colono-centric' psychopaths will divide their time between the 'health colonies', the spas which specialize in colonic lavage, and a variety of quacks. The doctors have little chance and little hope of curing them.

SUMMARY

The whole gut is under autonomic nervous control, so emotion and stress will alter its smooth functional efficiency. Constitutionally, certain people seem to be more liable to develop uncomfortable patterns of gut behaviour, and, in some, gastro-intestinal activities are nearer to consciousness than in most. The interaction of constitutional proneness and emotional stress provokes discomforts and disabling symptoms. Diagnosis implies thorough knowledge of these root causes and mechanisms by both doctor and patient, and to the latter, understanding is therapeutic. Drugs of sedative, antispasmodic, and relaxant properties are used to alleviate symptoms, to promote confidence, to take the edge from anxiety, and the hopelessness from depression.

FURTHER READING

ALVAREZ, W. C. (1956), *Nervousness, Indigestion and Pain*. London: Staples Press.
BROWNE, K., and FREELING, P. (1967), *The Doctor-Patient Relationship*. Edinburgh: Livingstone.
PALMER, E. D. (1967), *Functional Gastro-intestinal Disease*. Baltimore: Williams & Wilkins.

Chapter 2

The Mouth and Salivary Glands

ONLY THOSE aspects of oral disease which reflect or cause disorders of the gastro-intestinal tract are of paramount interest to the gastro-enterologist, and it is these which form the subject of this chapter.

THE TONGUE IN HEALTH AND DISEASE

There are great variations in the appearance of the tongue and not all are significant of disease. Those changes not indicative of nutritional deficiency and not apparently caused by general diseases are listed below. They can present diagnostic problems and the patient may need to be assured of their benign nature.

1. Prominence of Fungiform Papillae

These show up as pink dots which stipple the tip and lateral borders, and, if set against a background of white fur, the appearance is described as a 'strawberry tongue'.

2. Denudation or Stripping of Filiform Papillae

a. Median rhomboid glossitis. This is a developmental anomaly which appears as a reddish diamond-shaped area in the centre of the dorsum of the tongue.

b. Benign migratory glossitis. This condition in which the lesions change their location from day to day and give the tongue a map-like appearance is known as a 'geographic tongue'.

3. White Fur

'Fur' is dead epithelium which has not yet separated from the lining surface, and in it are entangled yeasts and other saprophytes. It is prominent in those who are feverish or anorexic, for in such cases the tongue is insufficiently active for the fur to be rubbed off. In apparently healthy people the presence of an adherent fur is more difficult to explain, though it is more common in smokers. It seems to be a physically harmless state of affairs, but one which may nevertheless cause unnecessary mental anguish to an introspective or obsessional patient.

4. Black Hairy Tongue

This is due to overgrowth of the filiform papillae, and the cause is unknown. Occasionally those taking broad-spectrum antibiotics grow a black mould on the tongue.

5. Indentation of the Sides of the Tongue by the Teeth

This may be an innocent abnormality, but is also associated with various systemic disorders. It is found in vitamin B deficiency glossitis, uncontrolled diabetes, iron deficiency, and in myxoedema. Any condition in which the tongue becomes enlarged, including acute inflammatory involvement, may give rise to indentation.

6. Fissuring

This is the commonest developmental abnormality of the tongue and usually follows a symmetrical pattern. It is quite benign though sometimes associated with chronic glossitis or lingual atrophy.

CHANGES IN THE TONGUE INDICATIVE OF DISEASE OR NUTRITIONAL DEFICIENCY

Acute Superficial Glossitis

This is characterized by: (1) Excessive redness and sometimes by a deep magenta colour; (2) Atrophy of lingual epithelium; (3) Shrinkage of the tongue; (4) Fissuring.

The condition may be caused by mineral or enzyme deficiencies which interfere with epithelial regeneration, or by acute infections and physical damage to the surface of the tongue.

1. GLOSSITIS DUE TO NUTRITIONAL DEFICIENCY

Glossitis may be due to depleted body stores of: Iron; cyanocobalamin (vitamin B_{12}); folic acid; riboflavin; nicotinic acid (niacin); thiamin.

It is not usually possible to determine the type of deficiency from the appearance of the tongue, although riboflavin deficiency is said to cause a glossitis of deep purple colour—'magenta tongue'.

Both iron and riboflavin deficiency can cause angular stomatitis, and the latter causes roughening of the mucocutaneous junctions (cheilosis). Cyanocobalamin, thiamin, and nicotinic acid deficiencies may be associated with mental confusion, neurological abnormalities, or anaemia.

There are many gastro-intestinal disorders which can cause multiple nutritional deficiencies, and thus the symptoms and signs of acute superficial glossitis may draw attention to the underlying disease. Gastric mucosal atrophy, which leads to malabsorption of cyanocobalamin, can be responsible for depleted body stores of that vitamin, the earliest manifestation of which may in some patients be sore tongue. This may be noticeable for some years before anaemia is apparent, although in such cases megaloblastic erythropoiesis can usually be detected in the marrow, and the serum vitamin B_{12} level is always low. Similarly, the patient with coeliac disease may notice little change of bowel habit at a time when malabsorption of both iron and folic acid is causing acute glossitis. The reddest and sorest tongues of all are found in those with gastro-jejunocolic fistula and other forms of spontaneous enterocolic fistulae.

Acute glossitis due to deficiency can be cured by repletion of the body stores of either iron or the missing vitamins, but so often it is impossible to tell which particular deficiency is responsible for the glossitis. Parenteral administration of vitamin B complex, with or without oral folic acid and iron, is necessary in most types of malabsorption, but parenteral vitamin B_{12} is necessary in ileal lesions and various blind-loop syndromes.

If a deficiency is of long standing, as, for instance, in chronic sideropenia or untreated vitamin B_{12} deficiency, the tongue may become generally shrunken and fissured, and the mucosa, which becomes incapable of specialized regeneration, remains smooth and atrophic even after treatment.

2. ACUTE SUPERFICIAL GLOSSITIS DUE TO INFECTION AND TRAUMA

This may be due to: (*a*) Irritation by drugs and oral antibiotics; (*b*) Local irritation by sharp tooth edges, dental calculus, and faulty prosthetic appliances. These cause bad 'tongue habits' which keep the glossitis active. Contact allergy from lipstick or toothpaste is a rare cause of glossitis; (*c*) A dry mouth and metabolic changes in untreated diabetes mellitus; (*d*) The failure of salivary flow, as in Sjögren's disease; (*e*) Part of a generalized stomatitis. This is particularly common in elderly people suffering from general infections.

Acute glossitis may occur without any clearly defined cause, but in these cases any source of local irritation should be removed, and a search made for intestinal deficiencies which can be corrected. Patients may complain of painful or burning sensations on the tongue without apparent clinical changes. In vitamin B_{12} deficiency such sensations may precede visible lesions of the tongue or marked anaemia. Thus, all such patients should be investigated carefully before considering a psychogenic origin. Many patients prove in the end to have psychological problems.

Other Diffuse Conditions of the Tongue

The tongue is larger than normal in acromegaly and in many cases of primary amyloidosis. A dry tongue may call attention to dehydration, mouth breathing, or hyperpnoea. In uraemic states, all three factors combine to make the tongue dry and wrinkled and to be covered with a brown fur.

Local Lesions of the Tongue

These rarely cause or relate to disease of the gastro-intestinal tract, and the subject is well covered in textbooks of surgery and surgical pathology. Ulcers or malignant growths of the tongue may, when very advanced, interfere with appetite and digestion, but as a rule patients seek attention long before this stage is reached. Leucoplakia characterized by deformity and metaplasia of the lingual epithelium is a rare but visible example of a premalignant condition.

THE TEETH AND GUMS

It is wise to have a good set of teeth. Many a case of dyspepsia or loss of weight can be ascribed to the bolting of insufficiently chewed meals, or to the inability to eat with pleasure and contentment. Insufficient teeth with which to chew, painful gums or teeth, or badly fitting dentures may all be responsible.

Gingivitis is common in those with a poor bite or dental gaps, especially if the diet is mainly bread and soft foods. Constant bleeding may cause positive faecal occult-blood tests, and if the diet is poor, iron-deficiency anaemia.

The role of chronic periodontal disease in the causation of dyspeptic symptoms is less certain. If septic material from the mouth is swallowed, it is unlikely that it will cause harm to a healthy stomach producing acid and pepsin enough to destroy and digest bacteria. The achlorhydric stomach may be more defenceless, and gingivitis can also impede mastication enough for food to be swallowed in hard lumps. Thus it seems reasonable in the presence of a non-specific type of dyspepsia to hope for improvement after thorough treatment of the chronic periodontal condition by a dental surgeon. The treatment consists of complete removal of dental calculus, polishing of the teeth, and instructions on the correct use of the toothbrush. Gingivectomy may be necessary, or if the condition has advanced to a periodontitis, flap surgery may be preferable. If the condition has gone too far, affected teeth must be extracted and resulting spaces within the dental arches must be made good with fixed or removable prostheses.

OTHER DISEASES OF THE GUMS

Bleeding gingivitis with visible granulations is seen most typically in scurvy, but in edentulous patients this manifestation of ascorbic acid deficiency is never seen. Bleeding gums also occur sometimes in leukaemia or diabetes.

Hypertrophied gums occur sometimes in patients who habitually take large doses of phenytoin for the control of epilepsy, or it may be a familial condition.

DISEASES OF THE BUCCAL MUCOUS MEMBRANES

Stomatitis

This is usually a reflection of lowered body resistance such as may occur in severe pyrexial illnesses, leukaemia, and agranulocytosis, or of altered conditions within the mouth in patients who fail to breathe through the nose, who are semi-comatose, or dehydrated as a result of diseases such as diabetes, uraemia, intestinal obstruction, or gastro-enteritis. Stomatitis may be caused by mercury, bismuth, or lead poisoning, and both penicillin lozenges and broad-spectrum antibiotics so alter the bacterial flora of the mouth that stomatitis may develop. In agranulocytosis the infection may be bacterial or spirochaetal. Vincent's organisms commonly cause a particularly severe and necrotizing stomatitis. More commonly, thrush (*Candida albicans*) infection occurs in patients with diabetes or in those with ulcerative colitis treated with corticosteroids.

Angular Stomatitis

This may be a manifestation of sideropenia, riboflavin deficiency, or untreated diabetes. It sometimes occurs in denture wearers, in which case it may be associated with *Candida albicans* infection. More simply it may be due to loss of the vertical dimension of full dentures which have been used for a long time. If no dentures are worn the folds at the corners of the mouth become even deeper.

Aphthous Ulcers

Small ulcers, without specific histological characteristics, form in the mucosa of the cheeks, lower lip, and underside of the tongue. They are painful when touched or rubbed, so that chewing of fruit and hard vegetable matter causes considerable discomfort. Isolated ulcers may be due to trauma from a toothbrush, or following dental treatment, but more commonly the ulcers tend to occur in crops of three or four. They heal spontaneously in ten to twenty days but further crops appear. On inspection, the active ulcer is about 2 mm. in diameter, has a greyish-white base, and a raised red margin.

No causative organisms have been found and antibiotic therapy does not cure. All clinicians who have attempted to ascertain the aetiology have been impressed by the susceptibility to aphthous ulceration of tense and worried people, and by the fact that fresh crops break out at times of exceptional stress. Nutritional deficiency seems to play no part, and food trauma is only of secondary importance in prolonging the life of the ulcer. Two measures help to reduce pain and hasten healing. First, and most effectively, hydrocortisone hemisuccinate in the form of a pellet (Corlan) can be closely applied to the base of the ulcer and held there by the tongue or finger. An alternative is triamcinolone in Orobase paste. This always relieves pain and shortens healing time. The older, less certain, and more painful remedy is to cauterize the base of the ulcer with a pledget soaked in surgical spirit.

In order to mitigate the mental and physical anguish caused by attacks of aphthous ulceration, some form of simple psychotherapy is helpful. This usually means the exhibition of sedatives, reassurance, practical measures to relieve pain, and some readjustment of the patient's life. As with other psychosomatic nuisances, a measure of success in relieving symptoms breeds confidence and promotes that relaxation of emotional tension which is necessary for cure.

The prognosis varies. Some patients are relieved for years at a time while others suffer from sporadic relapses. Chronically anxious patients may suffer continuously from successive crops of ulcers.

Behçet's Syndrome

This resembles severe aphthous ulceration, but conjunctivitis and some-times corneal ulceration, urethritis, and often vaginal or perineal ulcera-tion, also occur. Rarely, the central nervous system is involved. Although some believe that a specific virus is responsible, there is, in fact, no certain cause for this disabling and persistent disease. Only palliative treatment can be given.

DISEASES OF SALIVARY GLANDS

Many general diseases may involve all the salivary glands, but duct disease, septic lesions, calculi, and the mixed parotid tumour can occur in one gland only. The parotid is the chief salivary gland and some of the diseases which affect it are of interest to the gastro-enterologist.

Epidemic Viral Parotitis

This is of interest because of the rare complication of acute pancreatitis.

Suppurative Parotitis and Parotid Abscess

Often a complication of dehydration and stomatitis in a patient whose bodily resistance is low, this disease may also occur as a result of ascending infection from gingivitis or tonsillitis, or by blood-stream spread in cases of pyaemia. The predominant organism is usually *Staphylococcus aureus* or *Streptococcus pyogenes*. The patient, though febrile and ill, may suffer surprisingly little pain from the inflamed gland. An abscess may form and discharge to the outside or into the mouth. Treatment is by rehydration and by hot saline or antiseptic mouthwashes, local heat to the outside of the gland, and antibiotics. The causative organism should be isolated from the pus expressed from the parotid duct, and either a broad-spectrum antibiotic or a combination of penicillin and streptomycin is given as early as possible and without waiting for the culture report. Later, when the causative organism and its sensitivity are known, the antibiotic régime may be altered. Surgical treatment is only required if antibiotic therapy has been delayed or ineffective.

Chronic Parotid Infections and Swellings

Bilateral painless enlargement of the parotids may occur in many circum-stances, but particularly in patients with sarcoidosis or chronic alcoholism and cirrhosis. In the former, other signs of the disease are usually found in the eyes or lungs, but in the latter, the diagnosis may be obscure until a full social history has been obtained and liver function ascertained. The mechanism by which alcohol causes parotid enlargement is unknown and the histological picture is not specific. In obscure cases of recurrent parotid swelling sialograms may reveal calculi and sialectasis of the ducts. *Streptococcus viridans* may be grown from the duct saliva, but it is uncertain whether the infection is primary or secondary. The relationship of recurrent parotitis to asthma and chronic bronchial chest disease suggests a possible allergic basis.

Deficiency of Saliva

In Sjögren's syndrome, or kerato-conjunctivitis sicca, there is a drying-up of saliva and tears due to a chronic disease, probably of auto-immune character, which involves the salivary and lacrimal glands. This syndrome is sometimes associated with other diseases such as rheumatoid disease, thyroiditis, and 'immunological' liver disease. The clinical picture is one of painful joints, a gritty and troublesome conjunctivitis, rhinitis, a dry mouth, and a red, sore tongue. Recurrent infections of the salivary glands may occur. Patients may complain chiefly of a dry nose, or they may have an eczematous condition around the mouth and nose. Some have mainly oral symptoms and complain of dysphagia while others have thirst and polyuria. Chronic gastritis frequently coexists. So varied are the initial symptoms that the diagnosis may be missed. It can be confirmed by measuring the flow of saliva or of tears. There is no satisfactory treatment, but if joints and other organs are involved, corticosteroids may be given, and antibiotics as and when necessary to control infection.

MOUTH SYMPTOMS NOT DUE TO ORGANIC DISEASE

Anxiety causes a dry mouth and foetor oris. This is natural, but when the anxiety state is neurotic these symptoms become a focus of discomfort. Anxious obsessional people may be much distressed by an awareness of halitosis and unpleasant sensations in the mouth and tongue for which no organic disease can be held responsible. Often in such cases the tongue is furred. Still others become obsessed by the alleged 'bigness' of the tongue, or they may be worried by a pricking and tingling sensation from the surface of the tongue. On examination, it is obvious that these patients are continually licking their lips and passing their tongues over their palates, and it is not unreasonable to ascribe some of their discomfort to this self-inflicted trauma.

In treating them, it is important not to prescribe local remedies which may only worsen the soreness and, by focusing the patient's attention on his tongue, make him more difficult to cure, but thorough dental treatment with smoothing of sharp tooth edges and cleaning up of chronic periodontitis is a useful first step. He should be told of the absence of organic disease, and the mechanisms of anxiety must be explained. He should then be given some general treatment of a sedative or even merely of a placebo character, and he should be told firmly to try to forget about his mouth and tongue. This simple approach often succeeds, but sometimes mental investigation and deep psychotherapy are necessary.

FURTHER READING

The Tongue
KAPLAN, B. J. (1961), 'The Clinical Tongue', *Lancet*, **1**, 1094.

Aphthous Ulcers
SIRCUS, W., CHURCH, R., and KELLEHER, J. (1957), 'Recurrent Aphthous Ulceration of the Mouth', *Q. Jl Med.*, **50**, 235.

Behçet's Syndrome
DOWLING, G. B. (1961), 'Behçet's Disease', *Proc. R. Soc. Med.*, **54**, 101.

Sjögren's Syndrome
DENKO, C. W., and BERGENSTAL, D. M. (1960), 'The Sicca Syndrome (Sjögren's Syndrome)', *Archs intern. Med.*, **105**, 849.

Chapter 3

The Oesophagus

ANATOMY AND PHYSIOLOGY

THE TOPMOST part of the oesophagus is controlled by striated voluntary muscle, but the body of the oesophagus is composed of a circular and a longitudinal layer of smooth muscle. The whole is innervated by the vagus, and cholinergic endings motivate the normal peristaltic contractions. The adrenergic innervation, however, is complex with α-receptors transmitting contractile impulses and β-receptors mediating relaxation; there is some evidence that the upper oesophagus is somewhat differently innervated from the lower parts where adrenergic receptors mediating relaxation predominate. High section of the vagus paralyses effective peristalsis and prevents relaxation of the cardiac zone.

Because there is no anatomically distinct sphincter at the cardia, there is great interest in the mechanisms which control the entrance of food into the stomach and which prevent the reflux of gastric contents into the oesophagus.

The evidence from studies of intraluminal pressure in man indicates that above the cardia there is a short zone of increased muscle tone which maintains a high intraluminal pressure. This acts as a physiological sphincter. The voluntary act of swallowing sets in motion a propulsive wave of peristalsis preceded by a wave of inhibition which travels down the oesophagus until the high-pressure zone above the cardia is reached. A slight delay above the sphincter causes widening of the lumen, known at this point as the phrenic ampulla. The high pressure then falls so that food passes through the cardia into the stomach.

MECHANISMS PREVENTING
GASTRO-OESOPHAGEAL REFLUX
(*Fig. 2*)

The high-pressure zone above the cardia (or physiologic internal sphincter) is capable of withstanding moderate increases of intraluminal pressure, and its tone is controlled by circulating levels of gastrin. It is only one of the mechanisms which prevent gastro-oesophageal reflux. Two others, the comparative importance of which is differently assessed by various authorities, are as follows.

The gastro-oesophageal sling of oblique muscle which maintains the sharp angle of oesophageal entry into the stomach keeps the mucosa of the subphrenic oesophagus flattened in apposition with itself. This enables the subphrenic oesophagus to act as a flap-valve which can open only when an increase of intraluminal pressure forces the mucosal folds away from each other. In the healthy person, this only happens when a bolus of food passes through from above, because the intra-abdominal pressure, which is higher than the intrathoracic, keeps the flap-valve from admitting anything from below. Distension of the stomach by gas or fluid may, however, cause the intraluminal pressure within the cardia to rise beyond

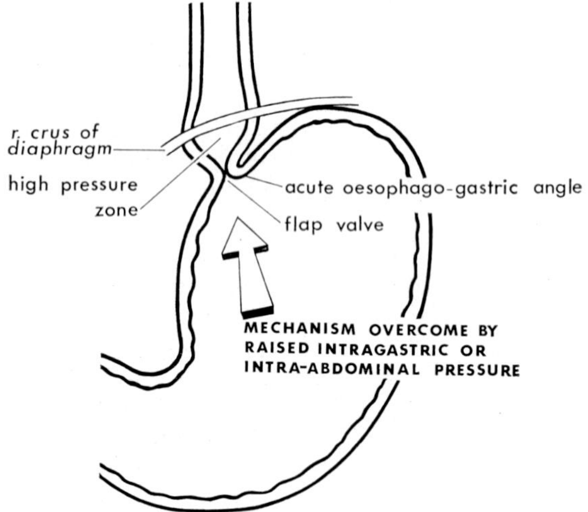

Fig. 2. Oesophageal closure mechanisms.

the levels within the thoracic oesophagus, in which case the valve opens and regurgitation occurs. The mechanism is similar to that of the rubber flap-valve used to inflate tyres and bladders.

It is the view of most authorities that the flap-valve mechanism, depending on the short segment of subphrenic oesophagus, can only operate efficiently if the oblique angle of oesophageal entry into the stomach is maintained, and if the stomach is wholly below the diaphragm.

The third mechanism is the so-called 'pinch-cock' action of the diaphragmatic crura on the lower oesophagus. This is certainly lost when the stomach herniates through the diaphragmatic hiatus, but its importance in normal physiological activity has probably been exaggerated by those who find the tightening of the crural ring a satisfactory surgical exercise and a means of maintaining the reduction of a hiatus hernia. Pressure studies in normal humans indicate that the action of the diaphragmatic crura is only important during forced and, to a much lesser extent, during normal inspiration.

Oesophageal Mucosa

The oesophagus is lined by squamous epithelium and the mucosa is thin compared with that of the stomach. Islands of columnar epithelium and secretory glands of gastric type may occur in the oesophagus, but these rarely secrete enough acid to cause serious trouble. However, in the very rare short oesophagus, gastric mucosa may extend as high as the arch of the aorta, and then peptic ulceration is liable to occur within the thorax.

Achalasia and Other Peristaltic Disorders

AETIOLOGY AND PATHOLOGY

Achalasia, sometimes called 'cardiospasm', is a disease of unknown aetiology characterized by weak oesophageal peristalsis and inability of the physiological internal oesophageal sphincter to relax in response to the peristaltic wave of swallowing (*Fig. 3*). The disease has been noted at all

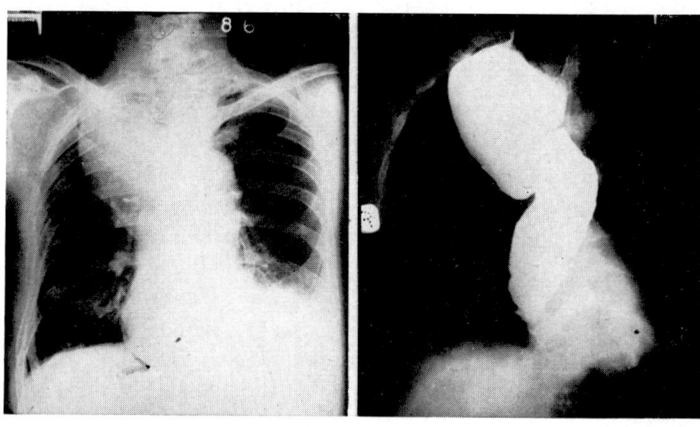

A   B

Fig. 3. Achalasia: A, Straight radiograph; B, Barium-filled oesophagus.

ages from 10 to 60 years, but mostly occurs in young adult life, and is slightly commoner in females. There is a deficiency throughout the oesophagus of the ganglion cells of Auerbach's plexus, but no other anatomical abnormality. The physiological fault is similar to that produced by section of the vagus nerve. In accordance with Cannon's Law that a denervated organ responds with greater force to the appropriate chemo-transmitter, the achalasic oesophagus contracts violently in response to acetyl-B-methylcholine, but peristalsis does not occur. Inhalation of smooth-muscle relaxants such as amyl or octyl nitrite will open the internal sphincter sufficiently for soft food and liquid to pass through into the stomach, but the diameter of the oesophagus may be as much as 15 cm. and the lower part may be so stretched by stagnant food and drink that it may fall down in a sigmoid loop above the cardia. In these circumstances, the food ferments and a retention oesophagitis develops. Fever, joint pains, and periosteal tenderness similar to that of hypertrophic pulmonary osteo-arthropathy occur rarely in those with severe oesophagitis.

In Chagas's disease, which occurs in South America, there is degeneration of ganglion cells in the wall of the oesophagus caused by a neurotoxin
liberated from dead *Trypanosoma cruzi*. The resulting clinical picture is
very similar to that of achalasia, but other hollow viscera may be similarly
affected. The neuropathy of diabetes can produce a similar picture.

CLINICAL PICTURE

Dysphagia is the most constant symptom, the difficulty being an inability
to swallow effectively rather than, as in the case of stricture, an inability
to swallow solid foods. Meals are interrupted by the discomfort of food
retained in the oesophagus or by the necessity to regurgitate, and consequently sufferers from this disease prefer to eat alone. The regurgitation
of fluid and food debris is interpreted by the patient as vomiting, but the
alkalinity of the vomitus indicates its oesophageal origin. Loss of weight
is often much less than one would expect, so that in spite of the regurgitation much food must find its way through the stomach.

Many patients with mild achalasia hardly ever regurgitate, and they
complain solely of discomfort or 'indigestion'. Dysphagia can be relieved
by eating in the standing position or by drinking cold water. Patients with
mild achalasia who but rarely suffer from dysphagia and regurgitation
may have a surprisingly large dilatation of the oesophagus.

DIAGNOSIS

A clear history, extending over several months, of regurgitation during
meals with comparatively little loss of weight suggests the diagnosis, but
there are no abnormal signs. A straight radiograph of the chest may show
a long, straight, oesophageal shadow above the heart and great vessels, and
extending behind them. When barium is swallowed, the peristaltic wave is
weak, the barium collects in the lower oesophagus, and the obstructing

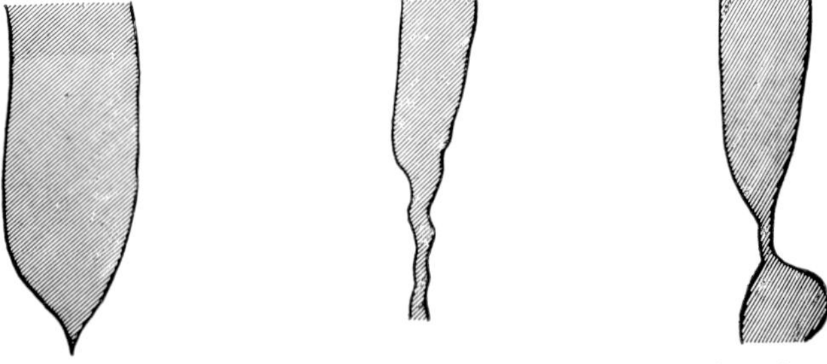

Fig. 4. The appearance of the barium-filled oesophagus in achalasia compared
with other forms of obstruction.

sphincter gives it a smooth funnel-shaped outline (*Fig. 4*). Some general
thickening of the oesophageal wall can often be detected, but there is no
soft-tissue shadow around the obstruction. There is no gas bubble in the

stomach. When octyl nitrite is inhaled the sphincter relaxes and lets the barium through. 1·5 mg. of the parasympatheticomimetic drug, Mecholyl, causes a violent contraction of the lower oesophagus in these patients.

A simple stricture can be distinguished by the fact that it is rarely placed exactly at the cardia, and that an associated hiatus hernia is often present below it. A carcinomatous narrowing is usually irregular, the oesophagus above is not much dilated and its wall not thickened, the soft-tissue shadow of the growth can often be seen, and nitrite inhalations cause no relaxation.

COMPLICATIONS

Spill-over of oesophageal contents into the bronchial tree may cause bronchitis and pneumonitis, but the condition is not so severe as that which results from inhalation of acid gastric juice in a case of hiatus hernia.

Oesophagitis may cause fever and arthralgia. Achalasia should be regarded as a precancerous condition, for there is a 10 per cent incidence of carcinoma of the oesophagus in long-standing cases, the growth usually occurring well above the cardia.

TREATMENT

Believing that emotional strain provokes the disease, some physicians have used psychotherapy, but the poor results offer little support for the psychosomatic theory. Temporary relief can be given to patients who inhale octyl nitrite vapour just before or during a meal, and in very mild cases with intermittent symptoms this may be enough to keep them comfortable.

Eventually most patients need either dilatations or operative treatment.

Dilatations

Two methods of dilatation are in use, mainly in North America:

1. STARCK'S DILATOR

This is a mechanically operated instrument which is passed until, under radiological control, it is seen to be correctly situated in the narrowed area of the oesophagus, when manipulation of the controls causes the expansion of the segment within the lower oesophagus. This powerful method probably ruptures many of the circular muscle-fibres, and one dilatation may last a year.

2. MOSHER BAG

Under local anaesthesia and with full radiological control, the bag is inflated to a pressure of 15 lb. per sq. in. for 15 sec. The dilatation which is to approximately 3 cm. is repeated two or three times.

Operative Treatment

Cardiomyotomy, or Heller's operation, is a delicate but essentially simple operation performed after thoracotomy. The region of the sphincter is dissected out and the circular muscle-fibres are divided for a distance of 5 cm. leaving the mucosa intact. This relieves the obstruction permanently, but the oesophagus remains dilated and ineffective as a peristaltic organ. It also abolishes one of the mechanisms guarding against gastro-oesophageal reflux, thus exposing the lower oesophagus to the risk of peptic digestion. In practice, peptic oesophagitis and stricture are rare after Heller's operation, but all patients who have had the operation are warned to avoid obesity, stooping, straining, and other activities which raise intra-abdominal pressure, and they are advised to sleep with the head of the bed raised on blocks. They should have regular medical supervision for several years after the operation.

In cases of long-standing obstruction due to achalasia, retention oesophagitis may render the delicate cardiomyotomy operation both difficult and dangerous, and in such severe cases a feeding gastrostomy may be made and used for 3 months to allow the oesophageal mucosa to recover.

In many centres, cardiomyotomy is the standard treatment for achalasia, and dilatations are never advised unless the patient refuses operation.

Tonic Oesophagus (Diffuse Spasm)

Manometric studies have revealed that a small number of patients suffering from dysphagia and oesophageal pain without organic narrowing have a diffuse high-pressure zone throughout the lower oesophagus. Hypertrophy of the muscle walls may occur but there is no degeneration of ganglion cells nor any increased sensitivity to acetyl-B-methylcholine. Pulsion diverticula are often caused by this neuromuscular disorder, and the radiological appearance of irregular spastic rings which can be made to relax by intravenous propantheline (30 mg.) is characteristic. If conventional barium studies show no abnormality, bread soaked in barium can bring out the characteristic irregular contractions of the oesophagus.

There is some evidence that lower oesophageal spasm may in some instances be caused by reflux of acid from the stomach. Certainly, pain and spasm can be produced by the infusion of $N/10$ hydrochloric acid into the oesophagus.

Corkscrew Oesophagus

This is a radiological diagnosis which has no specific symptomatology. Rings of circular muscle-fibres contract asynchronously down the oesophagus and there is no smooth peristaltic wave. The oesophageal muscular response to swallowing has been described as 'too soon, too much, and too long'. The radiological appearance of the barium-filled oesophagus is characteristic (*Fig. 5*). It is found commonly in old people, many of whom have organic lesions in the gastro-intestinal tract, chiefly peptic ulcer or gall-stones, but occasionally carcinoma of the stomach or bowel.

There is no radiological difference between those with and those without oesophageal symptoms.

Gastro-oesophageal reflux sometimes occurs in association with tertiary contractions.

Lower Oesophageal Ring

Some patients with dysphagia develop a tonic ring contraction in the lower oesophagus (Schatzki ring).

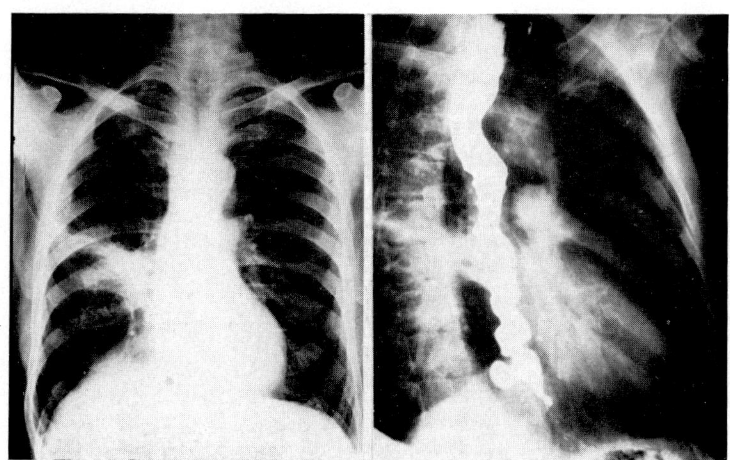

Fig. 5. Corkscrew oesophagus in patient with carcinoma of the bronchus.

Hiatus Hernia

For many years this condition, which is difficult to recognize at post-mortem, which rarely kills, and which causes a variety of symptoms, was thought to be a rarity. In spite of good clinical and radiological descriptions written in the early part of this century, it was not until intrathoracic surgery began to flourish and radiological techniques were refined that its prevalence was appreciated. Perhaps the pendulum of medical interest has already swung too far, so that those unfortunate enough to allow part of their stomach to slip through the hiatus while virtually standing on their heads under the watchful eye of a radiologist have attracted the interest of surgeons, both thoracic and abdominal, each of whom, in friendly rivalry, claims superior methods of hernial repair. In fact, minor degrees of hiatal herniation are probably physiological when intra-abdominal pressure is raised by obesity, pregnancy, or the head-down position. Certainly the incidence of hiatal herniation depends very much on the criteria adopted by the examining radiologist, and some would find an incidence of 20 per cent in middle-aged obese females while others would find less. Clinically, hiatus hernia causes symptoms most frequently at two different stages of life—infancy and after 40 years of age.

AETIOLOGY

Herniation and gastro-oesophageal reflux may occur commonly in infancy because of a weak diaphragm, or because air-swallowing may raise the intragastric pressure and so force open the flap-valve.

In later life, it is the conditions which raise intra-abdominal pressure, such as pregnancy and obesity, which either provoke herniation or symptoms of reflux. It is therefore most common in middle-aged obese females, and the gross incidence in females is three times that in males.

Hiatus hernia and peptic oesophagitis are commonly associated with duodenal ulcer, and many believe that pylorospasm may raise intragastric pressure sufficiently to open the flap-valve and allow regurgitation of strongly acid peptic juice.

PATHOLOGY

There are two distinct types of hernia and a combined form (*Fig. 6*).

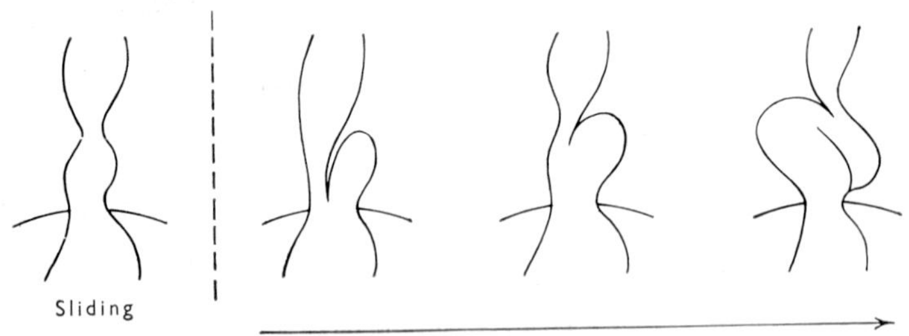

Fig. 6. Varieties of hiatus hernia.

1. *Sliding Hernia*

The gastro-oesophageal junction protrudes upwards through the hiatus and a bag of stomach below the junction comes to lie within the chest. This is the commonest form (70 per cent).

2. *Rolling Hernia*

The junction remains anchored below the hiatus, and a part of the cardiac end of the stomach prolapses through the hiatus alongside the oesophagus. This is less common, but gross lesions of this sort are found in aged people (20 per cent).

3. *Combined Sliding and Rolling Hernia*

This is also an uncommon type of lesion (10 per cent).

The Relationship of Hiatus Hernia to Gastro-oesophageal Reflux

Clearly, the displacement of the gastro-oesophageal junction to a position some distance above the hiatus will prevent the operation of a valve, nor can the crura of the diaphragm forced apart by the herniation play any useful part. Even so, the physiological internal oesophageal sphincter may remain competent against moderate increases of intragastric pressure, and thus it is that a patient may have a hiatus hernia without symptoms and without peptic oesophagitis.

Patients with the 'rolling' or para-oesophageal types of herniae who retain the gastro-oesophageal junction in its normal position do not usually suffer from reflux or its consequences.

On the other hand, patients without any hiatal herniation whatsoever may suffer from considerable reflux with or without oesophagitis. Presumably in these cases there is either a failure of the physiological sphincter or the flap-valve, or both together. Later, oesophagitis may lead to inflammatory fibrosis and shortening of the oesophagus, so that the gastro-oesophageal junction moves upwards. The truth is that hernia may exist without reflux, that reflux may occur without hernia, and that oesophagitis may occur in either situation. The intensity of the oesophagitis will depend not only on the degree of reflux but also on the character of the gastric contents and the factor of local tissue resistance. Minor degrees of subacute oesophagitis may occur from alcoholic or dietary trauma without either reflux or hernia. Cases of oesophagitis have been described in those suffering from ulcerative colitis, and here presumably the factor of mucosal resistance is all important.

COMPLICATIONS

Peptic Oesophagitis

This is commonly found in the oesophagus just above a sliding hernia. The early stage is hyperaemia, scattered superficial ulceration, oozing of exudate, and bleeding. Later there is a leucoplakic appearance, bleeding may be more severe, ulceration may coalesce, and deep fibrosis occurs. Peri-oesophagitis may cause a considerable soft-tissue swelling and occasionally mediastinitis. Later still, fibrosis causes shortening of the oesophagus and a stricture.

Peptic Ulceration

In a rolling hernia the prolapsed gastric mucosa may ulcerate, and a true chronic peptic ulcer forms, either in the thoracic part of the stomach or at the point of herniation through the diaphragm. These ulcers may cause no pain and are liable to bleed insidiously or acutely.

Anaemia

With or without iron deficiency this may cause symptoms which bring the patient to the doctor; careful inquiry and barium studies are necessary to disclose the primary lesion which may be oesophagitis or peptic ulcer in the hernial sac.

Inhalation Bronchitis and Recurrent Pneumonitis

Gastric contents regurgitating freely into the oesophagus during sleep may be inhaled and set up bronchitis, peribronchial infection, pneumonitis, and fibrosis of the lower lobes. Episodes of frank pneumonia or haemoptysis may call attention to the underlying condition.

CLINICAL PICTURE

Symptoms vary greatly and signs other than those complicating anaemia are not clinical but radiological. Consequently, diagnosis and assessment are full of pitfalls.

The following groupings may be found helpful.

1. *Asymptomatic*

Most rolling herniae, and many sliding herniae, with neither reflux nor oesophagitis cause no symptoms.

2. *Rolling Hernia*

(*a*) Intermittent dysphagia with borborygmi due to a hernia full of food and gas pressing into the lower oesophagus. (*b*) Iron-deficiency anaemia from insidious blood-loss from a symptomless gastric ulcer within the herniated stomach. (*c*) Haematemesis from such an ulcer.

3. *Sliding Hernia with Reflux but no Oesophagitis*

Occasional heartburn. Acid regurgitates into the mouth while stooping or when lying in bed. Discomfort on exercise after a heavy meal.

4. *Sliding Hernia with Reflux and Early Oesophagitis*

Reflux symptoms, heartburn, and lower substernal pain which comes on a few seconds after swallowing solid food, hot drinks, or alcohol, or a similar pain when stooping or lying flat.

5. *Ill-understood and Inconstant Symptoms*

Some patients experience quite severe attacks of pain which radiate from the sternum to the back, shoulders, and upper arm. This pain may occur during or after exertion, and bears a superficial resemblance to that of coronary insufficiency, even to the point where trinitrin may be expected to give relief. However, rest does not, as in angina pectoris, promptly relieve the pain, and indeed, the pain may well come on immediately after, rather than during, exertion. These attacks may be due to painful contractions of the oesophageal musculature brought on by exacerbations of oesophagitis. On this basis, the relief of pain by a smooth-muscle relaxant such as trinitrin can be understood.

DIAGNOSIS AND ASSESSMENT

A radiological diagnosis of hiatus hernia must be placed in clinical perspective. Air-swallowing and colon-spasm cannot be cured by attributing them to a hiatus hernia discovered radiologically, nor can surgical repair of a hiatus hernia be expected to cure a sick mind. The anatomical abnormality must on no account be made a scapegoat for other disorders.

In the first place, the type and degree of hiatal herniation must be determined from the radiologist's report, scrutiny of films, and discussion. Few radiologists are likely to make the elementary mistake of reporting a temporarily dilated phrenic ampulla as a hiatus hernia, but, to be certain, gastric mucosa must be seen above the diaphragm. Small sliding herniae may cause greater reflux and oesophagitis and therefore worse symptoms than huge and impressive rolling herniae. Secondly, the degree of reflux must be ascertained from the clinical history, from radiological studies in the head-down position, and from oesophagoscopy. Thirdly, the degree of oesophagitis must be assessed from symptoms and oesophagoscopic findings. Fourthly, anaemia, occult blood-loss, and iron deficiency should be ascertained. There are difficulties sometimes when clinical radiological and oesophagoscopic evidence does not tally. For example, the oesophago-scope may detect oesophagitis when there are no symptoms of it, or the patient may tell a convincing story of reflux which the radiologist cannot demonstrate.

An oesophagoscopic diagnosis of reflux should be treated with a certain amount of reserve as it is probable that the presence of the instrument in the oesophagus may interfere with the function of the physiological sphincter.

More difficulties arise when pathological conditions other than the hiatus hernia are present. Coronary insufficiency, gall-stones, and hiatus hernia are not uncommon in obese patients. A duodenal ulcer is frequently associated with sliding hernia and a gastric ulcer with rolling hernia. The history should always be taken very carefully so that the symptoms can be disentangled and correctly attributed. Radiological studies of the gall-bladder, electrocardiography, and gastric secretory studies are required in every case of doubt. When chest pain has some of the characteristics of coronary insufficiency and some of oesophagitis, an intra-oesophageal infusion of $N/10$ hydrochloric acid may throw light on its source. It has been shown that where the source of pain is oesophageal it can be repro-duced in most patients by such an acid infusion, and that oesophageal spasm appears to play only a secondary role in the mediation of the pain.

Information obtained by such means must be interpreted with reserve, and used simply as a guide to the best means of alleviating the patient's symptoms. Coronary insufficiency and oesophagitis frequently coexist, and the pain experienced may be the result of summation in the central nervous system. Thus, in such cases, relief may come from antacids and the usual methods for palliating oesophagitis, but this does not stop the patient from dying of a coronary artery occlusion a few months later.

TREATMENT

Conservative and Medical

Symptomless herniae require no active treatment, but the patient should be encouraged to keep slim, to abstain from fatty foods which stimulate gastric secretion, to avoid stooping, straining, and raising intra-abdominal pressure, and to sleep on a firm mattress with the head of the bed higher than the foot.

Patients with sliding hernia who have symptoms of reflux need similar advice, and they may be prepared to go further in the way of dietary restriction, slimming, and avoidance of stooping. Keen gardeners should be advised to do their work at least one and a half hours after a meal, and to use long-handled tools or to weed while sitting on a low stool. There is no doubt that a reduction of weight by about 10 per cent is the most effective medical treatment. Antacids, by raising pH in the antrum, cause gastrin release and tightening of the internal sphincter. Metaclopramide (Maxolon) also tightens the sphincter by sensitizing its smooth muscle to endogenous acetyl choline. Another method of reducing intra-oesophageal acidity is to give a 'barrier' preparation which floats on the gastric contents. Lastly, antacid-local anaesthetic mucilages can give relief from lower oesophageal pain.

Anticholinergic drugs, such as propantheline or poldine, may help to relieve symptoms by reducing gastric secretory activity and consequently lessening peptic irritation of the lower oesophagus. Preparations containing local anaesthetics and alkalis in a mucilage, if taken by mouth, may relieve heartburn and thus make the patient more comfortable.

The patient with symptoms of oesophagitis, but with only minor changes seen at oesophagoscopy, may safely be treated conservatively for a trial period. The avoidance of spirits, hot drinks, and hard, hastily chewed food is most important in these patients and also those with reflux alone.

Patients who do not respond to medical measures and who continue to suffer from embarrassing reflux and pain, or who have oesophagitis of more than slight degree, are candidates for surgical treatment. It is important to remember, however, when considering surgical treatment that in the words of Davidson 'a fat woman of 55 who has let herself go . . . may seek comfort from the priest, the psychiatrist, the beautician, or the surgeon' and that it is very difficult to know 'when an oesophagus is being digested by acid, and when it is blushing for shame, pining for love, quivering with anxiety, desolate with grief or merely reflecting downward trends on the stock market'.

Surgical

THE INDICATIONS FOR SURGERY ARE:

i. Persistence of genuine symptoms in spite of a carefully maintained conservative régime, and the presence of oesophagitis.

ii. A large rolling hernia complicated by attacks of pain or of strangulation.

iii. A penetrating gastric ulcer at the point of herniation.

iv. Recurrent blood-loss.

v. Development of a stricture.

The number of operations devised testifies to the occurrence of unsatisfactory results. Poor results may be due to:

1. Poor selection of cases.

a. Neurotics with functional or peristaltic disorders of the gut continue to complain of heartburn and belching after a technically successful repair.

b. Coexistent disease more important than the hernia which has been repaired, e.g., duodenal ulcer, gastric ulcer, gall-stones, coronary insufficiency, or relapsing pancreatitis.

2. Failure to repair the hernia, to prevent reflux, or to cure oesophagitis. Few patients have a detectable hernia immediately after operation, but within two years, 1 in 5 may have recurred. Occasionally, reflux may continue even though the hernia seems to be adequately reduced, and if oesophagitis has involved the whole thickness of the oesophagus it may be incapable of complete healing.

3. Post-thoracotomy intercostal neuralgia.

There are two main approaches to surgical repair.

TRANSTHORACIC

Advantages: good exposure, ability to inspect oesophagus some way above the hernia, ability to narrow oesophageal hiatus by approximation of diaphragmatic crura. It is essential to use this approach if there is severe oesophagitis or stricture.

Disadvantages: inability to inspect gall-bladder for coexistent disease. Post-thoracotomy pain.

ABDOMINAL

Advantages: ability to detect and deal with coexistent conditions such as pyloric obstruction, gall-stones, etc. No liability to post-thoracotomy pain. (One in 4 patients with hiatus hernia have associated intra-abdominal lesions.)

Disadvantages: probably not so good an exposure. Inability to proceed to oesophagogastrectomy if degree of oesophagitis renders this necessary.

SPECIAL OPERATIONS

A left phrenic crush or ablation to paralyse the left half of the diaphragm and so accentuate the gastro-oesophageal angle, though ingenious and promising, has not produced strikingly good results and often aggravates dyspepsia.

Attempts to sharpen the gastro-oesophageal angle by direct suturing have also not given reliable results.

The procedure of reduction and repair of the hernia from below, vagotomy to reduce gastric secretory activity, and either pyloroplasty or antrectomy is the logical answer to the patient with hiatus hernia, a duodenal ulcer, and some pylorospasm, but it is also done by some surgeons as a primary procedure for all cases of hiatus hernia, for they believe that gastric retention and reverse peristalsis may be equally important causes of reflux. A gastro-enterostomy may be done instead of a pyloroplasty. In cases of oesophagitis in patients with hyposecretion of acid and thought to be due to reflux of duodenal enzymes and bile into the oesophagus a vagotomy with gastro-jejunostomy and Roux-en-Y drainage of the afferent loop may be done.

OTHER NON-MALIGNANT DISEASES OF THE OESOPHAGUS

Pharyngeal Pouches and Oesophageal Diverticula

There is a weak spot between the oblique and circular fibres of the crico-pharyngeus muscle through which the mucosa and submucosa of the pharynx may herniate and form a pouch. This is particularly liable to occur when there is any peristaltic disorder of the oesophagus or inco-ordination of the swallowing muscles. The pouch may enlarge in such a way that food and liquids lodge in it and spill over into the oesophagus or trachea. Such a pouch can cause no symptoms, but dysphagia, regurgitation of undigested food, cough, and inhalation bronchitis may occur in time. A soft swelling anterior to the sternomastoid enlarges after eating and can sometimes be emptied by pressure. The radiological diagnosis is straightforward if films are obtained of the upper oesophagus filled with barium. Cineradiography is particularly valuable. If the oesophagus is displaced, dysphagia becomes troublesome, and weight is lost. The pouch should then be removed surgically after thorough attempts to cleanse it and to improve the patient's general condition. Tube feeding or gastrostomy is occasionally necessary.

In a tonic oesophagus, pulsion diverticula may develop as a result of a congenital muscle defect or because there is a peristaltic disorder which raises the intraluminal pressure. They are not common, occur as a rule just below the pharynx or above the diaphragm, and rarely cause symptoms. Traction diverticula caused by lymphadenitis are occasionally found at the bifurcation of the trachea. Surgical excision of a diverticulum should only be attempted if: (1) Other lesions causing raised intraluminal pressure within the oesophagus have been excluded or cured. (2) There is complete certainty that the symptoms—dysphagia or regurgitation of stale food, inhalation bronchitis, or chest pain—are due to the diverticulum and not to some other cause.

Spontaneous Rupture of the Oesophagus

This sudden catastrophe may occur during a bout of vomiting, often after a heavy meal. The oesophagus tears just above the cardia and the patient is seized by severe *abdominal* pain. The upper abdomen is rigid and signs of shock suggest that a peptic ulcer has perforated. However, bowel-sounds persist and radiographs show no free gas under the diaphragm. Air in the mediastinum may show up the heart in double outline. A hydro-pneumothorax may develop rapidly and surgical emphysema may be found in the neck, but, if possible, the diagnosis should be made and the tear sutured before this becomes clinically obvious. A small amount of fluid may give an appearance of haziness in one costophrenic angle of a straight radiograph of the chest, which together with negative findings in the abdominal film may clinch the diagnosis. A water-soluble contrast given by mouth may help in diagnosis.

Sideropenic Oesophagitis

Iron deficiency may cause not only a sore tongue but a sore gullet with dysphagia. Correction of the deficiency usually cures the condition, but occasionally mucosal webs are left in the upper oesophagus and these can be divided oesophagoscopically. This is a condition which should be rare in a population with a good standard of nutrition and medical services, and this seems to be the case in Britain. Nevertheless, it should always be suspected in a middle-aged woman with dysphagia; a blood-count is always necessary. Some patients with an oesophageal web are not iron deficient and in them an immunological basis is suspected.

Traumatic Oesophagitis

The swallowing of hard, unchewed foods, hot drinks, or strong alcohol may cause a short-lived oesophagitis, which provokes substernal pain a few seconds after eating. The discomfort is greater if alcohol and hot drinks are taken, but a soft diet and abstinence usually cure the condition within a month.

Traumatic Stricture

Very hot fluids or corrosives may cause such a severe oesophagitis that deep inflammation and fibrosis follow. Typically strictures due to corrosive fluids develop in the mid-oesophagus and are multiple, but if they are single it may be difficult to distinguish them from those caused by intense peptic oesophagitis or peptic ulceration complicating the congenitally short oesophagus.

Traumatic strictures may be treated by repeated dilatations, by insertion of an indwelling funnel and tube, by a permanent feeding gastrostomy, or by oesophagogastrectomy, using if necessary a colonic or jejunal transplant to bridge the gap between the upper oesophagus and stomach remnant.

Systemic Sclerosis—Scleroderma

Principally affecting the intercellular collagenous ground substance of the skin, joints, and muscles, this disease may involve in a similar way the kidneys, lungs, and smooth muscle of the gut. The lower oesophagus is affected more frequently than any other part of the gut, but the disease may cause very little in the way of symptoms. More often the oesophageal lesion is discovered accidentally or looked for systematically in patients with obvious scleroderma of the face and hands. The radiological behaviour of the barium-filled oesophagus is quite characteristic; the lower oesophagus tends not to propagate normal waves of peristalsis, the physiological sphincter does not close, and the oesophagus is shortened, thus dragging the gastric cardia up into the chest. The whole gives the appearance of a wrinkled and baggy tube which does not empty in the supine position. Regurgitation of acid and pepsin may set up a secondary oesophagitis (*Fig. 7*).

Heartburn, variable dysphagia, and acid regurgitation are all inconstant symptoms. Corticosteroids are sometimes given, but there is no cure for the disease. The usual measures to prevent gastro-oesophageal reflux should be adopted, and heartburn may be treated by alkaline mixtures. The oesophageal lesion, though it indicates the widespread distribution of the disease, does not in itself threaten life. It is the degree of renal involvement which determines the prognosis.

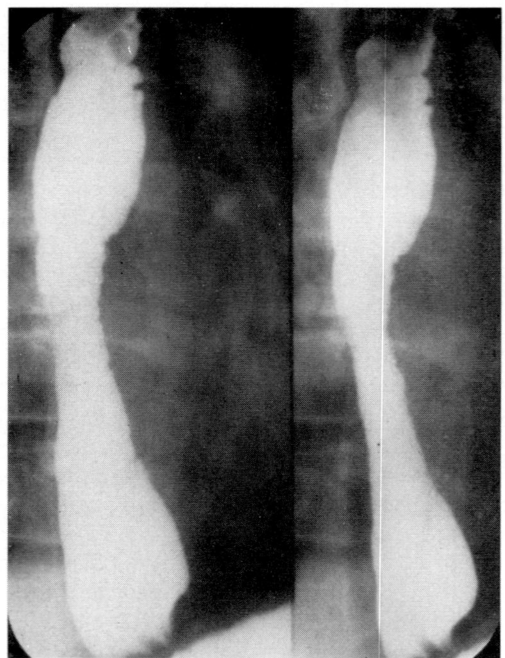

Fig. 7. The oesophagus in scleroderma.

Peptic Ulcer of the Oesophagus

This rare lesion usually occurs in the middle to lower oesophagus of patients with a short oesophagus or large islands of ectopic gastric mucosa. It may also occur in those with gross hypersecretion of acid gastric juice (e.g., Zollinger-Ellison syndrome), particularly after an insufficiently radical partial gastrectomy has been done. The symptoms vary, but severe pain on swallowing, or a constant and boring pain in the back or beneath the shoulder-blade, can be considered as characteristic. Haematemesis or insidious anaemia may occur, and ultimately the ulcer causes a stricture.

Gastric secretory studies must be made before treatment is planned, for it is sometimes more important to reduce hypersecretion by a subtotal gastrectomy or by subtotal pancreatectomy than to resect the ulcer-bearing tissue. The position of the ulcer as well as the gastric secretory state will determine the best type of operation, and in some cases conservative treatment may be best. Carbenoxolone can be tried.

Atresia of the Oesophagus

Babies may be born with a developmental anomaly of the foregut causing varying degrees of oesophago-tracheal abnormality. Failure to suck, cyanosis after attempts at feeding, and a straight radiograph of the abdomen which shows the absence of air in the stomach should lead to an early diagnosis. Occasionally, if a tracheo-oesophageal fistula is present, the stomach may be distended by gas. A surgical attempt must be made to repair and remedy the particular defect found.

NEOPLASTIC DISEASE OF THE OESOPHAGUS

Benign

A leiomyoma may occur in the oesophagus and cause dysphagia. Barium examination shows the typical appearance of a sausage-shaped sub-mucosal swelling. The lesion is rare, but bleeding may occur and the treatment is surgical.

Malignant

Though for reasons of surgical anatomy it is customary to group carcinomata into those involving the upper, middle, and lower thirds of the oesophagus, squamous-celled growths can involve any part of the gullet, and adenocarcinomata can invade from below or arise in aberrant gastric mucosa within the lower oesophagus. The malignant grade varies widely and it is not easy to predict the invasiveness of a growth or the prognosis from the histological study of a biopsy, but, in general, the squamous carcinomata do better than the adenocarcinomata. Carcinoma may spread widely beneath the mucosa and involve more than half the oesophagus. Multiple growths may occur. The condition is commoner in males, in alcoholics, in coeliac disease, achalasia, and congenital ichthyosis. In certain areas of the world such as the Transkei in South Africa and in north China oesophageal carcinoma is extremely common.

CLINICAL PICTURE AND DIAGNOSIS

The usual symptoms are pain and dysphagia provoked by solid foods. In many cases there is no early pain, and consequently the slight dysphagia noticed at first is often ignored. It is not until restriction of his diet causes rapid loss of weight that the patient seeks medical advice. He is often able to drink or to eat semi-solid foods for months or years after he is unable to swallow solids, but sometimes the oesophageal obstruction becomes complete in a few weeks, or suddenly after swallowing a piece of meat or vegetable. Vomiting and regurgitation take place soon after eating, and because the oesophagus is not dilated and capacious, inhalational bronchitis is rarely a problem.

Uncommonly, if the growth necroses or spreads outwards, pain and discomfort after food are the chief complaints, and dysphagia is not noticed. Invasion of the pericardium or pleura may cause blood-stained effusions; penetration into the trachea or main bronchi also occurs occasionally. Anaemia is common, and is sometimes severe. Metastases occur most commonly in the regional lymph-nodes, but occasionally in distant organs. Adenocarcinomata of the lower oesophagus frequently metastasize to the liver.

INVESTIGATIONS

A barium meal, faecal occult-blood test, and haemoglobin are the essential screening tests, and if a diagnosis of carcinoma is considered, an oesophagoscopy and biopsy must follow.

Barium in the oesophagus may outline the irregular and jagged upper edge of the carcinomatous obstruction and will show no dilatation above. The soft-tissue shadows of the growth may be seen, and lack of peristalsis with thickening of the wall may indicate submucosal carcinomatous infiltration upwards. An early carcinoma of the upper oesophagus is best shown by cineradiography.

TREATMENT

Radical Surgery

If possible, the growth should be excised and continuity of the foregut re-established. Usually surgical cure is attempted as soon as possible, but if the patient is very wasted, protein-deficient, and anaemic, time must be sacrificed to improve his condition. Oral hygiene is essential. Blood and plasma transfusions and parenteral iron may do much, but in some cases it is necessary to pass a feeding tube through the oesophageal lumen by means of an oesophagoscope or even to make a gastrostomy in order to improve nutrition.

Thoracotomy, followed by oesophagogastrectomy, is sometimes feasible for growths at the lower end and even for those in mid-oesophagus, but in the latter, colonic transplants are sometimes used to maintain continuity.

At the upper end, skin tubes are fashioned from the neck to replace the resected oesophagus, but if a colonic transplant can be brought up, this is better.

Palliative

Sometimes it is clear from the clinical picture that radical surgery cannot be attempted. Aged, frail patients with advanced cardiovascular disease will not stand such a severe operation. More frequently there is evidence of spread, either beforehand or at the time of thoracotomy, which precludes a radical excision. Even then some surgeons will attempt an oesophagectomy purely to prevent an uncomfortable death from complete dysphagia and starvation. Radiotherapy is to be preferred for growths of the upper oesophagus, and has a place in other situations if surgery is not possible.

In some cases, a plastic tube can be passed from an oesophagoscope through the growth and be maintained in place by a funnel-shaped top. Such tubes encourage necrosis and bleeding and may eventually slip through or cause ulceration and mediastinitis. A permanent feeding gastrostomy is occasionally the only answer, but an unsatisfactory one, to a most difficult situation.

When pain is a major symptom, oral pethidine 100 mg. and chlorpromazine 50 mg. given every 4 or 6 hours often induce tranquillity and relief, but sometimes injections of morphine or diamorphine are required. The latter is less liable to cause nausea and vomiting. Refreshing mouthwashes and gargles are soothing, and if the obstruction is incomplete, nutrition can be maintained by glucose-fortified drinks, fruit juices, meat juices, and milk foods.

THE CAUSES OF DYSPHAGIA

The function of the oesophagus may be impaired or rendered painful by disease elsewhere and it is well to consider the causes of dysphagia on both a regional and a symptomatic basis.

A. PHARYNX AND UPPER OESOPHAGUS

1. *Psychogenic*

Fear, anxiety states, and globus. These may cause drying of the mouth and inability to initiate the swallowing reflex. Over-awareness of the throat and neck is common in women, particularly those who are conscious of a thyroid enlargement and who have been told by helpful neighbours that they have 'gland trouble'. This leads to constant swallowing movements and a feeling of dysphagia. Their hands constantly stray to their throat and anxiety worsens the symptoms.

2. *Neurogenic*

Dysphagia is more troublesome with liquids than solids, because palatal palsy so frequently accompanies neurological lesions, and liquids more easily regurgitate into the nasopharynx.

a. Diphtheria may cause paralysis of the palatal muscles and thus inability to swallow without regurgitation. *Myasthenia gravis* may cause difficulty in swallowing towards the end of a meal or when tired.

b. Bulbar palsy from diseases of the medulla affecting the nuclei of the 9th, 10th, and 11th cranial nerves, e.g. motor neuron disease, thrombosis of small arterioles, gliomata, ependymomata, and syringomyelia.

c. Pseudo-bulbar Palsy. Arteriosclerotic, thrombotic lesions affecting the areas supplied by perforating branches of the anterior cerebral arteries cause variable dysphagia and dysarthria associated often with emotional lability and pyramidal tract lesions. Common in old and hypertensive persons.

3. *Mechanical and Traumatic*

Without realization of the event a fish-bone may impale itself in the tonsillar bed, posterior fauces, or pyriform fossa and cause painful dysphagia.

Intervertebral disk degeneration may cause anterior osteophytic outgrowths which may press on the oesophagus. A bolus of food then squeezes the posterior wall of the pharynx against the cervical spine and discomfort is felt, but the state of the patient's nervous system probably determines his sensitivity to this type of discomfort.

4. *Inflammatory*

a. Tonsillitis, pharyngitis, and peritonsillar abscess may cause intense dysphagia for a short while.

b. Sideropenia may cause atrophic glossitis and oesophagitis which may lead to the formation of mucosal webs (Plummer-Vinson syndrome).

5. *Neoplastic*

Leiomyoma or carcinoma of the pharynx and upper oesophagus.

B. MID-OESOPHAGUS

1. *Pressure from without*

Rarely, aberrant great vessels or dilated aorta may press on the oesophagus enough to cause dysphagia.

2. *Simple Stricture*

This may be due to:

a. Trauma (e.g., corrosive burns).

b. Peptic oesophagitis or peptic ulcer usually associated with short oesophagus.

3. *Neoplasia*

a. Squamous-celled carcinoma of the oesophagus.

b. Carcinoma of the bronchus involving and invading the oesophagus.

C. LOWER OESOPHAGUS

1. *Stricture*

This may be due to:

a. Corrosives.

b. Peptic oesophagitis.

2. *Neoplasia*

a. Squamous-celled carcinoma of the oesophagus.

b. Adenocarcinoma of columnar cells in the oesophagus.

c. Adenocarcinoma of gastric cardia invading the oesophagus.

3. *Rolling Hiatus Hernia*

4. *Peristaltic Disorders*

a. Achalasia.

b. Tonic oesophagus.

c. Corkscrew oesophagus.

d. After high vagotomy.

5. *Systemic Disease involving the Oesophagus*
Scleroderma or systemic sclerosis.

FURTHER READING

The Oesophageal Closure Mechanisms
ATKINSON, M. (1962), 'Mechanisms protecting against Gastro-oesophageal Reflux: A Review', *Gut*, **3**, 1.

Achalasia of Cardia
ADAMS, C. W., BRAIN, R. H., ELLIS, F. G., KAUNTZE, R., and TROUNCE, J. R. (1961), 'Achalasia of the Cardia', *Guy's Hosp. Rep.*, **110**, 191.

Incoordination of Oesophageal Motor Activity
ATKINSON, M. (1968), *Post-grad. med. J.*, **44**, 575.

Hiatus Hernia
DAVIDSON, J. S. (1968), 'Hiatal Hernia', *Post-grad. med. J.*, **44**, 579.
EDMUNDS, V. (1957), 'Hiatus Hernia: A Clinical Study of 200 Cases', *Q. Jl Med.*, **50**, 445.

Neoplasms
TANNER, N. C., and SMITHERS, D. W. (1961), 'Tumours of the Oesophagus', *Neoplastic Disease at Various Sites*, Vol. IV. Edinburgh: Livingstone.

Peptic Oesophagitis
WOOLER, G. (1961), 'The Diagnosis and Treatment of Peptic Oesophagitis', *Gut*, **2**, 91.

Systemic Sclerosis
DORNHORST, A. C., PIERCE, J. W., and WHIMSTER, I. W. (1954), 'The Oesophageal Lesion in Scleroderma', *Lancet*, **1**, 698.

Diffuse Oesophageal Spasm
BENNETT, J. R., and HENDRIK, T. R. (1970), 'Disorder with More Than One Cause', *Gastroenterology*, **59**, 273.

Chapter 4

Gastric Physiology

BY L. R. CELESTIN

GASTRIC MUCOSA

THE STOMACH is a powerful secretory organ lined by a gastric mucosa about
1 mm. thick lying over a muscularis mucosae which is responsible for
much of the motor power behind gastric emptying.

The superficial cells from cardia to pylorus all look alike microscopically,
have the same staining properties throughout, and are damaged equally
by the same chemical or physical agents. The turnover of these cells is
high and they secrete muco substances.

The deep cells show no such uniformity (*Fig. 8*).

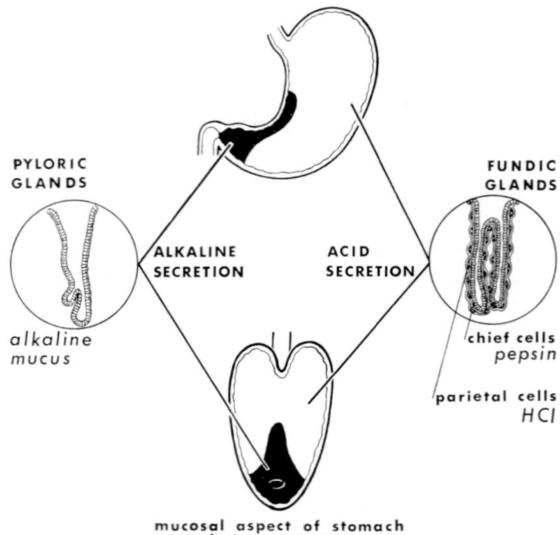

Fig. 8. Distribution of fundic and antral mucosa.

In the fundus and body they are made up mostly of chief cells and
parietal cells responsible for the elaboration of pepsinogen, hydrochloric
acid, electrolytes, and intrinsic factor. The turnover of these cells is slow.
They are the target organs of a multitude of gastro-intestinal hormones,
excitatory as well as inhibitory. Their mass is fairly constant over short

intervals of time, and bears a certain direct relationship to body-weight, but under the continuous influence of hormonal factors this mass may alter in time. The surface reaction in this area is acid.

The deep cells of the cardia and antrum have much in common. They do not contain chief cells or parietal cells. Their exact function is still unsolved.

Two main cells characterize the antro-pyloric region:

a. An argentaffin or enterochromaffin cell (the EC cell).

b. A cell showing all the staining properties of the delta pancreatic islet cell (the cell to be found in gastrin tumours of the pancreas) and exhibiting 'protein granules' under electron microscopy. Evidence so far suggests that this cell is a gastrin-producing one (the G-cell).

The surface reaction in the antrum is neutral to alkaline and a sharp pH border can be demonstrated between antrum and body of the stomach.

It is pertinent to note that gastrin-producing cells are also to be found in small numbers in the corpus and fundus, and therefore antrectomy does not lead to the total disappearance of gastrin output.

When the mucosa of the fundus and corpus is damaged H ions fail to be secreted and appear to be replaced by Na ions. The result is an alkaline surface reaction. The 'alkaline area' of the stomach can therefore alter and must not be taken to be synonymous with the antrum.

The mucosa receives a generous supply of blood and lymph and comes under strong nervous impulses of sympathetic and parasympathetic origin, transmitted via a rich submucosal plexus. Generally speaking the lesser curve comes under parasympathetic dominance, while the greater curve has a predominantly sympathetic supply

A wide network of arteriovenous shunts permeates the mucosa. These intramucosal shunts are mainly under nervous control and dictate the mucosal blood-flow. Both blood-flow and lymphatic drainage control the volume and quality of the mucosal secretion and are important regulators of that secretion. Closing of the shunts leads to an increase in gastric secretion, and opening to the reverse (as in vagotomy). Sympathetico-mimetic, parasympatheticomimetic drugs and gastro-intestinal drugs may all affect these shunts about which much is still unknown.

THE ROLE OF THE FOREGUT IN GASTRIC PHYSIOLOGY

Gastric peptic digestion results from an exocrine secretion of the fundus and body of the stomach in response to endocrine secretions, both ex-citatory and inhibitory, derived from the foregut mucosa stimulated directly by the chemical nature of its luminal contents.

The integration of exocrine and endocrine secretions is best appreciated by an understanding of the embryology of the foregut and a knowledge of the polypeptides elaborated in mucosal cells with a common ancestry.

EMBRYOLOGY OF THE FOREGUT

In the earliest stages of its development the stomach lies in the neck in close association with the heart and lung buds at the very site of the outflow of the vagus from the central nervous system. All three groups of viscera, as early as the third embryonic week, inherit a unique vagal dowry that will dominate their actions in the adult state.

Meanwhile at the junction of the yolk-sac and the midgut a totipotent endodermal outgrowth is becoming clearly delineated (*Fig. 9*). This is the hepatic diverticulum. It overlies the septum transversum, an intensely proliferating mesenchymal complex—the forerunner of the liver. From this hepatic diverticulum epithelial trabeculae sprout out to give rise to the duct systems of the hepatic tree, the gall-bladder, and the pancreas. They also produce the cells that carpet the bulb and the proximal portion of the second part of the duodenum and possibly the antrum. From the ductal arborization of the pancreas solid processes grow into the surrounding mesenchyme to form the acini of the pancreas—both endocrine and exocrine.

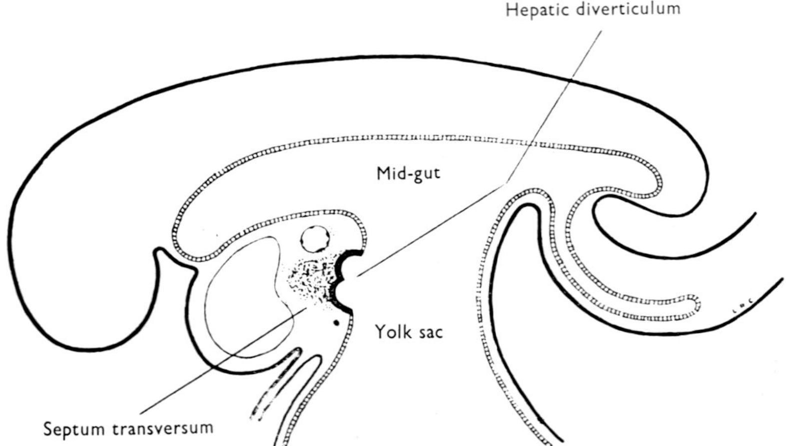

Fig. 9. Embryological origin of foregut cells.

As the result of this common lineage a parentage exists between antral, duodenal, hepatic tree, and pancreatic cells. This is well reflected in the chemistry of their secretion.

CHEMISTRY OF THE FOREGUT HORMONES

Five hormones elaborated by the foregut have been fully documented. Their precise chemistry has been decoded. The histological and cytochemical characteristics of their cells of origin are known. The hormones are:

1. Secretin.
2. Glucagon.
3. Insulin.
4. Gastrin.
5. Cholecystokinin-pancreozymin (CCK-PZ).

6. Gastric inhibitory polypeptide (G.I.P.).
7. Motilin.

The amino-acid sequences of secretin and glucagon are listed below in their correct order:—

Glucagon: HIS-SER-Gln-GLY-THR-PHE-THR-SER-Asp-Tyr-SER-Lys-Tyr-Leu-
ASP-SER-Arg-ARG-Ala-GLN-Asp-Phe-Val-GLN-Trp-LEU-Met-Asn-Thr

Secretin: HIS-SER-Asp-GLY-THR-PHE-THR-SER-Glu-Leu-SER-Arg-Leu-Arg-
ASP-SER-Ala-ARG-Leu-GLN-Arg-Leu-Leu-GLN-Gly-LEU-Val-NH$_2$

Their resemblance is striking. They have the same important N-terminal histidine-serine group and share 14 amino-acids in the same sequences (underlined capital letters).

Both secretin and glucagon are straight-chain compounds. Insulin, on the other hand, is made of two chains interlinked by two disulphide bonds and at first sight seems totally unrelated to the two previous hormones. If, however, the glucagon chain is so placed that its N-terminal histidine–serine group falls opposite the same amino-acids in the β-chain of insulin and the rest of the molecule is 'wrapped' across the disulphide bond on to the α-chain, then three serine sequences, a threonine and a tyrosine coincide. Furthermore the distances between the α-carbon atoms in the chain

His-Ser—Thr-Ser—Ser—Tyr

are almost identical, once more reflecting a distant blood tie.

G.I.P. an enterogastrone type polypeptide, is similarly related to secretin and glucagon.

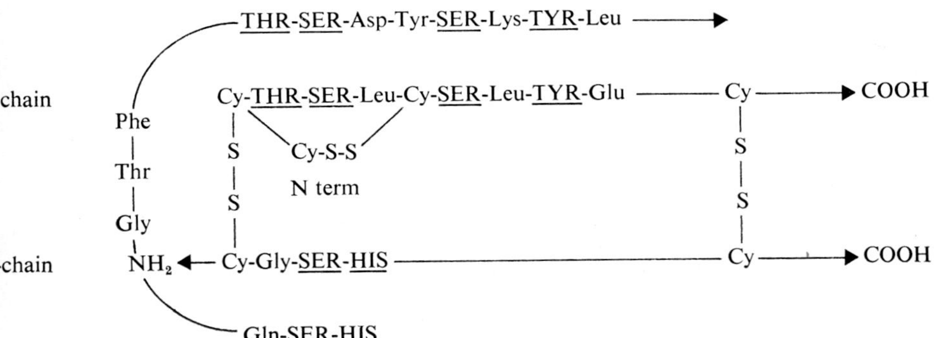

Insulin and Glucagon

Similarly, when the molecules of gastrin and CCK-PZ are compared the same ancestry is reflected this time in the C-terminal peptides, as shown below:

Gastrin: Glu-Gly-Pro-Trp-Leu-Glu-Glu-Glu-Glu-Glu-Ala-Tyr-
GLY-TRP-MET-ASP-PHE-NH$_2$

CCK-PZ: (21) ←——Leu-Sev-Asp-Arg-Asp-Tyr-Met-GLY-TRP-MET-ASP-PHE-NH$_2$

Antrum, duodenum, and pancreas thus show from the polypeptides they elaborate that they are cytogenic siblings of the same forebear and form a family of cells with an oligarchy of purpose: the control of digestion.

These cells in turn belong to a larger family of endocrine polypeptide-producing cells (EPP) with common cytochemical and ultrastructural features: these are the APUD cells, the name being derived from three of their initial characteristics, namely that they are *A*minergic and display amine *P*recursor *U*ptake properties as well as *D*ecarboxylation. They all take up and decarboxylate the amino-acid precursors DOPA and 5-HTP converting them to dopamine and 5-HT, which can be demonstrated by a fluorescent technique. Hence immunofluorescence is another feature of these cells. They all have a bearing on gastric physiology and physio-pathology since the parietal and chief cells of the stomach are directly or indirectly influenced by the polypeptides they elaborate. This is shown in *Table 1*.

Table 1. EFFECTS OF POLYPEPTIDE HORMONES ON GASTRIC ACID
SECRETION

CELL	POLYPEPTIDE	EFFECT
Pituitary corticotrophs	ACTH	+
Pancreatic α-cells	Glucagon	−
Pancreatic β-cells	Insulin	+
Pancreatic δ-cells	Gastrin	+
Stomach G-cells	Gastrin	+
Thyroid C-cells	Calcitonin	+ (via G cells)
Intestinal small granule cells	Secretin	−
Intestinal large granule cells	Enteroglucagon	+ or −
Intestinal entero-chromaffin (EC) cells	Serotonin	−
Intestinal D-cells	G.I.P.	−

CONTROL OF GASTRIC SECRETION

It can therefore be seen that the control of gastric secretion is highly complex and is governed by a number of interdependent factors aiming at producing the optimal pH required for efficient digestion. These factors are both nervous and humoral (*Fig. 10*).

1. ROLE OF THE VAGUS

The vagus consists mostly of afferent fibres bringing back visceral informa-tion to the C.N.S. Little is known about this aspect of the vagus.

The efferent fibres (10 per cent) constitute a preganglionic nerve arboriz-ing on cells in the intramural ganglionic plexuses of the stomach, chiefly in Auerbach's plexus. Vagal stimulation releases large doses of acetylcholine which then mediates the effect of this stimulation across synapses that spread the vagal impulses throughout the whole plexus. From there motor and secretomotor commands reach the mucosa. Vagotomy leads to a complete eclipse of acetylcholine production, leaving only local impulses to influence Auerbach's plexus.

Vagal stimulation and cholinergic action have three main effects on gastric mucosa:

a. They release gastrin from the antrum.

b. They produce pepsin secretion.

c. They sensitize the parietal cells, thus augmenting the action of gastrin on these cells.

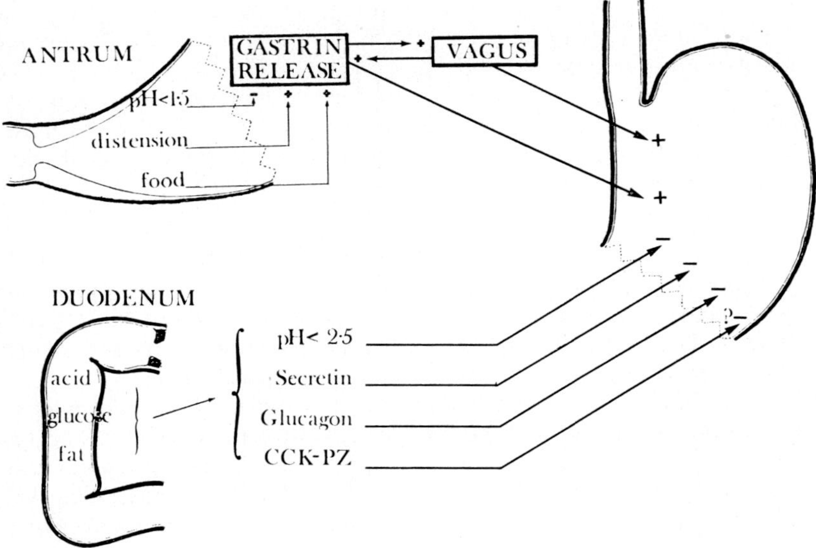

Fig. 10. Control of gastric acid secretion.

Though vagal excitation produced by insulin hypoglycaemia or electrical stimulation will induce acid secretion, it would seem that this is unlikely to occur under normal physiological conditions which require the presence of small doses of gastrin for oxyntic cell activity. Peptic cells, on the other hand, will secrete under vagal excitation alone. Gastrin in small doses affects but little this excitation, while in large doses it inhibits vagal action on these cells. Gastrin, however, will induce pepsin secretion without vagal influence. The vagus therefore plays a permissive role in normal physiology, its action being, in many ways, a synergistic one. Vagotomy will lead to a marked upset in this synergism, decreasing both peptic and acid secretion sufficiently to reduce a state of hypersecretion to one below normal, if not occasionally to one of total secretory suppression.

2. ANTRAL MECHANISMS

Distension, the presence of meat extracts, an alkaline *p*H, and acetylcholine, all fire off the gastrin-producing cells. This effect is via both a cholinergic reflex and a direct physicochemical effect on the G-cells that lie on the luminal aspect of the mucosa. The cholinergic reflex can be either a short or local one within the gastric wall, or a vagovagal one via both afferent and efferent vagal pathways. Acetylcholine is thus a mediator of gastrin release.

Regardless of the excitatory influences at work, gastrin release is invariably inhibited by a pH below 1·5, the inhibition becoming total as the pH falls to 1. On the other hand, high pH levels stimulate gastrin release. It is not strange, therefore, to find that serum-gastrin levels are very high in patients suffering from pernicious anaemia.

The role of the antrum therefore is to regulate the acid secretion so that it remains preferably above pH 1·5 in the normal stomach thereby favouring optimal proteolytic activity.

The presence of gastrin seems essential to the cholinergic release of acid by the parietal cells, and as such it is a mediator of the fundic 'vagal phase'.

Hence 'antral phase' and 'vagal phase' cannot be dissociated, both having the same mediators—gastrin and acetylcholine.

3. DUODENAL MECHANISMS

The presence in the duodenum of emulsified fats, of hyperosmotic substances, and of acid at a pH below 2·5 leads to suppression of gastric secretion. This is through a humoral pathway as both vagal and sympathetic denervation do not abolish this inhibitory mechanism.

Four definite hormones have been isolated from the duodenal mucosa: glucagon, secretin, G.I.P., and cholecystokinin-pancreozymin. The first three—with many common amino-acid sequences—inhibit gastric secretion to an equal degree (about 50 per cent) and in a similar manner. The exact effect of CCK-PZ is not as yet fully determined, but it shares with gastrin the important C-terminal pentapeptide.

In the duodenum, as in the antrum, an autoregulatory mechanism therefore exists whereby the constitution of the chyme expelled by the stomach into the duodenum determines the level of gastric secretion.

4. OTHER MECHANISMS

There is evidence that the pancreas plays a part in gastric secretion. Total pancreatectomy causes an increase in secretion suggesting an inhibitory role of the pancreas—perhaps through the loss of the α-cells. At the same time this viscus is the favourite site of the gastrin-producing tumours (δ-cells hyperplasia or adenoma).

Almost all endocrine systems have an effect on gastric secretion via their APUD relationship as already shown in *Table 1*. Whether these glands partake normally in the physiology of secretion or influence it only in pathological states is not yet ascertained.

Pathophysiology

HYPERSECRETION is to be expected in excessive vagal and endocrine influences.

The vagal or cephalic phase of secretion is undoubtedly influenced by psychological factors and is reflected usually in the nocturnal hypersecretion. There is no proof that a primary vagal lesion exists. Brain tumours and coma from head injury are associated with hypersecretion, but this could be due to the stimulation of parasympathetic pathways in the posterior hypothalamus and brain stem (Cushing). The most likely cause of the hypersecretion seen in the majority of duodenal ulcer sufferers is probably a combination of vagal hyperactivity and an inborn or an acquired large parietal cell mass. Vagotomy reduces secretion by an acetylcholine deprivation. The exact nature of this mechanism is not clear. It could work either by diminishing fundic cell reactivity to stimulating hormones or by allowing free play to the inhibitory ones.

A very small group of duodenal ulcers are associated with endocrine tumours of the APUD series, and are part of a series of syndromes hitherto known as the pluriglandular or multiple adenoma syndromes (*see* pp. 239, 241).

In this group would be included the gastrinoma (Zollinger-Ellison), the multiple endocrine tumours (the pluriglandular syndrome), and similar tumours associated with lung endocrine adenomata like bronchial carcinoids, or parathyroid tumours with intractable peptic ulceration. A high calcium level stimulates the G-cells to release their gastrin and this stimulation may well be the explanation of G-cell hyperplasia seen in association with such tumours.

HYPOSECRETION

Gastric antibodies and an antibody to the C-terminal tetrapeptide of gastrin are known. They both lead either to hypo- or achlorhydria, at least experimentally. The association of achlorhydria and gastric antibodies in P.A. is strongly suggestive of a cause–effect relationship. With achlorhydria the antral pH is high—a state that leads to gastrin release. It is therefore interesting to note that in P.A. there is a high serum level of gastrin. Gastrin stimulates gastro-intestinal motor activity. Again in P.A. rapid gastric emptying time and rapid intestinal transit time are observed.

Gastric Motility and Emptying

The stomach is a hopper in which food is mixed by strong peristaltic waves occurring every 20 sec. Peristalsis is strongest in the antral 'mill' by virtue of the funnel shape of the stomach. There is near the cardia a pacemaker that emits electromotive potentials which spread all over the fundus and body of the stomach, regrouping themselves as they are funnelled down towards the antrum. A build-up of potentials takes place in the latter and reaches a level at which a peristaltic wave is fired off—hence the triturating power of the antrum. These waves are under the influence of nervous mechanisms as far as gastric tone is concerned. Motility depends not only on this tone but also on those physical and chemical factors that affect the endocrine background of the stomach. Tone and motility in turn decide the rate of gastric emptying, which therefore results from the interaction of many factors, some of which are listed in *Table 2*.

Table 2. GASTRIC EMPTYING

RAPID	SLOW
Big meal	Small meal
Fluid meal	Solid meal
Proteins and carbohydrates	Fats
Aggressive emotions	Depressive states
Excitatory hormones	Inhibitory hormones
Hunger	Hypo- or hypertonic fluids
	Pain
	Mechanical disturbance of pylorus

Recently a new hormone named Motilin has been extracted from duodenal mucosa. It is stimulated by an alkaline pH in the duodenum and causes marked gastric contractions. Such a high duodenal pH is to be found in patients with pernicious anaemia and Motilin may be concerned in the rapid gastric emptying characteristic of this disease.

FURTHER READING

IRVINE, W. T. (ed.) (1972), *Scientific Basis of Surgery*. Edinburgh & London: Churchill Livingstone.

Chapter 5

Gastritis, Gastric Ulcer, and Gastric Carcinoma

INTRODUCTION

THOUGH CHRONIC gastritis is undoubtedly associated with both gastric ulcer and gastric carcinoma, the cause of the gastritis is shrouded in mystery and its precise relationship to ulcer and cancer is uncertain. Chronic gastritis causes no easily recognizable symptoms, but leads, as life progresses, to a gradual atrophy of the glandular structure of the stomach and failure of its normal secretory function. Intestinal metaplasia and polyposis may develop and in such a disorganized mucosa, carcinoma occurs with greater frequency than in normal mucosa. It can be said, therefore, with reasonable truth, that chronic gastritis is a precancerous condition. Its relationship to chronic gastric ulcer is even less clear. Though acute erosive gastritis causes small erosions or ulcers they are quick-healing and leave no scars; but repeated attacks of acute gastritis may be the cause of chronic gastritis, and chronic gastritis is found in most stomachs which are chronically ulcerated. It is true that this gastritis occurs more frequently in the antrum than in the body of the stomach, but at least a quarter of stomachs containing a chronic gastric ulcer on the lesser curvature have widespread chronic gastritis. We may, therefore, conceive of chronic gastritis either as a predisposing cause or as an accompaniment of gastric ulceration.

The next link in the aetiological chain is between ulcer and carcinoma. Allowing for the pitfalls of histological interpretation—the epithelial heterotopia so easily mistaken for early cancer and the peptic ulceration which may complicate the erosion of the mucosa by a carcinoma, factors which have undoubtedly magnified the risk in the eyes of some pathologists and of clinicians in North America—and paying most heed to the clinical facts, we would say that a chronic gastric ulcer is a precancerous condition, the risk being of the order of 1 per cent if a lesser curvature ulcer remains unhealed for a year or more and 3 per cent if an antral ulcer remains unhealed for a similar period.

Finally, the acute gastritis which may accompany both ulcer and cancer, particularly if there is gastric retention, is possibly the cause of symptoms such as nausea and anorexia. We can look on these three diseases, therefore, as linked in many ways (*Fig. 11*).

Gastritis

AETIOLOGY

Acute erosive gastritis is probably caused by two things: dietetic insults, such as the consumption of large quantities of alcohol, foods to which the subject is allergic (e.g., shellfish, mushrooms), drugs such as aspirin, or staphylococcal toxin from prepared meats and creams which have acted

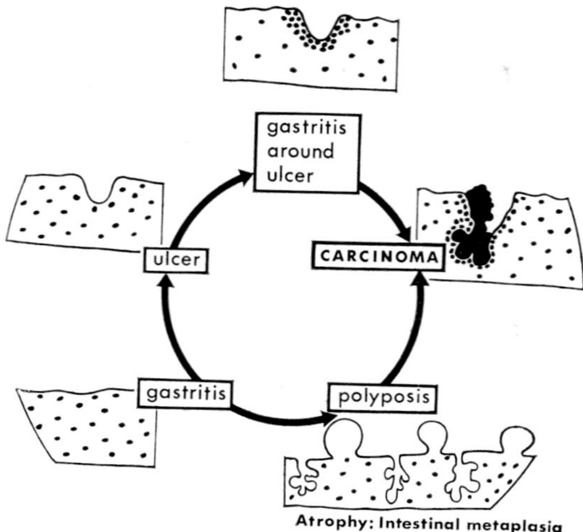

Fig. 11. The gastritic cycle.

as a culture medium, and also by viral infections which frequently cause enteritis at the same time. In these cases the patient is acutely ill and suffers from epigastric pain, nausea, and vomiting. Acute erosive gastritis may also be found in gastric biopsy specimens taken from patients who have no symptoms whatsoever. Chronic gastritis of varying degrees of severity also seems, from biopsy studies, to be a disease which causes no clearly defined symptoms, and apart from some rather tenuous evidence which suggests that the chronic form of the disease is due to repeated attacks of acute gastritis, we have no inkling of the cause. It is, however, commoner in those who smoke or drink heavily, in the lower income groups, and in older people. Auto-immune mechanisms do not seem to be the prime cause of chronic gastritis, though gastric mucosal atrophy which develops insidiously over many years is often due to the effects of antibodies against parietal cells. Reflux of duodenal contents into the stomach either due to an incompetent pylorus or to surgical operations such as gastrojejunostomy, partial gastrectomy, or pyloroplasty may be the cause of chronic gastritic changes and a shrinkage of the acid-secreting area of the fundus. The irritant effect of bile-salts may undermine mucosal resistance.

PATHOLOGY

Acute erosive gastritis may be diffuse or localized to the antrum. The mucosa is red and oedematous, and there are many small erosions 1–5 mm.

in diameter, the floors of which are covered with fibrinous exudate. Polymorphs, plasma cells, eosinophils, and lymphocytes infiltrate the stroma beneath the epithelium. Gland cells, particularly the chief cells, are necrotic. The epithelial cells of the surface become cuboidal and are separated by vacuoles containing polymorphs. If an erosion extends through the muscularis mucosa it is regarded as an acute gastric ulcer.

Chronic atrophic gastritis is of all degrees of severity, but can be divided arbitrarily into two groups: (1) Partial atrophic gastritis; (2) Complete gastric atrophy.

In the first, although glandular atrophy and destruction have advanced far, the mucosa is not substantially thinned, because the intestinal tissue is heavily infiltrated by cells, of which plasma cells predominate in the outer layers, and lymphocytes close to the muscularis. Chief cells are destroyed more than the parietal cells and surviving islands of glandular tissue may grow in a sea of collagen. At the surface, intestinal metaplasia occurs.

In the complete gastric atrophy of pernicious anaemia the gastric mucosa is thinned to about a fifth of the normal depth, and there is a loss of the glandular structure in the body of the stomach. The antral mucosa is always of normal thickness. There is good evidence from serial biopsy studies to suggest that partial atrophic gastritis may in time progress to a state of complete mucosal atrophy. Many such cases are due to the operation of antibodies against parietal cells, and some patients with such antibodies may also develop antibodies against intrinsic factor which hastens the development of pernicious anaemia; and against thyroglobulin which will lead to thyroiditis and hypothyroidism.

CLINICAL PICTURE

Acute gastritis may cause epigastric distress, pain, nausea, and vomiting of limited duration, but there is a poor correlation between histological gastritis and well-defined symptoms. This is even more true of complete chronic gastritis, which in its total atrophic form may cause no gastric distress whatsoever. Many patients with chronic gastritis and parietal cell hypofunction are found to be suffering from iron deficiency, and it is now thought that the iron deficiency is due to inadequate iron intake, poor absorption, recurrent bleeding from minor gastric erosions, or combinations of all three. It seems unlikely that the iron deficiency causes the chronic gastritis though secretory function may improve after repletion of iron stores. A widespread bodily disturbance associated with atrophic gastritis is due to the failure of secretion of intrinsic factor, and consequently to a gradually increasing deficiency of vitamin B_{12} in the body—pernicious anaemia. The symptoms of such a deficiency are not only those of anaemia, but also a sore tongue, nausea, anorexia, vomiting, and depression. Such symptoms are cured rapidly by the repletion of the body's vitamin B_{12} stores by parenteral administration of the vitamin, yet the gastric atrophy is unaffected by the treatment. Damage to the spinal cord (subacute combined degeneration), to the eyes, and to the brain caused by vitamin B_{12} deficiency is less easily made good.

As there is a poor correlation between histological gastritis and symptoms, so there is with gastroscopic signs. A discredited gastroscopic diagnosis is hypertrophic gastritis, which proves to be only a mucosal mamillation often associated with hypersecretion. The gastroscopist should be capable of diagnosing antral gastritis by noting the rigidity, the lack of normal regular peristaltic activity, and the exudate on the mucosa. Antral gastritis seems to cause symptoms similar to those of peptic ulceration, and it frequently accompanies duodenal ulcer.

The radiologist can diagnose gastric mucosal atrophy by noting an absence of rugal markings in the fundus. Such a 'bald' stomach often empties much faster than a normal stomach.

Some clinicians believe that recurring episodes of epigastric distress, nausea, and a feeling of distension may be due to attacks of acute-on-chronic gastritis; and yet again the diagnosis may be made when the food–pain–food–relief–pain sequence usually regarded as typical of ulcer is accompanied by a negative barium meal and achlorhydria.

We must also mention the clinical syndrome of gastric retention usually associated with pyloric stenosis, but sometimes with carcinoma or in vagotomized patients. In these cases there is a particularly severe erosive gastritis, blood and pus can be recovered from the gastric aspirate, and sometimes frank haematemesis or black vomits occur. These patients invariably have a poor appetite, complain of nausea, feeling of fullness after meals, and loss of weight. Gastritis, usually without symptoms, may occur due to the reflux of bile-acids and pancreatic enzymes into the stomach in cases of pyloric valve incompetence or after gastric surgery.

DIAGNOSIS

Antral gastritis which causes rigidity of the mucosa and slowing of the antral peristaltic mill is detectable radiologically, but raises suspicion of either carcinomatous or peptic ulceration close to the pylorus. Gastroscopy may resolve these doubts, and it is not usually necessary to confirm the diagnosis by biopsy of the antral mucosa. If there is any question of a simple or malignant ulcer complicating gastritis in the antrum, an E.S.R., faecal occult blood-tests, and the cytological examination of gastric washings may help to clear the picture; but exploratory laparotomy is sometimes necessary.

The clinical diagnosis of diffuse partial chronic gastritis is as often wrong as right, and since gastroscopy and radiology are so often misleading, the decision rests on biopsy of the gastric mucosa (*see Chapter 26*). The diagnosis of complete atrophic gastritis may be made radiologically, and confirmed by the finding of achlorhydria after maximal stimulation, malabsorption of oral cobalt-labelled radioactive cyanocobalamin, and a low serum B_{12} level.

Hyper-rugosity of the stomach is seen in hypersecretory states, commonly duodenal ulcer, and also in the rare Zollinger-Ellison syndrome (*see* p. 45). Hyper-rugosity is also found in the protein-losing gastropathy, Menetrier's disease, and in reticulosis.

Gastric Ulcer

There are four clinical groups separated by differences in causation, symptoms, and management (*Table 3*).

Table 3. FOUR CLINICAL GROUPS OF GASTRIC ULCER

TYPE OF ULCER	DEFINITION	SYMPTOMS	CAUSE
Acute gastric ulcer	An erosion which penetrates through the muscularis May be multiple Occurs with equal frequency in all parts of the stomach Heals without scarring	May be none May be short-lived dyspepsia of the acute gastritis type Acute or chronic bleeding	A complication of acute gastritis May be caused by aspirin, corticosteroids, or phenyl-butazone
Gastric retention ulcer	Acute or chronic ulceration, often multiple, associated with delay in gastric emptying and found in all parts of the stomach	May be none, or masked by associated duodenal ulcer Acute bleeding	Associated with pyloric stenosis due to duodenal ulcer
Lesser curvature ulcer	Chronic ulcer which causes surrounding oedema and scarring on lesser curvature May be a giant ulcer	Pain after food, relieved by food, vomiting, or alkalis. Periods of remission even though ulcer unhealed	Unknown. Commoner in cirrhotics, bronchitics, and the aged. Relatively common in females and poorer classes
Antral ulcer	An ulcer in pyloric antrum associated with antral gastritis	Pain after food, relieved by food, vomiting, or alkalis Wasting, nausea, and vomiting if pylorus involved	Unknown

AETIOLOGY (*Fig. 12*)

The difference between the acute gastric ulcer and the chronic lesser curve ulcer is that the one heals without trace, and the other, if it heals at all, leaves a scar. There are some grounds for considering the latter as more than a chronic extension of the former, for acute ulcers, as we know from studies of patients bleeding from the stomach, occur over a far wider area than do chronic ulcers, and they also commonly affect a wider range of population. For example, at the age of 20 years acute gastric ulceration is a more likely cause of gastric bleeding than a chronic ulcer. But apart from these few facts we know very little about the incidence of acute gastric ulceration in the different age-groups, sexes, occupations, and populations of the world. Far more is known of the aetiological background of the chronic gastric ulcer which can so easily be detected radiologically or traced after death.

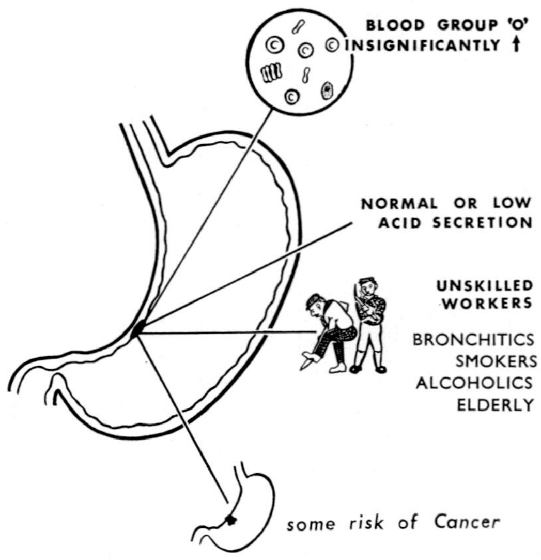

Fig. 12. Aetiology of chronic gastric ulcer.

It seems probable, though unproven, that acute gastric ulceration is conditioned by trauma, gastric in the case of foods, drugs, and poisons, but emotional and metabolic in other instances. A chronic gastric ulcer, on the other hand, forms because there is a failure of mucosal repair in particularly vulnerable parts of the stomach such as the lower lesser curvature, the posterior wall, and the antrum. We know that chronic gastric ulcers, often giant ones, occur most easily in the old, the poor, the alcoholic, the bronchitic, and others with chronic debilitating diseases, and we know that their healing is encouraged by physical rest and abstinence from tobacco. We know that though peptic self-digestion is partly the cause of chronicity, hypersecretion of acid-pepsin is not a factor in their development; indeed, those with chronic gastric ulcers secrete less than the average amounts of acid, both at night and after maximal stimulation by pentagastrin. We know that chronic gastritis is frequently associated with a chronic gastric ulcer.

From these facts it is possible to build up an aetiological concept in which acute gastric ulceration is seen as a response to trauma, both local and general, and chronic gastric ulceration as a failure to heal, conditioned by age, debility, and constitution. Bile reflux into the stomach may be important too in the aetiology of chronic gastric ulcer. A suggested mechanism is destruction of epithelial integrity and 'back' diffusion of H^+ ions into the mucosa which is damaged.

PATHOLOGY

The chronic gastric ulcer penetrates down to the muscular coat and its base consists of fibrin, pus cells, and necrotic granulation tissue. Beneath the floor and around the ulcer is live granulation and scar tissue. There are no living nerve-fibres at the base of the ulcer, but it is surrounded by a considerable zone of inflammatory oedema in which nerve-fibrils may be seen. Disorganized glandular tissue (heterotopia) around the ulcer may lie in the muscular coat and lead to unfounded suspicions of malignancy. The serous coat may be thickened and fibrinous or may be adherent to surrounding organs such as the pancreas. In some cases the muscle coat has been eaten away and the floor of the ulcer is the pancreas. Large blood-vessels may be exposed.

CLINICAL PICTURE

One of the strangest things about peptic ulceration in general is the symptomatology, and, in particular, the unpredictability of the pain response. There are those with large and chronic gastric ulcers who will admit to no present pain, and yet, on the other hand, there are patients without demonstrable peptic ulceration who complain of classic ulcer pain. Pain, however, is the most consistent feature of chronic gastric ulceration, and it is a pain which is intermittent in any one day, rarely lasting for longer than two hours at a time, but rising to peaks of intensity, often about thirty to ninety minutes after a meal. Instillation of acid into the stomachs of patients with ulcers has been followed by typical ulcer pain, but such experiments cannot show the means by which the acid concentration provokes the pain. Gastroscopists who are used to seeing ulcers in their active and painful, as well as in their inactive or painless, phase cannot help but be impressed by the importance of surrounding oedema as an almost inevitable accompaniment of the painful ulcer. As the oedema subsides, so does the pain. It has been suggested that the relief of ulcer pain by food and alkalis, which occurs not at once but after a few minutes, is due not to neutralization of acid and consequent inhibition of the peptic digestion of the ulcer base, but to the diversion of blood-flow away from the painful ulcer surroundings to the secretory glands in the body of the stomach.

Whatever the mechanism responsible, food, drink, and alkalis usually relieve ulcer pain, but the aftermath is more pain, often accompanied by nausea and sometimes by vomiting. Vomiting may relieve the pain. Ulcers near the pylorus can cause gastric retention and thus the vomiting of stale food, but in many cases of lesser curve ulceration the vomiting is the result of a reflex stimulated by pain and conditioned by the state of the patient's nervous system. Some patients with large, painful ulcers never vomit, but others with less severe ulcers become nauseated and vomit easily. It depends more on the person than on the ulcer. Some lose their appetite from fear of pain or nausea, and if this happens they lose weight. Elderly patients with giant gastric ulcers may lose protein from the ulcer base and become very weak, thin, and oedematous.

Reflex disturbances, such as oesophageal spasm, excessive salivation and waterbrash, colonic pain, and flatulence, are probably less common in gastric than in duodenal ulcer, but there is no sure way of telling from the history whether a patient has a gastric or a duodenal ulcer. Indeed, it is difficult enough to distinguish the symptoms of peptic ulcer in general from those of nervous dyspepsia, gastritis, and recurrent cholecystitis (*Table 7*, p. 73).

There are no physical signs of uncomplicated gastric ulcer except an inconstant tenderness over the ulcer itself. If the ulcer becomes attached to the surrounding structures, not only does the pain tend to become more continuous or penetrate to the back, but also muscle rigidity may develop. In severe penetrating ulcers, pain may be made worse by movements of the trunk. If the ulcer involves the pylorus, signs of gastric retention (*see* p. 78) may develop. Bleeding from the ulcer may be acute or insidious, and in the latter case there may be signs and symptoms of anaemia or iron deficiency.

HELPFUL INVESTIGATIONS

Barium Meal

Radiological examination is the method of choice in the initial investigation of a patient with a suspected gastric ulcer. An accuracy of 90–95 per cent can be expected.

Difficulties in diagnosis arise in shallow ulcers and those occurring high on the lesser curvature or posterior wall of the stomach. The presence of food or blood-clot may obscure ulcers. Trapping of barium between large gastric folds may simulate ulceration but these appearances are usually inconstant.

Benign ulcers usually project beyond the outline of the barium-filled stomach whereas malignant ulcers frequently appear to be within the lumen. The malignant ulcer is often shallow or irregularly shaped and the floor of the ulcer may be nodular. The adjacent portions of the stomach are often irregular. Convergence of the rugae of the stomach towards the ulcer is not a helpful sign. It must be firmly stated that there are no unequivocal signs to differentiate a benign from a malignant ulcer. Careful follow-up in all patients with gastric ulceration is essential and if complete healing can be established it is likely that the ulcer was benign. With ulcers close to the pylorus, it is difficult to say whether they lie on the gastric or duodenal side of the sphincter, and though the radiologist thinks that the ulcer is gastric, fibre-endoscopy may place it in the duodenum.

Endoscopy

Endoscopy and barium-meal examination should ascertain the nature of nearly all gastric ulcers. Fibreoptic instruments of the end and side viewing types have revolutionized gastric endoscopy. They are easy to pass and their use is well tolerated by patients. Furthermore, there are no areas of the stomach that cannot be seen. Photography and biopsy of ulcers and polyps are possible, and cytological specimens can be obtained.

The place of the gastrocamera appears to be in the field of mass screening programmes, and it is not much used in normal clinical practice.

Gastric Analysis and Secretory Studies

Resting juice may contain blood or pus cells, and the nocturnal secretory pattern is usually a fall in acid concentration and output during the early hours of the morning. This pattern is different from that of duodenal ulcer. The presence or absence of free acid after maximal histamine stimulation is of no value in the differentiation between simple and carcinomatous ulcers.

E.S.R., Haemoglobin, and Repeated Faecal Occult-blood Tests

These are useful both in diagnosis and assessment for treatment.

DIFFERENTIAL DIAGNOSIS, ASSESSMENT, AND TREATMENT

There is only one condition which can be confused with a simple gastric ulcer and that is a malignant gastric ulcer (*Fig. 13*). The initial diagnosis must therefore exclude carcinoma (*Table 4*), and in doing so, the severity of the ulcer is assessed and treatment planned.

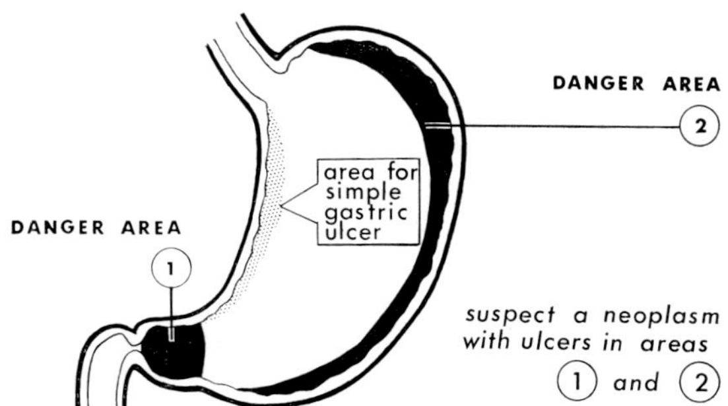

Fig. 13. Areas of predilection for ulcer and carcinoma.

Since antral ulcers are often malignant, and since differentiation may be difficult, it is wise to advise immediate treatment for all ulcers in this position if the radiological and gastroscopic findings are at all equivocal. Even if an antral ulcer has all the appearances of simplicity, medical treatment must be followed to a conclusion—complete healing of the ulcer within six weeks. If this is not achieved gastrectomy should be advised. If the ulcer is on the lesser curvature the same principle is followed, but since there is less likelihood of cancer, some physicians consider it permissible to persist with conservative treatment even though the ulcer has not healed. A strong cardiorespiratory hazard, or a patient's strong prejudice

Table 4. DIFFERENTIAL DIAGNOSIS BETWEEN BENIGN AND
MALIGNANT GASTRIC ULCER

	SIMPLE ULCER	CARCINOMA
Symptoms	Intermittent pain	Anorexia, and nausea prominent
Site	95 per cent on lesser curve or antrum	Anywhere
Radiology	Rugal convergence right into ulcer base	Irregular contour
	Contour not irregular	Ulcer often within the line of the lesser curvature
	Ulcer not within the line of lesser curvature	Rigidity
	Muscle spasm opposite	Indistensibility
		Lack of peristalsis
Gastroscopy	Oedema and spasm	Irregular margins Infiltration around
	Rugal convergence	Lack of peristalsis
Haemoglobin	May be reduced	Usually reduced
E.S.R.	Usually normal	Often raised
Faecal occult blood	Positive sometimes	Positive nearly always
Analysis of gastric aspirate	Sometimes achlorhydric	Red blood cells + + Pus cells + + Often achlorhydric Cancer cells may be found (but interpretation difficult)

against operation, would influence the decision. The basic principle is that all patients should, if possible, be treated until a conclusion is reached.

In Japan, where gastric carcinoma is at least ten times commoner than in England and where simple gastric ulcer is also common, the differential diagnosis between these conditions often requires endoscopy, air barium contract X-rays, four quadrant biopsies, gastrocamera surveys, and gastric cytology.

The authors' practice is to admit to hospital all patients with a gastric ulcer, to assess the general condition, anaemia, loss of blood in the stools, to make careful radiological and gastroscopic examinations, and to decide as soon as possible whether the ulcer is likely to be simple or malignant. Loose teeth or those surrounded by periodontal sepsis are removed. If the ulcer seems to be simple, then medical treatment is based on physical rest and recumbency for several hours each day, avoidance of smoking, and a dietary régime which avoids any strong stimulus to gastric secretory or motor activity. Although the value of the usual 'two-hourly milk feeds' and soft foods containing no cooked fat at the main meals is unproven, a strong prejudice in favour of such a régime exists in the minds of doctors, nurses, and patients, and it would be difficult to persuade patients to undergo the necessary periods of physical rest, to deny themselves the solace of tobacco, and to stay under observation, unless they were offered the supposed solid benefits of dietary treatment. The same may be said of conventional treatment with antacids. It is not believed that hypersecretion of the acid-pepsin mixture is an important factor in the causation of gastric ulcer, but the patient knows that antacids relieve symptoms, and the doctor believes that peptic digestion may be one of the causes of ulcer chronicity. Hence, in spite of the lack of any evidence that they quicken the healing of gastric ulcers, we are not prepared to recommend the abandonment of conventional antacids, though they could well be omitted as soon as pain has been relieved.

If there is any suspicion of an ascorbic acid deficiency from a diet deficient in fresh fruit and vegetables, ascorbic acid may be given, 200 mg. three times a day, for a week. In the case of iron deficiency, oral iron is sometimes badly tolerated, in which case iron may be given intravenously or intramuscularly. In very debilitated and anaemic patients, usually elderly, a blood transfusion may be necessary. Most patients with lesser-curve ulcers lose their pain, regain lost appetite, and begin to gain weight after less than a week of such a hospital régime. Unfortunately, however, further radiological and gastroscopic examinations after a month show that though oedema around the ulcer has subsided and spasm relaxed, the crater remains in about 70 per cent of cases. In these, surgery, which has been rendered safer by the improvement in general condition and the abatement of inflammatory reaction around the ulcer, is called for, and usually a partial gastrectomy with a Billroth-type of anastomosis is done.

Carbenoxolone (Biogastrone), a synthetic derivative of glycyrrhizinic acid, has been shown to promote the healing of gastric ulcers. The effectiveness of the drug has been proved by comparing the area of a barium-filled ulcer niche visible in a standard radiographic projection before and after treatment with carbenoxolone and a dummy preparation. Under this treatment without bed-rest and without antacids about 90 per cent of ulcer craters will shrink, and about 50 per cent appear to heal completely after a month's treatment. With placebo tablets about 50 per cent of ulcer craters shrink but only about 10 per cent appear to heal. The use of carbenoxolone is attended with some of the same risks which were noted when crude liquorice extracts were given—namely a tendency to salt and water retention causing headache and malaise, occasional hypertension, and a tendency to hypokalaemia. These side-effects are less noticeable with carbenoxolone than with crude liquorice extracts and can be minimized by giving only 50 mg. of the drug three times a day, and by using a thiazide diuretic and potassium supplements in all cases showing fluid retention. However, better healing of ulcers is achieved if doses of 100 mg. t.d.s. are given, and it appears that the healing effects of the drug are related not purely to a local action but to the general effects on the body, some of which are undesirable. A further attempt to utilize the healing effects of liquorice extract has been made by removing glycyrrhizinic acid from the extract. Such a deglycyrrhizinated compound of which 380 mg. have been added to various antacids has been made up into a tablet (Caved-S.) which has been tested by the same double blind technique as was used for carbenoxolone. The results suggest that this combination is capable of healing gastric ulcers in the ambulant patient, and that the side-effects noted with crude liquorice extracts and to a lesser extent with carbenoxolone do not occur. It has yet to be shown that the deglycyrrhizinated extract is effective on its own. The advantage of the liquorice-derived drugs is that they enable the gastric ulcer patient to be treated without putting him to bed. It is not, however, wise to attempt ambulant treatment in any case where there is a remote possibility of the ulcer being malignant, e.g., if it is an antral ulcer; and in all cases careful radiological or endoscopic follow-up and occult-blood tests on the stools are necessary. If a gastric ulcer recurs in the year after the patient leaves hospital he should be persuaded to have a gastrectomy.

Certain exceptions must be made. Patients with lesser-curve ulcers who have cirrhosis or serious heart and lung disease may not be fit enough to withstand gastrectomy, and operation is then usually avoided unless complications arise or symptoms are severe. Some patients, particularly middle-aged women, emphatically prefer to keep their ulcers, and since it is always unwise to force patients towards an operation which involves a degree of risk, it is better in these cases to accept the situation.

COMPLICATIONS

These are perforation, acute and chronic bleeding, penetration into surrounding tissues, obstruction of the pyloric valve by oedema, or fibrosis, and an hour-glass constriction by fibrosis of the mid-zone of the stomach.

Perforation

Anterior gastric ulcers perforate most rapidly and about 10 per cent of these prove to be malignant, the condition being less easy to recognize at operation than it is under the microscope. Most surgeons treat perforated gastric ulcers by immediate partial gastrectomy or else they take a biopsy from the ulcer, suture it, and perhaps proceed to a gastrectomy after an interval. The general surgical management of perforated peptic ulcer is dealt with in *Chapter 6*.

Bleeding

Acute bleeding is discussed in *Chapter 7*. Immediate partial gastrectomy is the treatment of choice.

Penetration

As with duodenal ulcers, penetration into pancreas, liver, or other organs may alter the symptoms. Intractable constant pain, pain in the back, and pain made worse by movement are the new features. Some relief can be obtained by rest in bed for a week or more, but a partial gastrectomy must be done as soon as the patient's general condition is good enough.

Pyloric Obstruction
This is dealt with in *Chapter 6.*

Hour-glass Stomach
This uncommon complication must be treated by gastrectomy.

Gastric Carcinoma

About one-half of all cases occur in the pyloric antrum and the rest in the body of the stomach. When the cardia is involved the symptoms approximate to those of carcinoma of the oesophagus. The cause is unknown, but there is a slight preponderance in males, a modal age of 60 years, and an excess in those of blood group A. Polyposis of the stomach, ulcer, and the gastric atrophy of pernicious anaemia are known precancerous conditions. Certain races seem to be more prone to this form of cancer, for example, Japanese, Icelanders, certain Dutch coast-dwellers, and the Welsh; it seems that dietary or soil factors may be important. Carcinoma occurs with significant frequency in the gastric remnant left after partial gastrectomy.

PATHOLOGY

The growth is an adenocarcinoma in which the relative proportions of glandular and fibrous tissue determine its type. The fungating polypoid carcinoma is usually a pure adenocarcinoma, the sessile ulcerated form has solid masses of tumour cells, while in the rarer scirrhous carcinoma, which may infiltrate the submucosa of the whole stomach, fibrous tissue predominates and tumour cells are scanty (*Fig. 14*). Many of the tumours are highly invasive and spread not only to surrounding organs but commonly to liver, ovaries, peritoneum, lungs, and less commonly to brain and bones.

CLINICAL PICTURE

The symptoms are extremely variable and in the early stages there may be none. Later, an insidious loss of weight, strength, and appetite may precede the specifically gastric symptoms of nausea, pain, and vomiting. The pain is sometimes worse after food, but may equally well be constant or affected by movement, depending on the invasive stage reached. Unfortunately, the growth may have spread to other organs before symptoms are appreciable to the patient; and even if the patient should consult his doctor early, the symptoms are usually so nondescript that investigation is delayed. Patients with recent dyspepsia, anaemia, or loss of appetite should be regarded with a highly suspicious clinical eye (*Fig. 15*).

Carcinoma of the stomach may not be suspected until the patient is breathless from the lymphatic spread of growth in the lungs, jaundiced from involvement of the liver, distended by the ascites provoked by peritoneal secondaries, or anaemic from insidious blood-loss. Haematemesis is not common as a first symptom and low-grade fever is a rare finding. The only physical signs of any importance are those of anaemia, a mass in the epigastrium, or gastric distension from pyloric obstruction. None of these may be present in patients who nevertheless have advanced carcinoma.

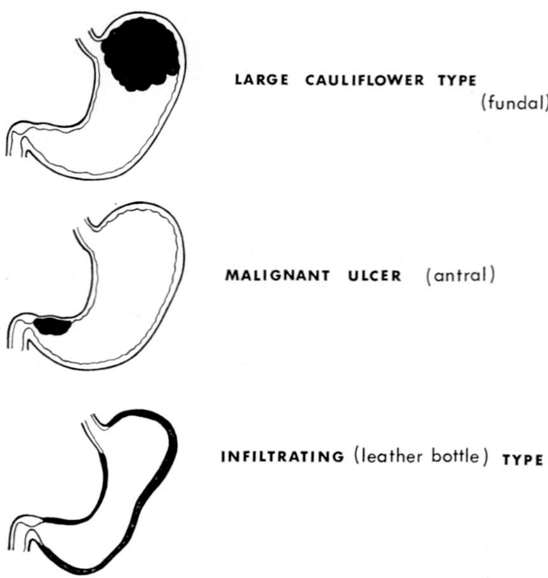

Fig. 14. Types of gastric neoplasms.

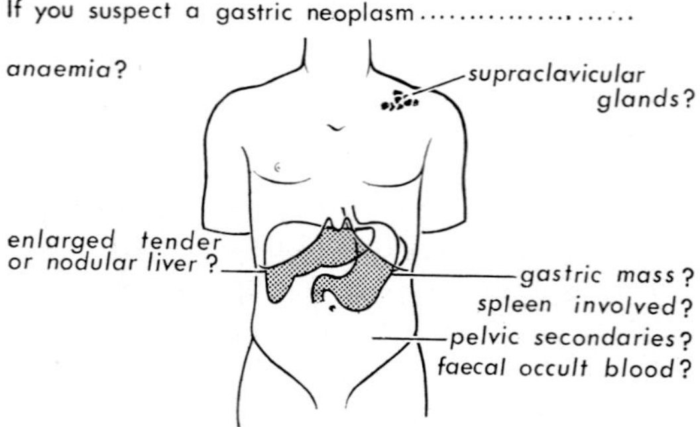

Fig. 15. Examination for gastric carcinoma.

DIAGNOSIS

Clinical suspicions must be aroused by any story of loss of appetite in a previously healthy person. Beyond this one symptom which is so characteristic of gastric carcinoma, there is little in the history or physical examination which can differentiate an early carcinoma from ulcer and a host of other conditions. Investigations are more helpful. The haemoglobin is usually reduced and the faecal occult-blood test is positive. A barium meal can demonstrate a gastric carcinoma in about 80 per cent of cases. In such patients destruction of the mucosa, intraluminal filling defects, rigidity of the gastric wall, and interference with peristalsis are common features. Infiltrative carcinoma may produce the classic leather-bottle appearance or linitis plastica. The mucosa is devoid of folds, the stomach is small, and peristalsis is absent. Emptying of the stomach is extremely rapid. Lesions of the fundus of the stomach may be difficult to diagnose and in such cases double-contrast studies can demonstrate the thickened gastric wall between air in the stomach and peritoneal cavity.

There remains a group of cases in whom the diagnosis is in doubt. In such patients tomography of the air-filled stomach sometimes assists in establishing the diagnosis.

If a negative barium study conflicts with a high index of clinical suspicions, fibreoptic endoscopy is invaluable. The instruments have attachments to enable direct-vision biopsy to be done, and it is also possible to photograph doubtful lesions. Gastrocamera pictures may be very valuable in cases of early or infiltrating carcinoma.

Exfoliative Cytology

Microscopical search for carcinoma cells in gastric washings obtained by a variety of methods from the simplest to the most complex depends for success on prompt examination, immaculate techniques, and considerable experience. The best results are obtained in cases of early cancer with small ulcerated lesions not easy to pick up radiologically. Direct exfoliative techniques using an endoscope have proved to be less tedious and more accurate than examination of bulk washings.

In all cases where the diagnosis remains doubtful it is customary to proceed at once to the final examination of laparotomy. It should be no disgrace to advise a laparotomy which proves that cancer is not present.

TREATMENT

Surgical treatment is desirable if feasible, but too often the disease at diagnosis has reached a stage in which neither palliative nor radical surgery has anything to offer. Radiotherapy is of no value, and palliative treatment in advanced cases must make use of pain-relieving and phenothiazine drugs. Old-fashioned mixtures such as Mist. Chlorof. et Morph., taken 4-hourly, are comforting to the patient. Blood transfusions and gastric lavage are of considerable temporary benefit.

The surgical treatment is a high partial gastrectomy with excision of drainage lymph-nodes and omentum, followed, if possible, by a Billroth-I reconstruction, but some surgeons prefer a total gastrectomy in spite of the higher operative mortality and the poor nutritional state which follows. When operating on a patient incapacitated by vomiting and pain, in whom the growth is found to have spread beyond the stomach, a palliative partial gastrectomy is done, or sometimes even a gastro-enterostomy.

Before operation, the patient's condition should, as far as possible, be improved by blood transfusion, repletion of iron, ascorbic acid, and electrolyte deficiencies, and by breathing exercises. Infected teeth should be removed and smoking should be forbidden Sometimes in cases of antral carcinomata, gastric lavage with normal saline twice daily will clean up the interior of the stomach and make the operation safer.

Growths at the cardia which are obstructing it can sometimes be removed by oesophagogastrectomy.

PROGNOSIS

If the history is long, yet at operation the growth proves to be both confined to the stomach and highly differentiated, then the outlook for the future is as bright as it can be. Patients with a short history and anaplastic growths already involving the omentum have almost no hope of survival. The prognosis in an individual case can therefore only be assessed by the surgeon at the time of operation and subsequently in the light of histological reports.

The usually quoted and easily remembered figure of 5 per cent survival at 5 years applies to all patients followed. The patients with least invasive and therefore the most resectable growths have a 20 per cent chance of surviving 5 years, and after this their chance of survival is good. In Japan, earlier diagnosis and treatment have led to even better results.

LESS IMPORTANT GASTRIC CONDITIONS

Adult Hypertrophic Pyloric Stenosis

Occasionally an adult develops hypertrophic pyloric stenosis similar pathologically to the well-known infantile form. The story is one of attacks of vomiting, and radiological studies show a rigid funnel-shaped antrum and pylorus. The treatment is surgical. There is often difficulty even on the operating table in distinguishing the condition from carcinomatous infiltration.

Leiomyoma

This is a locally invasive tumour of the muscularis which easily ulcerates and bleeds. It is rare, and the first manifestation may be a haematemesis. Radiologists can distinguish the smooth oval filling defect of this type of tumour from that caused by a cancer.

Sarcoma

May develop primarily or in a leiomyoma, and is very rare indeed. Bleeding is an early symptom.

Polyps

Single or multiple adenomatous polyps in the stomach are not very unusual. They are often associated with atrophic gastritis and achlor-hydria, and are considered by many to be a premalignant condition, but the evidence is conflicting. Though symptoms are few, gastrectomy is usually advised if the risk is reasonable.

Diverticula

These occur mainly in the fundus near to the cardia. Radiologically they are often large and impressive, and can be distinguished from penetrating ulcers by their position, narrow neck, and smooth walls (*Fig. 16*). Although

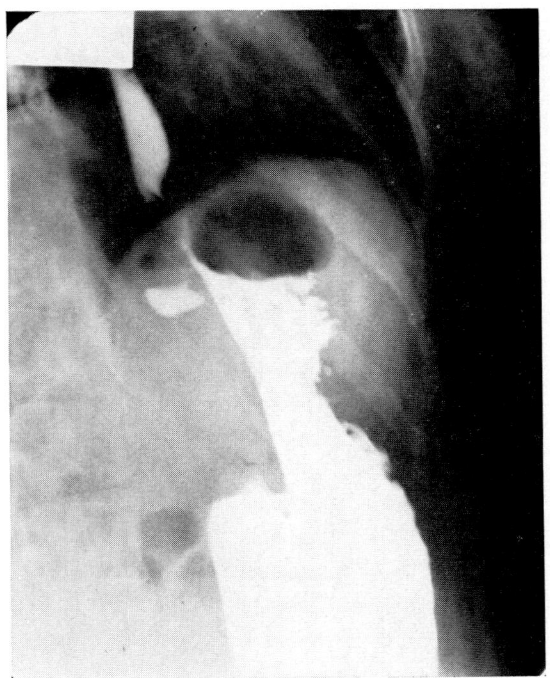

Fig. 16. Barium meal showing gastric diverticulum.

such a diverticulum may be the only radiological finding after a haematemesis, it is doubtful whether they do, in fact bleed. Other complications such as perforation, inflammation, and cancer formation are but medical curiosities. At operation they are most difficult to find.

FURTHER READING

Gastric Atrophy
GLASS, G. B., SPEER, F. D., NIEBURGS, H. E., ISHIMORI, A., JONES, E. LINN, BAKER, H., SCHWARTZ, S. A., and SMITH, R. (1960), 'Gastric Atrophy, Atrophic Gastritis and Gastric Secretory Failure', *Gastroenterology*, **39**, 429.

Gastritis
DOIG, R. K., and WOOD, I. J. (1952), 'Gastritis Study of 112 Cases diagnosed by Gastric Biopsy', *Med. J. Aust.*, **1**, 593.
MAGNUS, H. A. (1952), 'Gastritis', p. 323 in *Modern Trends in Gastroenterology* (ed. JONES, F. AVERY). London: Butterworth.

Giant Hypertrophic Gastritis
BUTZ, W. C. (1960), 'Giant Hypertrophic Gastritis', *Gastroenterology*, **39**, 183.

Diagnosis of Gastric Carcinoma
BURNETT, W., MACFARLANE, P. S., SCOTT PARK, S. D., and KAY, A. W. (1960), 'Carcinoma of the Stomach: An Evaluation of Diagnostic Methods including Exfoliative Cytology', *Br. med. J.*, **1**, 753.

Aetiology of Gastric Carcinoma
DOLL, R. (1956), 'Environmental Factors in the Aetiology of Cancer of the Stomach', *Gastro-enterologia, Basel*, **86**, 320.

Treatment and Prognosis of Gastric Carcinoma
BARBER, K. W., GAGE, R. P., and PRIESTLEY, J. T. (1961), 'Significance of Duration of Symptoms and Size of Lesion in Prognosis of Gastric Carcinoma', *Surgery Gynec. Obstet.*, **113**, 673.
MCNEER, G., LAWRENCE, W., ASHLEY, M. P., and PACK, G. T. (1958), 'End Results in the Treatment of Gastric Cancer', *Surgery*, **43**, 879.

Chronic Idiopathic Gastritis
COGHILL, N. F. (1969), *Fifth Symposium on Advanced Medicine (Royal College of Physicians)* (ed. WILLIAMS, R.), p. 10. London: Pitman.

Prognosis of Early Gastric Cancer
KASUGAI, T. (1970), 'Prognosis of Early Gastric Cancer', *Gastroenterology*, **58**, 429.

Chapter 6

Duodenal Ulcer

DESPITE A GREAT deal of research the cause of duodenal ulcer remains a puzzle. The results of radical gastric surgery, though good, are not good enough to provide the answer to the problem of treatment. Physicians, unable to find an effective medical alternative to the radical surgical approach, have directed their investigations mainly towards the basic aetiology, whereas surgeons, working on the assumption that the peptic hypersecretion is the critical factor, have concentrated on finding methods of reducing that hypersecretion. Neutralization of gastric juice by medical measures is so short-lived that antacids can only be valuable in relieving symptoms, and the whole basis of standard medical treatment by diet and drugs has been discredited by controlled trials of therapy. On the other hand, surgeons realize full well that there is no perfect operation for duodenal ulcer, and whether they be gastrectomists or gastro-enterostomists and vagotomists, they expect some of their patients to be dissatisfied.

AETIOLOGY (Fig. 17)

1. *Hypersecretion of Acid Pepsin*

All are agreed that duodenal ulcer—a peptic ulcer in the full sense—will not occur unless the stomach is capable of secreting acid and pepsin. It has been proved that most, but not all, patients with duodenal ulcer secrete greater quantities of acid in response to a maximal stimulation with histamine or pentagastrin than do normals. Their basal or nocturnal gastric secretion of acid is also greater (*see* p. 72).

It has also been shown that they have a larger mass of acid secretory (parietal) cells than normal (*Table 5*).

Furthermore, duodenal ulcer occurs nearly always in the first part of the duodenum, the part which is most exposed to the acid and peptic

Table 5. ACID SECRETORY CELLS IN DUODENAL ULCER PATIENTS AND NORMALS

	NO. OF CELLS IN BILLIONS	
	Males	*Females*
Normals	1·0	0·8
Duodenal ulcer	1·75	1·5

activity of the gastric juice, and this argues that ulceration is at least maintained, if not certainly provoked, by the acid-pepsin mixture. In the rare Zollinger-Ellison syndrome gross hypersecretion of acid associated with a gastrin-secreting adenoma in the pancreas or its neighbourhood leads to severe peptic ulceration not only of the duodenum but also of the jejunum.

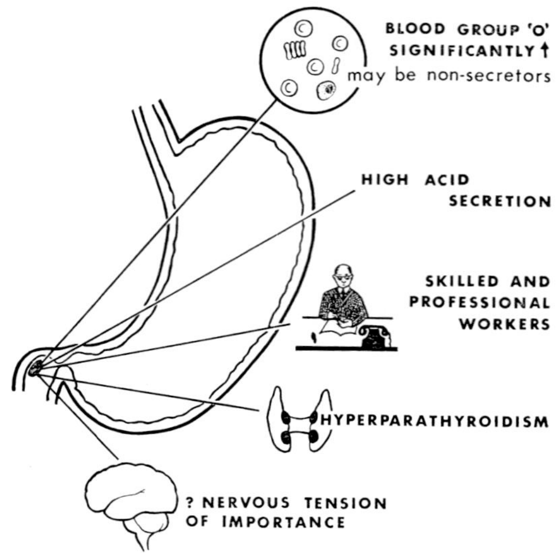

Fig. 17. Aetiology of chronic duodenal ulcer.

2. *Preponderance in Males*

In all countries males suffer more frequently, but the proportion varies. The usual ratio is 4 : 1. In England nearly 10 per cent of males aged 45–54 years have suffered from a duodenal ulcer, but of these only a quarter have symptoms which incapacitate them. From the age of 20 to 65 years the incidence in males is steady, but thereafter it declines. In females the highest incidence is after the menopause.

3. *Constitutional Background*

There is a familial predisposition, but no certain method of inheritance. Those with group O blood and those unable to secrete AB substances into their saliva and gastric secretions have a greater liability to duodenal ulceration. Patients with chronic anoxia and infection (namely, chronic emphysema) seem more liable, as do patients with rheumatoid disease and polycythaemia.

4. *Endocrine*

Patients with hyperparathyroidism and tumours of the G-cells are unduly prone to duodenal ulcer, whereas those with pituitary or adrenal failure are immune. Cortisone treatment often causes exacerbation of ulcer symptoms and complications.

5. *Social and Occupational*

Professional people, notably doctors, are unduly prone, whereas agricultural workers are the least liable to develop duodenal ulcer.

6. *Geographical and Dietary*

The very much higher incidence of duodenal ulcer in Southern India compared with Northern India correlates well with different dietary habits. In Northern India the diet is fibrous and requires much chewing whereas in Southern India soft rice is the staple food and is gulped down without being mixed with saliva. The theory has been propounded that thorough mixture of the food with saliva protects against duodenal ulcer by ensuring the proper buffering of the gastric contents.

Table 6. SPECIFICITY OF DUODENAL ULCER SYMPTOMS

| | | ALSO OCCUR IN | | |
DUODENAL ULCER SYMPTOMS	*Gastric ulcer*	*Gall-bladder disease*	*Gastritis*	*Nervous dyspepsia*
1. Pain—food relief	+	−	+	−
2. Intermittency	+	+ (longer gaps)	±	−
3. Pain—freedom on rising	+	−	−	−
4. Pain—relief by vomiting	+	−	±	−
5. Pain—relief by antacids	+	−	+	±
6. Night pain	±	Severe (bouts longer)	−	Patient wakes first; has pain later
7. Pain—provocation by fat	±	+	±	+
8. Pain—provocation by stress	+	−	±	+
9. Pain—localized in epigastrium	+	±	±	—

7. *Environmental*

It has been shown that the incidence of the complications of ulcer, such as bleeding and perforation, rises at times of stress to the population, as in the bombing of London in 1941 and again in 1944. Burns and physical trauma act in the same way. Individual patients can often relate exacerbations of ulcer symptoms to periods of mental strain or sleeplessness. Direct gastric trauma from drugs, e.g., aspirin, may precipitate bleeding in patients with chronic ulcer, and may cause acute peptic ulceration.

Conclusion

The general picture seems to be one of genetic and sex predisposition complicated by the environmental and local factors which cause acute ulceration. Once acute ulcers form the important question is why some become chronic. Some of the factors are sex, age, blood group, anxiety, smoking, and certain drugs. The intermediary mechanism may be a failure of the duodenum to neutralize the acid gastric contents squirted into it.

Pathology

In their histological characteristics duodenal ulcers do not differ from gastric ulcers (*see Chapter 5*). They may be single or multiple. They may penetrate deeply into the pancreas and they may erode major blood-vessels in the pancreatico-duodenal area. Rarely, the biliary or pancreatic ductal sphincters may be involved by the inflammatory oedema of an ulcer, and more commonly the pyloric mechanism is obstructed by oedema and fibrosis. Antral gastritis is frequently associated with duodenal ulcer.

CLINICAL PICTURE

The concept of a classic duodenal ulcer history is hallowed by tradition, by constant textbook repetition, and is associated in Great Britain with the name of that pioneer of gastric surgery, Lord Moynihan. Unfortunately, ulcer patients rarely complain of such textbook symptoms, and duodenal ulcer may occur without any at all. A certain pattern is, however, usually discernible, and the features which are both frequently noted with, and most typical of, duodenal ulcer are listed in order of their estimated importance:

1. A food–pain–food–relief–pain sequence, relief occurring immediately after food and pain about two hours later.

2. Periodicity of symptoms, bouts of trouble lasting for an average of three weeks.

3. Freedom from pain for about two hours after rising.

4. Relief of pain after vomiting of acid fluid.

5. Relief of pain by antacids.

6. Pain which wakes the sufferer in the night.

7. Provocation of pain by cooked fat in food.

8. Provocation of bouts of ulcer distress by mental or physical fatigue.

9. Ability to localize the pain to the epigastrium.

The choice of these nine features is made solely because they seem to the authors to be the most important in a large and varied symptomatology. In *Table 6* we attempt to indicate their specificity for duodenal ulcer. We are clear on two points: first, that it is impossible to distinguish gastric ulcer from duodenal ulcer by the history, and secondly, that periodicity of symptoms and freedom from pain on rising are the two features which are the most specific for peptic ulceration.

Atypical histories are given by patients in whom:

1. *There is a high pain threshold,* so that little or no pain is experienced.

2. *There is enhanced reflex activity* in the gastro-intestinal tract, so that a duodenal ulcer may produce:

a. Oesophageal spasm with regurgitation of fluid (waterbrash).

b. Pylorospasm and reverse peristalsis in the stomach with gastro-oesophageal regurgitation and heartburn.

c. Colon spasm causing left iliac fossa pain, diarrhoea, constipation, and narrow stools.

d. When other common conditions such as hiatus hernia or gall-stones coexist.

3. *Complications cause new symptoms:*

a. Penetration of ulcer may cause continuous pain, pain in unusual sites such as the shoulder region, the pectoral region, and the back, and pain made worse by movement or certain positions of the body.

b. Pyloric obstruction may cause nausea, anorexia, loss of weight, and vomiting.

c. Insidious bleeding may cause symptoms of anaemia.

d. Perforation of an ulcer into the lesser sac may cause back pain, fever, and malaise.

4. *Neurosis complicates the picture,* so that genuine ulcer symptoms are buried beneath a burden of emotional distress, which causes so many gastro-intestinal discomforts.

It is our impression that atypical histories are to be expected in children, in women, in those with a background of neurosis, and in those with a tendency to spasmodic or episodic disorders such as migraine and the irritable colon.

5. *Patients with postbulbar ulcers* may suffer chiefly from back pain or insidious bleeding.

Physical Signs

There are none in many patients with duodenal ulcer, but deep tenderness to the right of the midline in the epigastrium probably indicates an active ulcer with oedematous surroundings and involving the serosa. Deep localized tenderness must be distinguished from the more superficial and factitious tenderness which occurs in the epigastrium of highly strung people. These tend to wince, jump, contract their abdominal muscles, and remove the examining hand, but with patience they can be made to relax and then tenderness disappears.

A gastric splash sometimes suggests gastric retention due to a duodenal ulcer near the pylorus, but can also occur in narrow-chested nervous patients whose stomachs empty slowly. It may be elicited by firm flapping movements of the hand, the palm of which is pressed to the right of and below the epigastrium. It is of no significance if the patient has recently eaten. The patient with duodenal ulcer may be anaemic.

INVESTIGATIONS

Radiology

The barium meal is the one crucial investigation, but since techniques and skill differ, it is unsafe to rely entirely on a radiological diagnosis. To project the barium-coated first part of the duodenum in such a way that an ulcer crater can be seen is unfortunately sometimes impossible. This is particularly liable to happen when the patient has a transverse stomach.

In other instances, obesity, anatomical abnormalities, and lack of co-operation by the patient make for difficulties.

Postbulbar duodenal ulcers are particularly easy to miss because the barium-filled crater beyond the cap is either not seen or mistaken for normal duodenum. Nevertheless, in spite of these difficulties, it is probably near the truth to say that a competent radiologist can demonstrate an ulcer *crater* in 60 per cent of all cases of active chronic ulceration. In a further 30 per cent of cases he can infer the presence of a duodenal ulcer because the duodenal cap is distorted by spasm or by scar tissue. Some radiologists prefer to produce evidence of duodenal ulceration in films, while others rely on screening. To the clinician, films are of little value without the screening report.

Sometimes spasm of the duodenal cap can be caused by other diseases such as carcinoma of the stomach, the pancreas, and the liver, and thus a radiological diagnosis of duodenal ulcer may divert attention from the underlying pathology.

The radiological appearances of the ulcerated duodenal cap are illustrated diagrammatically and in films (*Fig. 18*).

There is no justification for repeated barium studies on patients with duodenal ulcer, as the radiological appearances do not change much even when the ulcer is quiescent or healed.

Endoscopy

Examination of the duodenal bulb by end-viewing and side-viewing instruments allows ulcers missed by barium examination to be visualized. A prior injection of N butyl hyoscine (Buscopan) facilitates the procedure by paralying the musculature of the bulb.

Gastric Secretory Studies (*see also* p. 87)

Excluding patients who have had gastric surgery, the main reasons for secretory studies are:

a. The investigation of those with a history suggestive of peptic ulcer, but a negative barium meal.

b. To assess the degree of hypersecretion, which may influence the choice of operation.

c. To differentiate secondary hypersecretion due to endocrine tumour (Zollinger-Ellison gastrinoma syndrome).

d. To assess prognosis in patients with proven duodenal ulcer. The rationale for this investigation is dubious, since there is no hard evidence that patients with higher levels of acid secretion do worse than those with lower.

The object is to assess the basal, unstimulated secretion in the fasting subject over a control period and then to put all the parietal cells into maximal activity by injection of a stimulus.

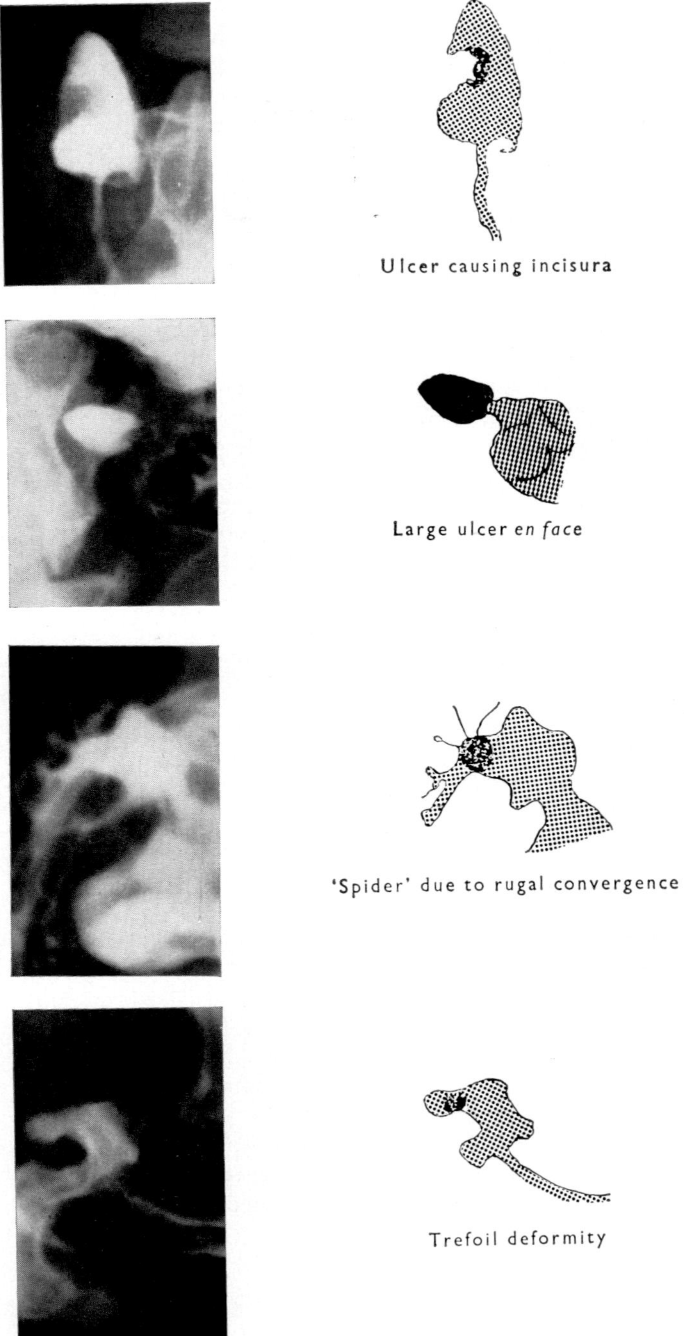

Fig. 18. Radiological appearances of duodenal cap in duodenal ulcer.

Basal secretion can be measured by continuous gastric aspiration over either a 12-hour night period or a 4-hour night period, or for a 1-hour period before the maximum stimulation. In all instances the result is expressed as volume, and mEq. HCl/hour. The longer periods of test, though marginally more accurate, are probably unnecessary in the vast majority of patients.

Maximal secretion can be achieved either by injection of pentagastrin 6 μg. per kg. body-weight i.m., or by injection of histamine acid phosphate 0·04 μg. per kg. body-weight i.m. 30 min. after injection of 100 mg. of mepyramine maleate i.m. to curtail the unpleasant side-effects of the large dose of histamine. Histalog is now no longer used. The gastric juice is aspirated for four successive 15-min. periods following the injection. Peak secretion usually occurs in the second and third 15-min. period, and results can either be expressed as the Peak Acid Output (that is double the sum of the two highest consecutive 15-min. outputs), or as the Maximal Acid Output (that is the output for the whole hour following the stimulant injection).

Continuous intravenous infusion of pentagastrin (6 μg. per kg. body-weight per hour) or histamine gives a more reproducible stimulus to gastric secretion but is not necessary for routine practice.

MEAN VALUES, WITH RANGE

	BASAL ACID OUTPUT	PEAK ACID OUTPUT
Normal	1–2 mEq. HCl per hour (range 0–5·0)	25 mEq. per hour (range 5–45)
D.U.	3·0 mEq. per hour (range 0·1–10+)	43 mEq. per hour (range 15–70+)

NOTES

a. Basal acid output. About one-third of D.U. patients have diagnostically high outputs (>10 mEq. per hour), but the rest are in the normal range.

b. Peak acid output. About one-third of D.U. patients have diagnostically high outputs (>45 mEq. per hour), but the rest overlap with the normal range. There is, however, a minimum level (12 mEq. per hour) below which D.U. does not occur.

c. A basal acid output greater than 15 mEq. per hour or a basal acid output/maximal acid output ratio of more than 0·6 suggests the possibility of a gastrinoma (Zollinger-Ellison syndrome).

Faecal Occult-blood Test

A rectal examination can be combined with examination of faecal smear for occult blood. This is sometimes positive if the duodenal ulcer is active.

Haemoglobin and Mean Corpuscular Haemoglobin Concentration
These tests are used mainly in order to assess the patient's general condition
preparatory to treatment.

ASSESSMENT FOR TREATMENT

Careful studies of the long-term results of both medical and surgical
treatment have taught us much about the virtues and limitations of each,
and in choosing a suitable therapy for a particular patient we have to
consider these alongside his social, psychological, and physical state.

It would be just as inappropriate to advise surgical treatment for a
cardiac cripple with a trouble-free duodenal ulcer as it would to suggest a
conservative régime in the face of evidence that an ulcer was penetrating
into surrounding organs and was causing not only physical distress but loss
of work and economic hardship for the patient. In some circumstances the
'whole' is more important than the 'hole', but in others the opposite is
true.

Generally speaking, medical treatment is chosen if the patient has a
short history of ulcer and has had no complications; surgical treatment if
he is middle-aged and gives a long history of ulcer and its complications,
and once again medical treatment if age and infirmity seem to presage a
hazardous operation. Surgery should, if possible, be a planned procedure
after medical treatment has brought the patient into the best possible
condition, with anaemia cured, vitamin deficiencies, if any, corrected, and
weight restored; but gastrectomy is an emergency after the complications
of perforation and severe bleeding.

Table 7. PROBABILITIES DETERMINING CHOICE OF TREATMENT

	MEDICAL		SURGICAL	
	Elderly or disabled by other diseases (per cent)	*Healthy (per cent)*	*Elderly or disabled (per cent)*	*Healthy (per cent)*
Expectation of temporary symptomatic relief	80	90	—	—
Healing of ulcer	5	15	95	98
Cure of complications				
Haemorrhage	75	90	90	96
Anaemia	100	100	—	—
Penetration	Nil	Nil	95	98
Perforation	25	50	90 (if early diagnosis)	95 (if early diagnosis)
Complete cure by surgery	—	—	88	90
Recurrent ulcer after surgery	—	—	2	3
Dumping, etc., after surgery	—	—	5	5
Death (immediate) after surgery	—	—	4	1

Table 7 attempts to express the probability that certain objectives of medical and surgical treatment will be reached, these estimates being based on published work and the authors' experience. It is on these probabilities that the physician or surgeon bases his judgement as to which treatment to adopt. Nowadays there is rarely any tendency for the surgeon or the physician to favour exclusively his own side of the treatment. On the contrary, both may fight shy of the same type of patient—the neurotic, for example, is not considered good for surgery because of the high risk of postgastrectomy symptoms, yet he may be an almost insoluble problem for the physician who is in the long run tempted to hand him over to the surgeon. Similarly, the cardiorespiratory cripple may have a severe and painful duodenal ulcer most unlikely to heal, yet, naturally, the surgeon would prefer him to be treated medically.

To summarize, we would say that medical treatment cannot be expected to heal chronic duodenal ulcers, and it certainly will not heal an ulcer which has penetrated into surrounding structures, but surgical treatment cannot be expected to heal a sick mind or a disturbed life. The patient who does well medically often does well after surgery.

MEDICAL TREATMENT

Many régimes have been advocated, but the one most commonly used in Britain combines physical and mental rest, with a soft diet low in cooked fat, and milk feeds 2-hourly. Controlled studies on the rate of healing of *gastric* ulcers have shown that it is the rest and not the diet which helps, though this is not necessarily true of duodenal ulcers. The dietary régime helps to free the patient of symptoms. Those who cannot afford to rest report that a careful diet alone will often relieve them. For this reason, and because it is difficult to enforce adequate rest without the stimulus of a special régime, it would, in the present state of our knowledge, be unwise to abandon dietary treatment. However, careful studies have shown that 2-hourly small meals chosen by the patient are as effective as fixed diets in controlling the pH of gastric contents.

The suppression of acid secretion is the aim of all medical treatment, but unfortunately the drugs which do this by interruption of vagal pathways also cause unpleasant side-effects (dry mouth, dilated pupils), and they cannot, of course, affect the hormonally mediated secretion which seems to depend on the integrity of the gastric antrum. Oral antacids have been shown to neutralize the gastric contents for a very short while (2–3 minutes at most), and the effectiveness of milk-alkaline tablets, which must be sucked continuously to keep the gastric contents neutral, is limited by the ability of the patient to co-operate in this way. The best compromise is to use antacids in tablet or powder form to relieve symptoms as they occur, to give heavy doses of an anticholinergic drug at night to suppress the nocturnal secretion, and to use milk drip neutralization for severe cases of ulcer pain which do not respond to lesser measures. Controlled trials have not shown any benefit from long-term use of anticholinergic drugs.

Suggested Régime for Severe Case

6.0 a.m.	Warm or cold milk on waking.
8.0 a.m.	Porridge, patent barley, or cornflakes with milk. Egg boiled or poached. Two cream crackers with honey, jelly, or butter. Milky tea.
10.0 a.m.	Milk, Ovaltine, or Horlicks. Alkaline powder or tablet (Mag. Trisil. Co.; Actal–Bayer) if pain occurs between meals.
Midday	Steamed fish or egg as main dish. Creamed potatoes and vegetables purée. Junket, rice, cornflour, semolina, or arrowroot flavoured with vanilla, coffee, chocolate, etc., or sponges, or fruit foods.
2.0 p.m.	Warm milk drink. Alkalis if pain occurs.
4.0 p.m.	Crisp bread, rusks, or cream crackers with jelly, syrup, or honey. Milky tea. Plain cake.
6.0 p.m.	Evening meal—a variation on midday meal.
8.0 p.m.	Warm milk drink.
10.0 p.m.	Warm milk drink and either propantheline 30 mg. or poldine 4 mg.

If the patient is restless, sodium amytal 200 mg., *or* phenobarbitone 60 mg., may be given at night. If the patient has been eating a poor diet for some time he may be given ascorbic acid 400 mg. daily for the first 5 days of treatment, or if there is anaemia he should be given ferrous sulphate 1·2 g. daily in divided doses with the main meals.

If there are symptoms of reflex spasm, such as oesophageal cramps, heartburn, or colon spasms, atropine or another anticholinergic drug may be given 3 times a day, or it may be combined with a barbiturate sedative in various proprietary preparations. These may also help the spastic type of constipation which sometimes accompanies duodenal ulcer. Alkaline mixtures containing magnesium salts are also helpful in this respect.

Finally, the patient should be helped with his emotional and social difficulties. Often the physician can suggest the right solution or can see things in better perspective than the patient. Simply to listen sympathetically is often enough to calm the agitated, and time must be found for this.

Not all patients can afford a month in which to rest in bed, and 'take the cure', and in advising him to do this the doctor is aware of his own weak position, since he can only offer a small chance of a permanent cure (*see Table 7*). However, it is as well to be firm and dogmatic in all young patients with 'young' duodenal ulcers (history one year or less), because these are probably less scarred and therefore more likely to heal soundly.

In disabled elderly patients with severe symptoms the full medical régime, often with a milk drip, is required.

Middle-aged males or females who, though suffering, are too occupied with their work to take kindly to a month's enforced rest must be treated as seems best for their circumstances. Often a strict diet, a week-end in bed, belladonna with barbiturates, and antacids as necessary will end a phase of ulcer symptoms. Coated preparations of carbenoxolone (Duogastrone) have been found by some workers to promote healing of duodenal ulcers, but a controlled trial with fibreoptic inspection of the ulcers shows that the preparation may give no permanent benefit.

Gastric freezing offers no lasting benefit for the ulcer patient.

SURGICAL TREATMENT

The aim of surgical treatment is to reduce or to neutralize gastric secretion. The operations in use are depicted in *Table 8*. All the operations have their zealous exponents, but it is evident that great attention is now being paid to more critical selection of the operation for each patient. Some of the factors that assist in this selection are as follows:

1. Mortality. This is greater for gastrectomy compared with simpler operations, especially in older age-groups.

2. Ease of performance.

3. Men are more prone to recurrence of ulcer than women.

4. Women are more liable to postgastrectomy symptoms than men.

5. The greater the amount of stomach resected, the greater is the risk of sequelae.

Vagotomy with pyloroplasty is the most popular at the present time. Generally speaking gastrectomy is avoided in the very young, the old, women, those underweight, and those with a previous history of tuberculosis. Vagotomy together with antrectomy, though it directly attacks the controlling mechanism of secretion and avoids the consequences of high resections, has not proved entirely satisfactory. A careful trial comparing the results of partial gastrectomy, gastro-enterostomy with vagotomy, and pyloroplasty with vagotomy has been made in which the patients were allocated to the three different treatment groups by almost random methods. This trial shows very little difference between the results from the three groups, but there is a slightly higher incidence of recurrent ulceration in the vagotomy groups and a slightly higher incidence of anaemia and minor nutritional disturbances in the gastrectomy group.

Super-selective vagotomy designed to denervate the fundus of the stomach while retaining the motor nerve to the antrum has been practised recently. The advantage of the operation is that it is unnecessary to do a stomach-drainage procedure at the same time, and there should be minimal interference with small intestinal and pancreatic function. However, it is much too soon to evaluate the full potential and disadvantages of this operation.

Approximately one in four of patients with duodenal ulcer come to surgery within four to five years of onset. The indications for operation are: Intractable pain. Pain occurring after bleeding and after perforation. Stenosis. Haemorrhage.

The operative mortality depends mainly on the age and physical status of the patient, and obesity particularly increases the technical difficulties and hazards. Nevertheless, risks may have to be taken. If, for example, a patient suffering from severe rheumatoid arthritis and bronchiectasis has a penetrating duodenal ulcer which causes intractable pain unrelieved by medical measures, then surgical treatment is inevitable.

Table 8. OPERATIONS FOR DUODENAL AND GASTRIC ULCERS

OPERATION		ADVANTAGES	DISADVANTAGES
Partial gastrectomy Billroth-I		Maintenance of normal food pathway guarantees minimum of nutritional disturbances afterwards. Less 'dumping'. Ideal for gastric ulcer	High rate (6 per cent in males) of recurrent ulceration if done for duodenal ulcer
Partial gastrectomy Polya type		Combines removal of large part of acid-bearing area and antrum with neutralization of anastomotic area by alkaline duodenal juices. Low rate of recurrent ulcer (1–2 per cent)	Poor mixing of food and enzymes. Loss of weight and anaemia are fairly frequent. 'Dumping' symptoms in about 10 per cent. Severe steatorrhoea rarely
Vagotomy and gastro-enterostomy		Simplicity. Low risk. Alkalinization of gastric contents by duodenal juice	Difficult to make vagotomy complete. Fairly high rate of recurrent ulceration (5–8 per cent)
Vagotomy and pyloroplasty		Cuts vagal acid secretion and drains stomach. Low risk. Maintains normal food pathway. Popular at present time	No alkalinization of gastric contents. Fairly high rate of recurrent ulceration
Vagotomy and antrectomy (limited resection)		Cuts vagally mediated and hormonally mediated (gastrin from antrum) secretion. Low risk	Removes pH monitoring function of antrum, so gastrin secretion from outside the stomach may be permanently high

COMPLICATIONS

Perforation

This occurs in only about 2 per cent of patients with duodenal ulcer, but sometimes quite early in the history. A patient may notice only a few days of epigastric pain and then the ulcer perforates. There is evidence to suggest that physical and mental stress may cause perforation.

The clinical picture is usually one of a sudden onset of abdominal pain and rigidity with sweating and shock. Movement is painful, and generalized peritoneal tenderness is associated with extreme muscular guarding. Bowel-sounds are absent. Acute pancreatitis, mesenteric infarctions, and volvulus of the intestine may cause difficulty in diagnosis, and certain conditions above the diaphragm, notably myocardial infarction and acute pneumonia, may cause a rather similar picture of shock, sweating, referred abdominal pain, and reflex rigidity.

Aspiration of gastric contents by tube and intravenous infusion of plasma and glucose-saline help to resuscitate the patient preoperatively, but surgery should not be delayed. The sooner the operation, the less the risk.

Whereas most surgeons prefer to treat perforated gastric ulcer by partial gastrectomy, it is not always feasible to do this, or to remove a perforated ulcer in the duodenum. But in favourable conditions a partial gastrectomy is done, since once a perforation has occurred, further trouble from the ulcer is likely. When the patient's condition is poor the surgeon satisfies himself with peritoneal toilet and simple suture of the perforation.

Elderly or high-risk patients whose condition is very poor owing to late diagnosis may be treated conservatively, in the hope that the perforation will heal itself. In this group the mortality from either medical or surgical treatment is over 25 per cent. The régime adopted is to give no food and to pass a Levine tube, to aspirate the gastric contents continuously, and to give intravenous fluids, their amount and composition depending on the state revealed by estimation of packed-cell volume and serum electrolyte levels, the object being to maintain a reasonable urinary flow of about 700 ml. per 24 hours without causing pulmonary oedema by fluid overload. Broad-spectrum antibiotics are given to limit the spread of peritoneal infection.

Pyloric Obstruction or Stenosis with Gastric Retention

It seems worth while to say that the exclusive use of the term 'pyloric stenosis' for this complication can be misleading. Many patients who have complete failure of the pyloric valve mechanism, causing severe gastric retention, have no stenosis of the pyloric area. Inflammatory oedema and muscular incoordination are enough to cause the valve mechanism to fail. Furthermore, the clinical picture of pyloric stenosis usually painted is that of a patient vomiting profusely and frequently. This also can be misleading, for the symptoms of pyloric obstruction are modified by dilatation and atony of the stomach and the development of a retention gastritis. It is most usual for a patient whose pylorus is obstructed to vomit rather infrequently, perhaps once a day or every other day. The vomitus is large, nasty-smelling, often black or dirty in appearance, and does not taste as acid to the patient as perhaps it has done in the past. The patient loses appetite, weight falls off rapidly, and he may notice thirst and scanty urine. Occasionally he may have diarrhoea but more usually is constipated. He may belch unpleasant gas. Sometimes he may complain of headache, lethargy, muscular weakness, and other symptoms of hypokalaemic alkalosis. He may even be mentally confused or violent. To his relatives, the patient appears to have lost a great deal of weight in a short while, but the doctor may elicit on examination signs of dehydration and salt deficiency. The skin loses its elasticity. The outline of the dilated stomach may be clearly visible when the abdomen is inspected in a good light, a gastric splash is often elicited, but visible peristalsis from left to right is seen less frequently.

Investigations reveal a scanty urine containing less than 1 g. chloride per litre, haemoconcentration, and a deficiency of chloride and potassium ions. There is a metabolic alkalosis which must always be allowed for.

On passing a stomach tube dirty brown or black fluid is aspirated which contains altered blood and fermenting food.

The management of this condition calls for prompt action and some skill, for the patient who has already developed considerable dehydration and alkalosis is in serious danger. Without waiting for the results of serum electrolyte estimations, intravenous therapy with normal saline is started and a tube is passed into the stomach. The contents are aspirated and if the tube blocks it should be washed through with normal saline. In any case, it is good practice to wash out the stomach with a litre of warm saline after aspiration of the contents. Even then the aspirate may not be clear until several washings have been done. Haematocrit and serum electrolyte readings now allow the fluid deficiency, the electrolyte position, and the degree of alkalosis to be estimated, and a programme of intra-venous medication for the next 12 hours is decided upon. Usually, normal saline is alternated with glucose saline, and 1 g. of potassium is given in each litre of fluid. It may be necessary to give as much as 6 litres in the first 24 hours. The patient's general condition improves dramatically, though if the alkalosis has been severe he may take several days to recover his normal mental faculty. Retention gastritis is an important cause of malaise and anaemia from blood-loss, and it is very important to recognize this and to wash out the stomach twice daily with saline until the washings are completely clear. This will also allow oedema in the pyloric region to subside and the patient will then begin to absorb fluids given by mouth. Milk and fruit juices, 50 ml. every 2 hours, can be given after the first 24 hours. It is important to remember that the patient should no longer be allowed to take alkaline powders or medicines. In two or three days it is usually safe to discontinue intravenous therapy in all but those with fibrotic stenosis of the pylorus. These patients must be brought into the best possible state of nutrition and metabolic balance, so that a gastrec-tomy or gastro-enterostomy can be done, the procedure of lowest risk sometimes being chosen of necessity. Well over half the patients with pyloric obstruction recover with the medical régime, and although gastric surgery will be required eventually, it can be planned at a time when the patient's nutritional state is at its best.

Penetration
Severe continuous pain, often in the back and made worse in certain positions of the body, suggests that the ulcer has penetrated, and this is a clear indication for surgical treatment.

Haemorrhage

Acute bleeding is dealt with in *Chapter 7*. Loss of occult blood or un-recognized melaena from a duodenal ulcer is a common cause of anaemia. If the faecal occult blood-test is strongly positive and the anaemia is normochromic, the bleeding has been recent, and the body's iron stores are probably sufficient to allow the marrow to restore the loss. Where, however, the mean corpuscular haemoglobin concentration is below 31 per cent, iron deficiency must be assessed and oral iron (ferrous sulphate 400 mg. 3 times a day) given.

Complications of Treatment

Faddy diets have sometimes given a patient scurvy, and the abuse of alkalis and milk has caused the milk-alkali syndrome. The latter is associated with hypercalcaemia, and the symptoms are lethargy, nausea, vomiting, polyuria, and pruritus. Albuminuria and uraemia often occur, and renal damage may be irreversible in severe cases.

PROGNOSIS

It is clear that duodenal ulcer is a disease with a high morbidity and a low mortality. In an individual person the outlook may be bright if the ulcer appears to have been caused by outside circumstances capable of correction, but if ulceration occurs early in life in a patient with a strong family history of the disease, then the prospects of cure or of long remissions are poor. In cases of uncomplicated duodenal ulceration it is often impossible to give anything approaching an accurate prognosis until the patient has been watched for five years. If, with conservative measures, he has only rare bouts of trouble which are easily controllable by a stricter régime, then he can be advised to 'live with' his ulcer. A permanently unsatisfactory domestic or occupational situation, onset of ulcer symptoms early in life, a family history, and the occurrence of one or more complications make the outlook for the future bleak.

SUMMARY

Constitutional and endocrine factors are important and the tendency to hypersecretion of acid in patients with duodenal ulcer is probably cause, not effect.

Signs are neglible and symptoms confusing, intermittency of pain being the most reliable. Radiology makes the diagnosis 95 per cent accurate, and medical or surgical treatment is chosen pragmatically. The former is valuable mainly in relieving symptoms, the latter, thoroughly successful in nine out of ten cases, none the less carries a distinct mortality and a morbidity of its own. The advantages and risks of the various operations are by now well enough known for the correct procedure to be chosen, and a firm assessment of physical and emotional background, together with acid secretory studies, determines the choice.

FURTHER READING

CLARKE, C. A., EVANS, D. A. P., MCCONNELL, R. B., and SHEPPARD, P. M. (1959) 'Secretion of Blood Group Antigens and Peptic Ulcer', *Br. med. J.*, **1**, 603.
JONES, F. AVERY (1957), 'Clinical and Social Problems of Peptic Ulcer', *Ibid.*, **1**, 719; 786.
PULVERTAFT, C. N. (1968), 'Incidence and Natural History of Gastric Ulcer and Duodenal Ulcer', *Post-grad. med. J.*, **44**, 561.

Treatment
KAYE, M. D., RHODES, J., BECK, P., SWEETMAN, P. M., DARUS G. T., and EVANS, K. T. (1970), 'A Controlled Trial of Glycopyrronium and L-Hyoscyamine in the Long Term Treatment of Duodenal Ulcer', *Gut*, **11**, 559.
KIRSNER, J. B., and PALMER, W. L. (1960), 'Treatment of Peptic Ulcers', *Am. J. Med.*, **29**, 793.
WELBOURN, R. B., and JOHNSTON, I. D. A. (1961), 'The Assessment and Selections of Elective Operations for Peptic Ulceration', p. 301, *British Surgical Practice, Surgical Progress* (ed. SIR ERNEST ROCK CARLING and SIR JAMES PATERSON ROSS): London: Butterworth.

Chapter 7

Haematemesis and Melaena

ONE OF THE commonest medical emergencies is acute bleeding from the gastro-intestinal tract, and though the final treatment may be surgical, the care and responsibility for correct decision rest with the physician. He must marshal both knowledge and experience to make the right decisions, for the comparative risks (or benefits) of medical and surgical treatment as estimated by him in a particular patient bleeding from a known cause will determine the choice, and this choice is crucial. If the bleeding comes from certain types of lesion, surgical treatment immediately after resuscitation may be less risky than a conservative approach, but in other circumstances a medical régime may be safer. Therefore, diagnosis of the source and cause of the bleeding is as important as an awareness of mortality statistics. The difficulty is heightened by the great age and decrepitude of some who suffer from haematemesis, and by other diseases which hinder their recovery and augment the surgical risk.

None the less, the mortality from haematemesis has fallen from 20 per cent to 7 per cent in thirty years, and this is due as much to the availability of blood for transfusion and the care in the maintenance of the body's homeostasis as to the appreciation of risks, skill in management, and low surgical mortality.

THE CAUSES OF HAEMATEMESIS AND MELAENA

In Britain chronic duodenal ulcer is responsible for more than half the hospital admissions for acute gastro-intestinal bleeding; acute and chronic gastric ulcers together account for another 30 per cent; anastomotic jejunal ulcers, hiatus hernia erosions, and oesophageal varices together for about 10 per cent; carcinoma and various rare conditions for about 4 per cent.

Something is known of the factors which provoke peptic ulcers to bleed. During the Second World War the highest incidence of haematemesis in London was during the two phases of aerial bombardment in 1941 and 1944. Patients will often attribute their haemorrhage to family or business worry, or to a period of overstrain. There is a high incidence of haematemesis after serious injuries and operation, particularly those on the genito-urinary tract and transplants. Exacerbation of chest or urinary tract infections may provoke bleeding from chronic ulcers. Haematemesis is commoner in winter. Local trauma from drugs such as aspirin or phenylbutazone may cause not only acute erosions to form and to bleed, but also haemorrhage from quiescent chronic ulcers.

Table 9. CAUSES OF HAEMATEMESIS IN ORDER OF FREQUENCY

ESTIMATED INCIDENCE OF THE VARIOUS CAUSES IN 100 HOSPITAL ADMISSIONS FOR INTESTINAL BLEEDING

Admissions

50 Chronic duodenal ulcer

15 Chronic gastric ulcer

20 Acute gastric erosions
- idiopathic
- due to aspirin
- due to phenylbutazone
- due to alcohol
- due to food allergy (e.g. mushrooms, shellfish)

4 Erosions and ulcers close to the anastomosis of gastro-enterostomy or gastrectomy

4 Erosions and ulcers associated with hiatus hernia

3 Bleeding from oesophageal varices

4
- Nose-bleeding into the stomach
- Carcinoma of stomach
- Sarcoma of stomach
- Other gastric tumours
- Blood diseases—leukaemia, purpura, haemophilia, thrombocythaemia
- Hereditary telangiectasia
- Pseudoxanthoma elasticum
- Mallory-Weiss syndrome

CAUSES OF MELAENA WITHOUT HAEMATEMESIS

All conditions listed as causing haematemesis may cause melaena alone. Additionally, certain diseases may cause melaena but not haematemesis, the chief of which are:

Meckel's diverticulum with ectopic gastric mucosa
Diverticulosis coli
Neoplasms of small intestine
Neoplasms of colon
Bleeding from biliary tract

The rarer causes of bleeding often cause great difficulty. For example, pseudoxanthoma elasticum can only be recognized if the skin of the neck and axillae is examined for extra folds and loss of elasticity and if angioid streaks are seen in the retina. Von Willebrand's disease may occur without a clear family history, and the combination of a prolonged bleeding time, a positive Hess's test, and a normal platelet count should suggest the diagnosis which can be confirmed by finding abnormal prothrombin consumption and absent Von Willebrand factor in the blood. More obvious general diseases such as uraemia, myelomatosis, or diffuse intravascular coagulation (D.I.C.) found in the late stages of pregnancy or after delivery can cause troublesome bleeding from the gastro-intestinal tract. Peritoneal dialysis checks the bleeding in uraemia, and epsilon aminocaproic acid may be helpful if excessive fibrinolysis has been demonstrated. Otherwise fresh blood or fresh frozen plasma should be used in all cases with prolonged clotting time.

The Mallory-Weiss syndrome can usually be diagnosed from the history of vomiting, coughing, or retching which is *followed* by the vomiting of bright blood.

CLINICAL PICTURE

Sometimes bleeding is so slight as not to be recognized, or, alternatively, slight melaena and subsequent symptoms are noted by a patient who does not feel very ill. One of the surprising things is that some patients who have suffered no pain from their duodenal ulcer may have a series of minor haemorrhages in a period of years. There is a poor correlation between the severity of the ulceration, i.e., the amount of pain it causes, and the liability to haemorrhage.

The symptoms are those of any haemorrhage: a feeling of weakness, faintness, or giddiness, sometimes a cold sweat and palpitations. Nausea may occur before the vomiting of stale black or brown blood, and if the bowels act soon after the haemorrhage, then bright blood may be passed, but usually the stool is dark and tarry. Pulse-rate rises, blood-pressure falls, and pallor is obvious. Some who have experienced a comparatively minor haemorrhage develop a marked shock reaction with profound pallor, sweating, tachycardia, and a drop of systolic blood-pressure, but this lasts only a short while. A fall of blood-pressure which lasts an hour or more is sure to reflect the severity of the haemorrhage.

Rapid bleeding in elderly patients may cause severe shock with diminished oxygenation of the brain, so that confusion and restlessness complicate the management. A few cases of blindness, retinal haemorrhage, or permanent dementia have followed severe exsanguination, and myocardial infarction may occur during the phase of hypotension caused by a haematemesis.

If the vomitus contains red blood, it may mean either that such a rapid haemorrhage has occurred that there has been no time for digestion, or that the bleeding has occurred into a hypochlorhydric stomach, as may happen in patients with oesophageal varices or acute gastric ulcers.

Patients usually complain of thirst, have a dry tongue and unpleasant breath, and pass small quantities of concentrated urine. They have little appetite for food, but will drink readily.

In the days when it was the custom to give the patient a little ice to suck during the first three days after a haemorrhage, serious dehydration and uraemia occurred, but nowadays, with better efforts to maintain the hydration of the body and to provide for the renal water requirements, it is unusual for the blood-urea to rise to over 60 mg. per 100 ml. in young and healthy patients. A rise of urea to over 100 mg. per 100 ml. may occur in the elderly or in those suffering from renal or prostatic diseases. Haematemesis may precipitate liver failure in those with pre-existing cirrhosis.

DIAGNOSIS

There is little difficulty in diagnosing a haematemesis once it has occurred, apart from occasional false alarms due to the vomiting of digested beetroot or raspberry cordial. Sometimes a haematemesis can be attributed to a minor cause such as the trickling of blood from the nose into the stomach during sleep. In cases of doubtful melaena, dark blood-containing faeces on the finger-stall used for rectal examination can confirm the diagnosis.

The main problem is to diagnose the cause of the haematemesis, for the policy of treatment will depend on this. There are five main sources of information from which diagnosis may come:

1. History
2. Examination of patient and vomitus
3. Barium meal
4. Endoscopy.
5. Gastric secretory studies.

1. *History*

A patient may give a classic history of duodenal ulcer, and he or his relatives may report that a barium meal has in the past shown a duodenal ulcer. From such information one cannot infer with certainty that a duodenal ulcer is the cause of the haematemesis, for the blood may be coming from a gastric ulcer which has developed in addition to the duodenal ulcer, but it is at least probable that the bleeding is related to *chronic* as opposed to *acute* peptic ulceration. Although some patients may deny having pain after food or dyspepsia they will admit to taking antacid tablets or medicines. Such an admission may be the only clue to chronic peptic ulceration. If there is no history of previous dyspepsia, if there has been recent emotional stress, or if the patient has been taking aspirin or phenylbutazone, then the haemorrhage may be from acute erosions. The patient should be asked about any previous disease or habits likely to damage the liver, e.g., alcoholism or jaundice.

2. *Examination*

If the vomitus is bright red it argues a lack of acid secretion to digest the blood, and this may be found in patients with acute, chronic, or malignant gastric ulceration or in those with cirrhosis and oesophageal varices. Very rapid bleeding from whatever cause results in bright red haematemesis.

A patient should also be examined carefully for stigmata of cirrhosis, especially spider naevi, atrophic testes, dilated abdominal veins, and splenomegaly. An enlarged spleen is easily missed unless the examination of the left hypochondrium is thorough. The skin should be inspected carefully for purpura, telangiectasia, and tested for elasticity. Localized tenderness in the epigastrium may have diagnostic value in patients with chronic peptic ulceration.

3. *Barium Meal*

At one time it was thought that to subject a patient to X-ray study during the first three weeks after a haematemesis was to risk a recurrence of bleeding, but it is now known that barium examinations can be carried out safely soon after the patient's admission to hospital. The advantages of obtaining valuable diagnostic information outweigh the disadvantages of moving the patient about, and the question is more of what is practicable in a collapsed or feeble patient. Some believe that useful information can be obtained from a series of supine and erect films taken after the patient has swallowed a cupful of barium while in his bed; 80 per cent diagnostic accuracy has been claimed for this method. Others maintain that it is possible to move even the most ill patient to the X-ray table, and so to make a further and more useful barium study of the stomach and duodenum. By using a tilting couch, on to which the patient can be strapped, and an image intensifier, it is possible not only to detect and displace filling defects due to blood-clot but to obtain some information on the degree of mucosal oedema and muscle spasm around an ulcer. Oesophageal varices if present can be detected. The clinician can, in these circumstances, witness the examination and take decisions on the spot. For instance, if no certain source of bleeding is detected he may decide to proceed forthwith to gastroscopy, or if a chronic gastric or duodenal ulcer is found, he may seek a surgical consultation right away.

The limited film examination at the patient's bedside requires a good portable apparatus, a radiographer and a nurse, and some radiological help in interpretation of difficult films, whereas the fuller examination in the X-ray department calls for the radiologist's whole time. The decision as to which method to adopt will depend partly on the local facilities and preferences, and partly on the patient's clinical state. There is a very small number of patients whom it is not practicable to move to the X-ray department, but it is, on the other hand, quite feasible to make a full radiological examination while blood is transfused. Patients are not upset by the procedure and often welcome all attempts to find the cause of the bleeding.

Many radiologists prefer gastrografin to barium in this situation, and certainly barium in the stomach may be an embarrassment to the surgeon who does an emergency gastrectomy. Gastrografin should also be used if a perforation is suspected.

4. *Endoscopy*

Oesophagoscopy using an end-viewing fibrescope is the safest way of assessing oesophagitis, varices, or mucosal tears (Mallory-Weiss ulcers) at the gastro-oesophageal junction. The main use of endoscopy is in the diagnosis of multiple acute ulcers or erosions, and in determining the main site of the bleeding. It is usually best to subject to endoscopy all patients who continue to bleed after X-ray studies if clinical data have tended to exclude chronic peptic ulceration and oesophageal varices. Acute ulcers or severe erosive gastritis which cannot be shown by X-ray may be obvious to the endoscopist, and sometimes a chronic gastric or duodenal ulcer which has not been detected radiologically may be found. Modern fibrescopes can be passed more easily and give a wider field of observation than the older gastroscopes, and therefore this form of endoscopy may in time supersede immediate radiology in the diagnosis of the cause of haematemesis.

The only preparation necessary is an intramuscular injection of diazepam 10–20 mg. half an hour before. If bleeding is continuous an intragastric tube should be passed to evacuate the stomach and wash it out with iced water just before gastroscopy.

5. *Gastric Secretory Studies*

If a tube is passed into the stomach and left there overnight after a haematemesis, something can be learnt from the aspirate. Fresh blood indicates renewed bleeding from the stomach, and high acid output throughout a fasting period suggests duodenal ulceration. Low acid outputs or achlorhydria are compatible with acute gastric erosions, and intermediate values with nocturnal neutralization are found typically with chronic gastric ulcer. This method of obtaining diagnostic information is less direct and less conclusive than radiology, and some patients will not tolerate intragastric tubes for any length of time.

6. *Arteriography*

In certain cases where doubt exists as to the cause of bleeding, selective arteriography of the coeliac axis has been shown to be a helpful procedure. The investigation may show leakage of contrast medium into the lumen of the bowel at the site of bleeding. In order to be helpful the patient must be bleeding at the time of the examination at a rate of 0·5 ml. per min. This examination may be of considerable importance in patients who continue to bleed after a blind gastrectomy. Small vascular malformations may be readily shown as well as aneurysms at the base of ulcer craters or indeed aneurysms of the aorta eroding into an abdominal viscus. Patients are disturbed very little by this procedure which can be carried out under local anaesthetic.

MEDICAL TREATMENT

The principles are those of giving physical and mental rest, while attempting to maintain the stability of the body's internal environment. Bleeding stops as a rule, but the factors responsible for its continuation are: (1) Ulcer has eroded a major blood-vessel. (2) Impairment of blood coagulability. (3) Possibly, hypertension and arteriosclerosis. (4) Possibly, emotional restlessness.

The patient is kept in bed, but it is not necessary for him to lie flat. Pulse and blood-pressure are measured and charted every half-hour. A central venous pressure line may be helpful in very shocked patients. Fluids are given *ad lib.* or in amounts of not less than 80 ml. hourly, usually milk or tea-flavoured milk—i.e., more milk than tea, or a proprietary milk beverage.

As some patients cannot tolerate milk, it is permissible to give them glucose-fortified fruit drinks. Food is allowed as soon as appetite permits, but it is usual to offer only soft foods such as boiled fish, rice, mashed potatoes, semolina, fine porridge, jelly, and sponge cake. The urine output is watched, and, if possible, fluid intake adjusted to maintain it at 1 litre daily.

It is customary to give antacids such as magnesium trisilicate or aluminium hydroxide every four hours, but it is doubtful whether this is necessary, and it is certainly not effective in maintaining neutralization of the gastric contents. Alkaline tablets or tablets containing both alkalis and milk powder may be sucked throughout the day, but again there is no proof that this is necessary. Pain usually disappears after a haematemesis, but if it does not, surgical treatment will often be necessary. Nevertheless, some physicians may attempt the ultimate in the buffering of gastric contents by giving a continuous milk drip. This has the advantage of maintaining the fluid intake at a high level, which may be necessary in elderly and feeble patients, but it is unwise to persist if the tube is badly tolerated.

Anticholinergic drugs, such as poldine 4 mg., propantheline 15 mg., or atropine, may be given to reduce gastric secretion, but their value is doubtful, and the side-effects, such as a dry mouth, may be annoying, while intestinal distension and retention of urine can be dangerous in elderly patients.

Sedatives are useful in maintaining physical inactivity and tranquillity, and the choice is wide. Morphine 20 mg. has been much used, but it causes nausea and vomiting in a few, and constipation in many. Phenobarbitone 200 mg. by injection, followed by 65 mg. twice a day orally, is recommended.

On admission, blood is taken for estimation of haemoglobin and cross-matching, and blood is transfused if the haemoglobin falls below 75 per cent (10 g. per 100 ml.), or if the systolic blood-pressure drops suddenly or falls below 110 mm. of mercury. It is usually possible to give the blood by needle into a superficial vein, but patients suffering from severe shock may develop venospasm which prevents adequate administration by such a route and it is then necessary to cut down to a major vein and insert a fine polythene cannula. Blood transfusion is continued slowly until the haemoglobin rises to about 90 per cent (12 g. per 100 ml.), and until there is no sign of further bleeding. When a patient has bled severely, the rapid infusion of large amounts of blood containing citrate may interfere with coagulation and so perpetuate the bleeding (calcium gluconate should be given intravenously if more than 1 litre of blood is transfused per hour).

Signs of Renewed Bleeding

Sweating; restlessness; rise in pulse-rate; sudden drop in blood-pressure; nausea; vomiting of blood, or loose stools.

If a central venous pressure line is available renewed bleeding can be detected early.

If bleeding stops for two days or more, then usually no further bleeding occurs. The patient should continue to rest for at least a week, but for a much longer period if the haemorrhage has been severe or the ulcer large and active.

SURGICAL TREATMENT

Indications

1. Bleeding from a chronic gastric ulcer.
2. Bleeding from a chronic duodenal ulcer (*a*) if the patient has a long history of ulcer troubles; (*b*) if no major contra-indication.
3. Renewed bleeding from a chronic duodenal ulcer after its initial cessation, if patient is aged over 50 years.
4. Very rapid bleeding from any cause other than oesophageal varices, e.g., transfusion at 1 litre per 2 hours does not control signs of shock.

Relative Contra-indications

1. Chest and spinal fixity.
2. Severe chronic bronchitis and emphysema.
3. Advanced hypertension and atherosclerotic disease of heart, brain, and kidney.
4. Pyelonephritis with blood-urea over 150 mg. per 100 ml.
5. Senile dementia.

The main difficulties arise in the following situations:

1. Uncertain cause of bleeding which is renewed after initial treatment.

This is sometimes due to the failure to detect a chronic peptic ulcer which is in a difficult situation, such as in the second part of the duodenum, and sometimes because the blood is coming from a number of acute gastric erosions. If the bleeding is rapid, or if the patient is a male aged over 45 years, it is wisest to operate, and if no source of bleeding can be found then to open and inspect the inside of the stomach. Occasionally a single open vessel which has failed to retract through a tiny erosion may be the cause of very severe blood-loss. Such a source of bleeding may only be detected at gastrotomy.

2. Renewed bleeding from a known chronic peptic ulcer in a very poor-risk patient.

The decision for or against surgery must be based on the patient's age and mental status, and it is sometimes best to continue a conservative régime even though the patient has bled twice or more since admission.

3. Rapid bleeding from known acute gastric ulcers or multiple erosions.

If the patient is young or female, it is best to continue a conservative régime for several days, even though this may necessitate the transfusion of up to 10 litres of blood. Repeated gastric lavage with ice-cold water may be helpful. In a few cases, particularly young males, the bleeding may be so severe and continuous that supply of blood becomes a problem and surgical exploration seems to be the lesser risk.

The objections to recommending emergency partial gastrectomy for all patients who continue to bleed after a trial of the conservative régime are that it is an operation with an appreciable mortality and morbidity, and that it may be an ineffective procedure if the bleeding arises from a mucosal tear at the gastro-oesophageal junction, erosive gastritis in the cardia, an isolated vessel sporting through the mucosa of the upper stomach, or a postbulbar duodenal ulcer. It is wiser to select patients carefully before seeking surgical advice and help, and the surgeon should be offered a firm conclusion as to the source of the bleeding so that he can plan the operative procedure.

Operative Procedure

If bleeding is from a gastric ulcer a Billroth-I type of gastrectomy is feasible, whereas if a duodenal ulcer is found, the alternatives are a Polya gastrectomy or vagotomy–pyloroplasty with undersewing the ulcer to check bleeding. Sometimes oedema, scarring, or the position of the ulcer make it impossible to remove it, in which case it is undersewn to occlude its vessels, but leaving enough blood-supply to make safe the closure of the duodenal stump. Gastro-enterostomy with vagotomy is sometimes indicated.

Where there is doubt as to the cause of the bleeding, some surgeons prefer to do a blind gastrectomy, and others to open the stomach and search its interior. This is neither a very safe nor a very easy procedure, for small mucosal bleeding-points are not easily visible in the cavity of the stomach or towards the cardia. The stomach also contains some debris even though it has been drained by a tube. It is best for the physician never to allow this situation to confront the surgeon, and herein lies the importance of thorough diagnosis. In cases of severe bleeding from gastric erosions, conservative and radical operative techniques have been compared and there is little to choose between the mortality in each group. Second operations are necessary more often in those having subtotal gastrectomy. The conclusion is that it is safest to adopt a conservative non-surgical policy in all cases of bleeding from known erosive gastritis but in the event of bleeding being severe and continuous, conservative surgery with undersewing of the main bleeding point is the safest procedure. Opinion is divided as to whether a vagotomy–pyloroplasty should also be done.

PROGNOSIS

It has been shown that the mortality from haematemesis increases with age, and this is partly due to the aged person's own difficulty in responding to stress and maintaining homeostasis, and partly to the fact that in the elderly haematemesis so often occurs as a complication of other diseases which in themselves threaten life or hamper resistance to sudden stress.

Bleeding from chronic gastric ulceration causes a higher mortality than that from acute ulcers or duodenal ulcer, and this difference is independent of the age factor. Bleeding from acute ulcers is less dangerous than bleeding from chronic duodenal ulcer.

A favourable outcome is to be expected in all cases under the age of 30 (*Fig. 19*), where the haemorrhage is mild enough to cause melaena rather than haematemesis, and where the source of bleeding is from a duodenal ulcer. Some mortality may be expected in those over 50 who have more severe bleeding, who have diseases of other systems, and in whom operation is postponed beyond 48 hours from the start of the bleeding. In fact

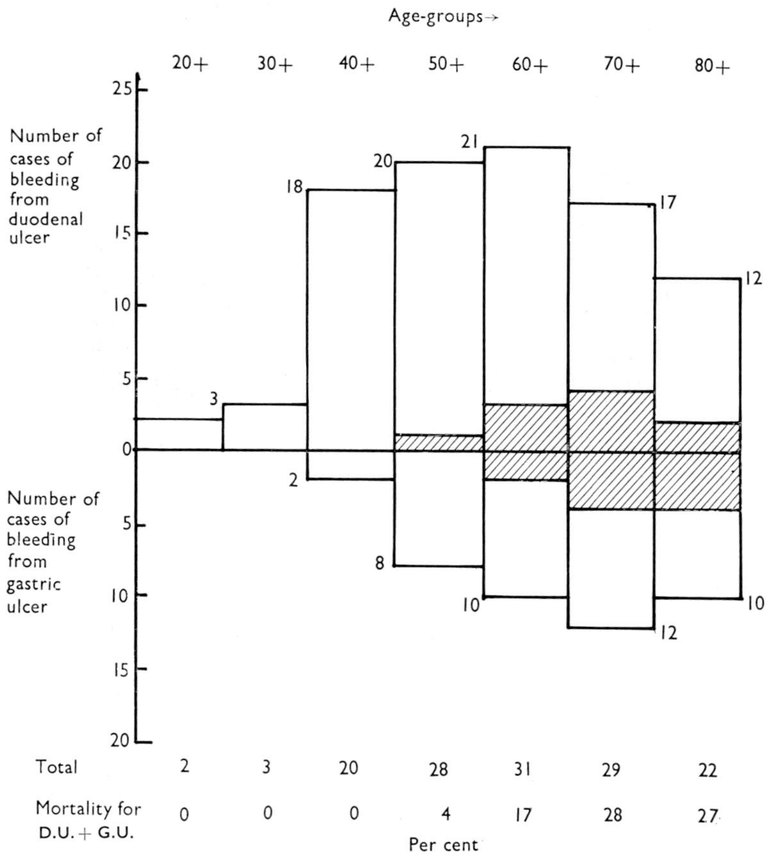

Fig. 19. Distribution of morbidity and mortality from bleeding gastric and duodenal ulcers (135 cases). (Deaths shown as hatched areas.)

statistics show a fairly constant mortality of 7 per cent of all cases admitted with haematemesis as the admission diagnosis, despite changing techniques of investigation and treatment.

From these facts it is apparent that the elderly patient with intercurrent disease and a chronic gastric ulcer has the worse outlook, and the young patient with an acute ulcer the best. There should, in fact, be no mortality whatsoever from acute ulcers. With duodenal ulcer the main risk is in the elderly or those with pre-existing disease, but occasional fatalities occur due to erosion of a major blood-vessel which causes so catastrophic a haemorrhage that resuscitation is hampered and surgical treatment is delayed. Errors in management occur most readily in such situations.

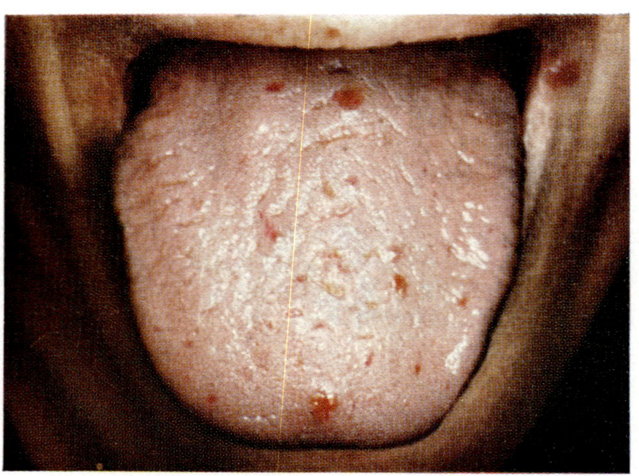

Fig. 20. The tongue in hereditary telangiectasia.

INSIDIOUS OR RECURRENT BLEEDING FROM THE GASTRO-INTESTINAL TRACT

Patients who do not bleed abruptly may seek medical attention for the acute symptoms of anaemia or for the more chronic manifestations of sideropenia. The main problem for the physician is to ascertain whether bleeding is due to the use of drugs such as aspirin, phenylbutazone, or corticosteroids and, if not, to find the source of the bleeding, having established from the history or from the results of serial faecal occult blood-tests that blood is being lost from the gastro-intestinal tract. In cases of doubt, blood-loss from the gut may be more accurately determined by first giving a dose of chromium-labelled red blood-cells and then measuring faecal radioactivity.

Hereditary telangiectasia should be considered first as a possible diagnosis in cases of obscure blood-loss, the family history should be ascertained and the lips and tongue carefully inspected for the small red lesions (*Fig. 20*). If this disease is excluded, and if gastroscopy, sigmoido-scopy, barium meal, barium enema, and small-bowel enema provide no evidence as to the source of the bleeding, then a Miller-Abbot tube may be passed into the small gut, and the aspirate from different levels in-spected and tested for blood. The procedure is laborious and often fruitless. Another manœuvre is to make the patient swallow a string and afterwards to give fluorescein intravenously. When the string has passed as far as the ileocaecal valve it is withdrawn and examined under ultra-violet light. The level at which fluorescence begins should indicate the position of the bleeding lesion (*see Chapter 25*).

These investigations are of little value if the bleeding is intermittent. In such cases the patient may be shown how to test for occult blood and be asked to report at the hospital whenever visible or occult bleeding occurs. An immediate laparotomy may then enable the surgeon to see the place in the gut from which the blood is coming, the intestine below the lesion being coloured by blood. This may be the only way of diagnosing and localizing an angioma of the small gut or similar small lesion. Angiography is currently under trial for the diagnosis of these difficult cases.

FURTHER READING

Haematemesis and Melaena
CLARK, C. G. (1968), 'Bleeding from Peptic Ulcer', *Post-grad. med. J.*, **44**, 590.
COGHILL, N. F., and WILLCOX, R. G. (1960), 'Factors in the Prognosis of Bleeding Chronic Gastric and Duodenal Ulcers', *Q. Jl Med.*, **53**, 575.
JONES, F. AVERY (1956), 'Haematemesis and Melaena with Special Reference to Causation and to Factors influencing Mortality from Bleeding Peptic Ulcers', *Gastroenterology*, **30**, 166.
— — (1970), 'Problems of Alimentary Bleeding', *Br. med. J.*, **2**, 267.
NORTHFIELD, T. C., and SMITH, T. (1970), 'Central Venous Pressure in the Clinical Management of Acute Gastro-intestinal Bleeding', *Lancet*, **2**, 584.
SCHILLER, K. R. F., TRUELOVE, S. C., and WILLIAMS, D. GWYN (1970), *Br. med. J.*, **2**, 7.
SPIRO, H. M. (1962), 'Stomach Damage from Aspirin, Steroids and Antimetabolites', *Am. J. dig. Dis.*, **7**, 733.
TUDHOPE, G. R. (1958), 'The Loss and Replacement of Red Cells in Patients with Acute Gastro-intestinal Haemorrhage', *Q. Jl Med.*, **51**, 543.

Surgical Treatment of Alimentary Bleeding
KAY, A. W. (1962), 'Management of Obscure Alimentary Bleeding', *Br. med. J.*, **1**, 1709.
ZAMCHEK, N., COTTER, T. P., HERSHORN, S. E., CHALMERS, T. C., RITVO, M., and WHITE, F. W. (1952), 'Early Roentgen Diagnosis in Massive Bleeding from the Upper Gastrointestinal Tract', *Am. J. Med.*, **13**, 713.

Chapter 8

Postgastrectomy and Postvagotomy Problems

By L. R. Celestin

It will be recalled from previous chapters that several types of gastrectomy are in common use (*see Table 8*, p. 77):

1. Partial gastrectomy—Billroth-I operation for gastric ulcer.
2. Partial gastrectomy—Billroth-II (Polya) operation for duodenal ulcer.
3. Total gastrectomy—for malignant disease of the stomach.

The results of partial gastrectomy for the treatment of peptic ulcer are good in 90 per cent (± 5 per cent) of patients. The remainder may have one or more unsatisfactory features.

Apart from the complications which may follow any operation there are particular sequelae of gastrectomy. Some of these occur in the immediate postoperative period, e.g., bleeding from the anastomosis, leakage from the duodenal stump, afferent loop obstruction, pancreatitis, enterocolitis, and delayed gastric emptying. Others occur later, e.g., retrograde intussusception, internal herniation, and obstruction. The most important postgastrectomy problems, however, are twofold: (*a*) Recurrent ulceration; (*b*) Special complications directly attributable to the altered alimentary function following resection.

These are to be the subject of this chapter.

THE PROBLEM OF RECURRENT ULCERATION

The 'acid test' of an operation for the treatment of ulcer is the ulcer recurrence rate. When a Billroth-I operation is done for gastric ulcer recurrence is very rare indeed; when used for duodenal ulcer recurrences may appear in approximately 10 per cent of patients. The Polya operation, on the other hand, has a 1–4 per cent recurrence rate for duodenal ulcer. It is particularly significant that this recurrence rate may rise to 20–30 per cent if any gastric antrum is inadvertently left behind. Some of the causes of recurrence are shown in *Fig. 21*.

Although the new ulcer may occur in the gastric remnant, usually it is found on the jejunal side of the anastomosis (anastomotic ulcer). *Table 10* shows the incidence of such recurrences following various operations on the stomach.

In general, ulceration following partial gastrectomy tends to occur during the first year and is manifest clinically by a return of symptoms. The pain, which occurs immediately after food, is frequently in the left side of the abdomen. Bleeding from the ulcer is a common feature.

Pathologically, the chief characteristic of the anastomotic ulcer is its tendency to penetrate and to adhere to neighbouring organs.

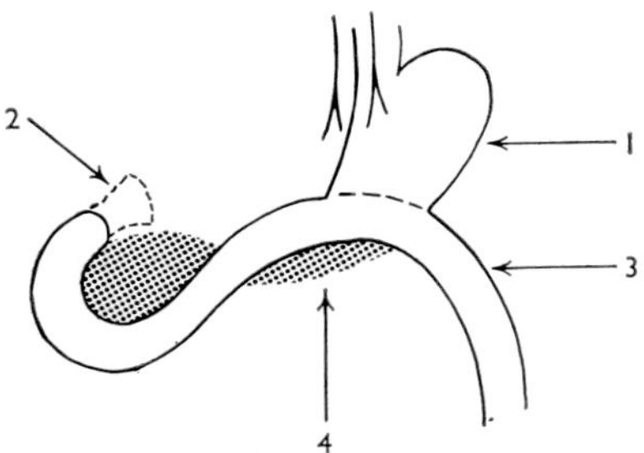

Fig. 21. Some factors in the causation of recurrent ulceration. 1, Remnant too large. 2, Retained antrum. 3, Anastomosis too low in jejunum. 4, Zollinger-Ellison syndrome.

Table 10. ULCER RECURRENCE RATE FOLLOWING GASTRIC OPERATIONS

	Per cent
Gastro-enterostomy	30
Vagotomy alone	13
Vagotomy + gastro-enterostomy	5
Gastrectomy ($\frac{3}{4}$)	1–4
Vagotomy + antrectomy (hemigastrectomy)	Less than 1

The patient must be assessed in exactly the same manner as in primary cases. Barium meal may show the ulcer, whilst gastroscopy may reveal the crater or an area of 'cellulitis' around it. Secretion studies must be repeated to determine whether or not hypersecretion is still present.

The subsequent management may be summarized as follows:

1. *Anastomotic Ulcer with Hypersecretion.* If the initial gastrectomy was adequate vagotomy is the treatment of choice. This may be done trans-thoracically, but an abdominal approach is essential if refashioning of the stoma is necessary, or if there is any doubt at all about the complete removal of the antrum at the previous operation.

2. *Anastomotic Ulcer without Hypersecretion and Ulcer in Gastric Remnant.* Secondary (subtotal) gastrectomy is indicated for these.

3. *Recurrences due to Ulcerogenic Pancreatic Tumours* (Zollinger-Ellison Syndrome). During the operation on these patients continuous gastric suction should be maintained as an aid to detection of the tumour. A sudden decrease in the aspirated secretion occurs when the tumour is removed. Classically, if the tumour can be located, its removal is all that

is necessary. Otherwise subtotal pancreatectomy and total gastrectomy may be the only procedure possible (*see Chapter 16*).

4. Gastric carcinoma can arise in a gastric remnant and if detected early enough a total gastrectomy must be done.

Gastrocolic Fistula

Apart from rare causes (carcinoma of stomach or colon or ulcerative colitis) gastrocolic fistula is essentially a complication of anastomotic ulceration. It is estimated that about 10 per cent of such ulcers develop this complication, more especially after gastro-enterostomy than gastrectomy. The actual fistula may be gastrojejunocolic in its course.

When it develops the ulcer symptoms may cease and be replaced by diarrhoea, weight-loss, faecal vomiting or eructations, borborygmi, fatigue, and dehydration. There may be evidence of severe malabsorption by the presence of cachexia, oedema, anaemia, steatorrhoea, and glossitis. The fistula is best demonstrated by barium enema, but some evidence of it may be seen on gastroscopy. Barium meal may fail to demonstrate the communication in more than half the patients.

Two pathological facts are of paramount importance in these patients:

1. There is gross inflammatory reaction around the fistula and adjacent structures, making reparative surgery hazardous.

2. The chief factor producing the deterioration of the patient's condition is the fouling of the jejunum by colonic contents. Recognition of this fact is the basis of doing a simple preliminary operation to improve the general nutrition of the patient prior to the main reconstructive operation.

TREATMENT

The aims of specific treatment are twofold: (1) Repair of the fistula. (2) Correction of the factors producing recurrent ulceration at the stoma.

On this basis, it will be appreciated that treatment in patients with a previous gastro-enterostomy is hopeful, whilst in those with a previous gastrectomy it will be difficult. The mortality-rate of surgical management is high—of the order of 30 per cent—and is a reflection both of the poor state of the patient and the difficulty of the procedure.

The first step is to correct as far as possible the malnutrition, anaemia, dehydration, and electrolyte defects by conservative means, e.g., blood transfusion and intravenous electrolytes. Intestinal antibiotics should be given. A one-stage operation can be contemplated in those improving with this régime and in those patients who are reasonably well when seen despite the presence of the fistula. The majority need a two-stage procedure:

1. Preliminary stage to correct the fouling of the jejunum and to improve the patient so that the second stage can be done more safely. This stage consists either of a proximal colostomy or an ileosigmoid anastomosis with division of the ileum.

2. The second stage is carried out some three months later, the patient being much improved and local pathology permitting direct attack with greater ease. The fistula is excised, the intestine repaired, and the

appropriate correction of the ulcer process carried out, e.g., gastrectomy, antrectomy and vagotomy, or vagotomy alone if previous gastrectomy was adequate. In all cases, however, the pancreas must be inspected to exclude ulcerogenic tumour.

COMPLICATIONS RELATED TO ALTERED FUNCTION

After gastric resection and the subsequent anatomical reconstruction, the following changes in function may be observed:

1. Rapid emptying of the stomach remnant.
2. Reduced secretion of hydrochloric acid and pepsin.
3. Reduced secretion of the intrinsic factor.
4. Reduced secretion of pancreatic enzymes.
5. Inadequate mixing of food with enzymes and bile.
6. Reduced absorption of certain food substances, especially protein and fat. Glucose is absorbed very rapidly.
7. Abolition of the normal *p*H gradient in the alimentary canal (*Fig. 22*).
8. Increased intestinal motility.
9. Altered bacteriological state of intestine occasionally.
10. Effects related to the creation of the afferent loop.

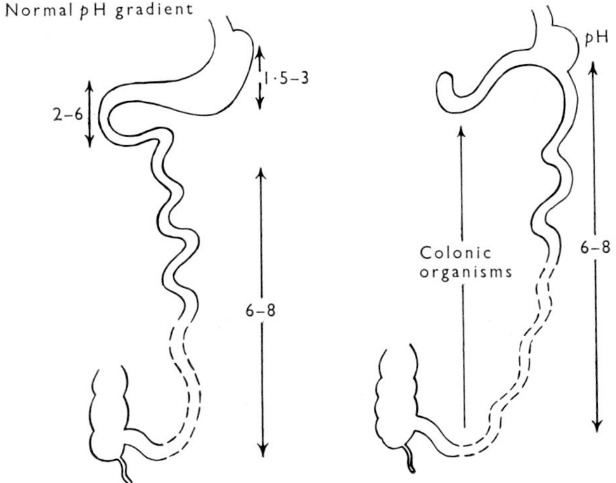

Fig. 22. Effect of gastrectomy on *p*H gradient of alimentary canal.

The clinical features related to some of these changes may appear directly after meals, and produce the 'post-cibal syndrome'. The effects of other changes, however, may appear very slowly after a long interval of time; these present as nutritional disturbances.

The various postgastrectomy syndromes may therefore be classified in the following manner:

A. Post-cibal symptoms
    1. Early post-cibal syndrome ('dumping syndrome')
    2. Late post-cibal syndrome (hypoglycaemic syndrome)
    3. Bile vomiting

B. Nutritional disturbances
  1. Weight-loss and steatorrhoea
  2. Iron-deficiency anaemia
  3. Megaloblastic anaemia
  4. Vitamin-B deficiency
  5. Severe malnutrition

A. Post-cibal Symptoms

1. EARLY POST-CIBAL SYNDROME

This occurs rather more often in women than in men, and is seen more frequently and in its more persistent form after the Polya operation. The symptoms occur towards the end of a meal or a few minutes after completion. Characteristically, the patient complains of epigastric fullness, drowsiness, muscular weakness, and sometimes faintness. He may be aware of a sensation of heat, with flushing and perspiration. Occasionally there is vomiting of bile or colic followed by diarrhoea. During the attack there is usually tachycardia, but blood-pressure changes are variable. The attack lasts for about thirty minutes.

The majority of patients experience some of these symptoms, especially the abdominal features, during convalescence, but they tend to abate during the first year after operation. In about 5 per cent of patients the syndrome may be persistent.

It is very difficult to be precise about the exact mechanism of production of this syndrome. In the simplest terms, one may regard it as the result of a reflex initiated in the jejunum in response to many possible stimuli, and mediated through the sympathetic system. Nevertheless, it is necessary to try to assess the cause in order to provide a basis of management. There is evidence that all the features of the syndrome are not due to the same cause. The abdominal component—epigastric fullness, borborygmi, etc.— is probably due to the precipitate emptying of the gastric remnant and increased motor activity of the small bowel. The vasomotor features seem to be related to a fall in plasma volume, of the order of 7 per cent or more, in patients who are susceptible to such a change. The work of Le Quesne has indicated that there may be an underlying primary disorder of glucose metabolism as a cause of the fall in plasma volume. It is well recognized that transient hyperglycaemia follows the ingestion of glucose after gastrectomy. Hyperglycaemia may reduce further glucose absorption from the jejunum and retained sugar in the intestine causes a shift of fluid from the blood into the intestine by osmosis. This may be responsible for the fall in plasma volume, and, in addition, may stimulate the increased bulk within the intestine, may augment peristalsis, and contribute to the abdominal symptoms. Despite its shortcomings, the importance of this concept of production of the syndrome lies in the fact that it provides the most satisfactory basis of treatment to date.

Management: Patience and perseverance are essential so that sufficient time is allowed to elapse for the symptoms to ameliorate. The bulk of the meals should be reduced and taken more frequently. The meals should be dry, and soups, milk, and sweets avoided. Drinks should be taken separately from the main meals. It is worth while lying down for a short period after meals. With reference to the use of drugs, two additions to the régime seem to be rational. The hyperactivity of the intestine may be reduced by the use of belladonna, codeine, or ganglion-blocking drugs. Insulin, or one of the oral hypoglycaemic agents, may be given before meals and deserves a trial. The use of a serotonin antagonist, cyproheptadine hydrochloride (Periactin), 4 mg. before food, may also be used. In some patients splanchnic block with local anaesthetics affords relief for long periods.

If symptoms persist despite this conservative drill, and especially if there is an associated decline in the patient's condition, surgical measures may be considered. Conversion of the Polya anastomosis to one of the Billroth-I type is the best procedure (*Fig. 23*).

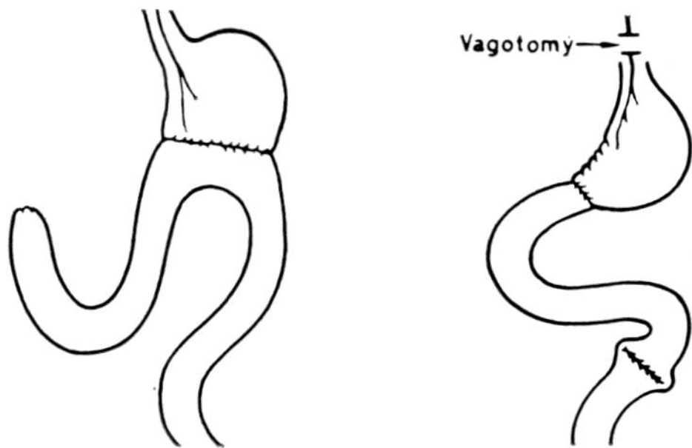

Fig. 23. Conversion of Polya anastomosis to Billroth-I type for severe post-cibal syndrome and malabsorption syndrome.

2. LATE POST-CIBAL SYNDROME

Following the hyperglycaemic phase after the ingestion of sugar, transient hypoglycaemia may occur, the blood-glucose level falling to 50 mg. per cent. Symptoms of faintness, tremor, sweating, and weakness may occur. The syndrome is seen in 5 per cent of patients after all types of gastrectomy. It is probably due to increased insulin sensitivity rather than to either delayed or increased output of insulin.

As a rule the symptoms are not serious. They are best controlled by dietary means—low carbohydrate and high fat and protein intake, to avoid wide fluctuations of the blood-sugar. Glucose, however, will relieve symptoms when they occur.

3. BILE VOMITING

This symptom may be seen as an isolated feature, but may occur in association with the early post-cibal syndrome. About 10 per cent (± 5 per cent) of patients may suffer from this type of vomiting, and it is probably seen more frequently after the Polya operation with antecolic anastomosis.

The vomit consists of bile unmixed with food. The vomiting occurs intermittently rather than after every meal. It is believed that the cause of this
symptom is transient obstruction of the afferent loop, which holds up the
bile and pancreatic secretion. It can be largely avoided if the afferent loop
is made as short as possible at the primary operation.

When surgery is necessary to correct this type of vomiting, conversion
to a Billroth-I is used if there are associated features of the post-cibal
syndrome. If, on the other hand, vomiting of bile occurs alone, conversion
to a Roux-en-Y anastomosis is preferable (*Fig. 24*).

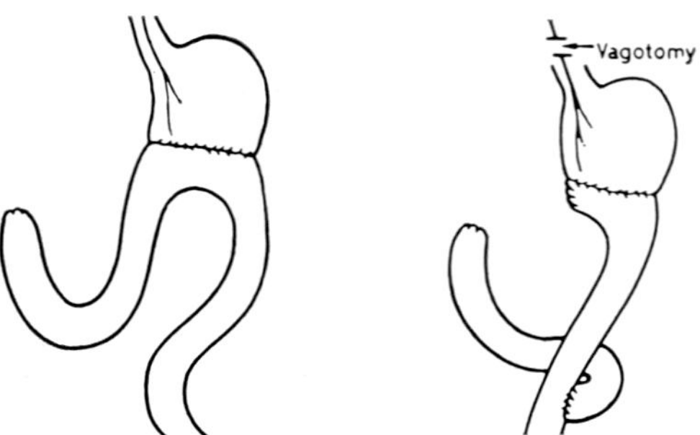

Fig. 24. Conversion of Polya anastomosis to Roux-en-Y type for bilious vomiting.

B. Nutritional Disturbances

1. WEIGHT-LOSS AND STEATORRHOEA

Weight-loss is a well-recognized feature after gastrectomy, and is seen
more frequently in women than in men, and most especially in patients
with post-cibal symptoms. It can be stated to be the rule following total
gastrectomy, common after Polya operations, and rare after Billroth-I
procedures. Overall, the incidence is about 60 per cent. It is not necessarily
a serious symptom; indeed, for a few it is beneficial. A reduced incidence
of coronary thrombosis has been recorded following gastrectomy, and is
possibly related to weight-loss.

The cause of weight-loss is reduced food intake, especially if there is
anorexia or post-cibal syndromes and reduced absorption of food. This
latter feature has been demonstrated for protein and fat, and the defect is
probably greater for protein than for fat.

Increased fat loss in the stools occurs in about 1 per cent of patients
after the Billroth-I operation, but may be observed in 20–60 per cent of
patients with Polya anastomosis, a greater incidence occurring with long
afferent loops. The causes of steatorrhoea are summarized in *Fig. 25*, but
the main factors are poor mixing of food and enzymes, reduced pancreatic
output, and inactivation of enzymes in the afferent loop. Although steatorrhoea may be manifest very soon after operation, occasionally it appears
slowly. In these cases, latent defects of intestinal absorption may be brought
into relief by the operation, or alternatively they may be due to changes in
intestinal flora dependent on the afferent loop (cul-de-sac phenomena).

The patient may have diarrhoea associated with the steatorrhoea. In about 1 per cent of patients it is episodic, attacks occurring every few weeks and lasting for a few days. Some 4 per cent complain of persisting diarrhoea. The majority of patients, however, observe that the regularity of their bowel habits is greatly improved. Metabolic bone disease, usually osteoporosis or osteomalacia, may be seen with or without accompanying steatorrhoea.

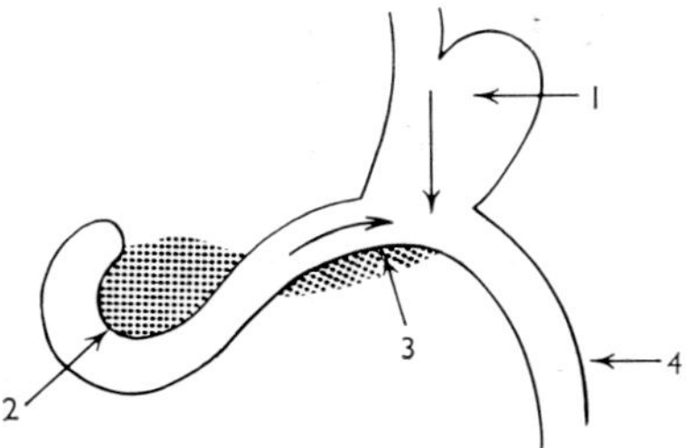

Fig. 25. Some factors in the production of postgastrectomy steatorrhoea. 1, Rapid emptying of gastric remnant—food particles too large for enzymes. 2, Inadequate pancreatic secretion. Afferent loop cul-de-sac. 3, Poor mixing of food and enzymes from afferent loop. 4, Intestinal hurry, altered bacterial state of intestine, latent intestinal defects.

Postgastrectomy weight-loss is treated when necessary by a high-protein, high-calorie diet, using frequent meals. Encouraging results may follow the use of anabolic steroids, e.g., methandienone 50 mg. daily. It is important to exclude pulmonary tuberculosis, as this may follow gastrectomy, especially in those with a previous history of the condition and in those with a poor nutritional state prior to operation.

2. IRON-DEFICIENCY ANAEMIA

This may follow all types of gastrectomy in about 40 per cent of patients, but is commoner after the Polya operation than the Billroth-I. It is seen more frequently in women than in men. The important feature is that the anaemia is slowly progressive. Although the uptake of inorganic iron does not appear to be reduced by gastrectomy the same may not be true of organic or food iron. It is certain, however, that gastrectomy deprives the anaemic patient of the ability to absorb iron according to his need.

It is obviously fundamental to exclude occult blood-loss in these patients. and if this is done, the anaemia can be readily corrected by the administration of iron. Indeed, in view of what has been said, it should be a constant supplement to the patient's diet—one tablet (180 mg.) of ferrous sulphate thrice daily after meals. (Only very rarely is the anaemia refractory to oral iron, and then intramuscular or intravenous iron may be given.)

3. MEGALOBLASTIC ANAEMIA

This type of anaemia is usual following total gastrectomy, but appears slowly after four to five years. This is due to the gradual depletion of liver stores of vitamin B_{12} (about 2000 μg.), which are used at a rate of approximately 1 μg. daily. When this form of anaemia follows partial gastrectomy it may be an isolated feature associated with atrophy of the gastric mucosa, or it may be part of a severe malabsorption syndrome (*see below*). Serum B_{12} levels are, however, often found to be low some years after partial gastrectomy, and in some patients its absorption is found to be impaired. Anaemia is corrected by giving intramuscular vitamin B_{12} (cyanocobalamin) twice weekly in a dose of 100 μg. until the blood is normal. Thereafter a maintenance dose of 250 μg. each month is necessary.

4. VITAMIN B DEFICIENCY

This may occur in approximately 10 per cent of patients, presenting as hyporiboflavinosis (angular stomatitis and glossitis), or as thiamine deficiency with peripheral neuritis. Vitamin B, like iron, is normally absorbed high in the intestine, maximally in the least alkaline part of the duodenum. A regular supplement in the diet is the best way of preventing deficiency.

5. SEVERE MALABSORPTION

It has been mentioned already that weight-loss and steatorrhoea are common after gastrectomy and are not usually associated with symptoms. Occasionally, however, they contribute to a well-established malabsorption syndrome with wasting, gross vitamin deficiencies, hypoproteinaemia, steatorrhoea, and anaemia. Such a state is seen in much less than 1 per cent of all patients undergoing operation. It usually follows the Polya operation, especially if the afferent loop is long, and usually takes many years to develop. Clinically these patients resemble those developing malabsorption effects after intestinal surgery which leaves culs-de-sac.

There is little doubt that some of the postgastrectomy patients develop this syndrome due to the afferent loop cul-de-sac, but others are due to a pre-existing defect of intestinal absorption being brought into relief by the increased load on the intestine following gastric resection. Indeed, some are gluten-induced syndromes, whilst others are due to ascent of organisms altering the bacterial state of the gut.

All need careful assessment. Temporary exhibition of chlortetracycline may result in improvement. The majority need conversion to a Billroth-I anastomosis, the results of which are very satisfying.

POSTVAGOTOMY PROBLEMS

The shortcomings of partial gastrectomy were reappraised when in 1948 Dragstedt and Camp showed that vagal nerve section with a drainage operation offered a better alternative operation. Amongst the many praises sung for vagotomy and enterostomy or vagotomy and pyloroplasty were:

a. A low postoperative mortality-rate.

b. No interference with the size of the gastric reservoir.

c. Fewer postoperative sequelae.

d. A lesser recurrence rate based on the technical ease of performance.

The latter point demanded complete vagal section at the time of surgery, and this completion was ascertained by the Hollander insulin test *after* the operation. This is obviously not an ideal test and Burge and Vane (1958) suggested a test at the time of the operation. However excellent this idea, it has not found favour since the test is a cumbersome one and incomplete vagal section is not always necessarily followed by a recurrence (Ross and Kay, 1964). In the hands of the experienced gastric surgeon incomplete vagotomy is uncommon and the recurrence rate is between 1 and 3 per cent; unfortunately the same results cannot be claimed for the inexperienced in whom incompleteness is to be found in some 10–25 per cent of cases. It cannot therefore be held that vagotomy is an easier operation than partial gastrectomy. On the other hand, the mortality-rate is very low and this makes vagotomy a safer procedure.

Time has shown that, like partial gastrectomy, vagotomy and pyloroplasty is followed by certain unpleasant sequelae. The main ones are:

1. Epigastric fullness   (45 per cent)
2. Flatulence   (30 per cent)
3. Nausea   (25 per cent)
4. Heartburn and dysphagia   (15 per cent)
5. Bilious and food vomiting   (15 per cent)
6. Diarrhoea   (20 per cent)
7. Dumping—early and late   (12 per cent)

These sequelae are equally present after vagotomy and gastro-enterostomy or vagotomy and antrectomy, but to a lesser or greater extent.

Epigastric fullness and flatulence are probably the result of the impoverished gastric tone after vagotomy with associated delayed gastric emptying. Most cases respond to the use of long-acting cholinergic drugs. Others may be due to too small a pyloroplasty, which should always be generous. Both symptoms are less common if gastro-enterostomy or antrectomy is used as a drainage operation.

Vomiting of bile and food and dumping are less frequently met after pyloroplasty than after the two latter operations, and are far less tolerated by the sufferers than post-cibal fullness and flatulence. Their treatment follows the same lines as when the symptoms occur after gastrectomy.

Diarrhoea has become the subject of much discussion. It can be episodic or continuous, the latter form being uncommon. The majority of cases suffer it only in a mild or moderate form, often associated with poor gastric emptying or with dumping due to a sugar intolerance. Such diarrhoea can be corrected by carefully avoiding offending foods; by the use of anti-diarrhoeal and cholinergic drugs. A small group of patients— less than 5 per cent of all total vagotomies—have a more severe form. It is characterized by its urgency and by its greater frequency. It is more common when vagotomy has been added to an existing partial gastrectomy, and some of these patients exhibit an inadequate personality. They either fail to discipline themselves as regards food intake and/or the regularity with which they take anti-diarrhoeal drugs. Their condition makes them still more indrawn and they become work shy and social recluses. This very small group may be amenable to only one form of treatment: the interposition of a reversed ileal segment in the mid-ileum, but the operation should not be lightly undertaken and should be reserved specially for those suffering severe malnutrition as a result of their previous surgery.

Prophylaxis against diarrhoea has taken the form of selective vagotomy, either anterior or posterior, or both. There is as yet no firm evidence that selective vagotomy alters this incidence; but the operation should be encouraged since only the stomach should be denervated and not the entire gastro-intestinal complex.

The malnutrition states that follow vagotomy are similar to those met with after partial gastrectomy but on the whole the metabolic ill effects are less.

In conclusion it can be said that both from the point of view of post-operative sequelae and mortality, vagotomy and pyloroplasty offers the best procedure for the majority of elective cases, with vagotomy and gastro-enterostomy closely behind, while the addition of antrectomy—though it reduces the recurrence rate—introduces the same technical problem as partial gastrectomy.

FURTHER READING

ILLINGWORTH, C. F. W. (1960), 'Post Gastrectomy Syndromes', *Gut*, **1**, 183.

Blood Changes
DELLER, D. J., and WITTS, L. J. (1969), 'Changes in the Blood after Partial Gastrectomy with Special Reference to Vitamin B_{12}', *Q. Jl Med.*, **55**, 71.

Vagotomy
BURGE, H., and VANE, J. R. (1958), 'Method of Testing for Complete Nerve Section during Vagotomy', *Br. med. J.*, **1**, 615.
DRAGSTEDT, L. R., and CAMP, E. H. (1948), 'Follow-up of Gastric Vagotomy alone in the Treatment of Peptic Ulcer', *Gastro-enterology*, **11**, 460.
ROSS, B., and KAY, A. W. (1964), 'The Insulin Test after Vagotomy', *Ibid.*, **46**, 379.
WILLIAMS, J. A., and COX, A. G. (1969), *After Vagotomy*. London: Butterworths.

Chapter 9

Jaundice

THE STAINING of the body tissues with bile-pigments is called jaundice. In its mildest form it is recognized clinically by yellow discoloration of the sclerotics, but in deeper jaundice the skin and mucous membranes are also stained. The normal serum bilirubin level is 0·2–0·8 mg. per 100 ml. Jaundice is detectable clinically when the serum level is about 3 mg. per 100 ml. or more. Three main varieties are usually recognized. These are *obstructive* jaundice, *liver cell* jaundice, and *haemolytic* jaundice. It must be remembered that sometimes more than one variety can occur at the same time.

BILE-PIGMENT METABOLISM

Bile-pigments (bilirubin and biliverdin) are produced by the breakdown of senescent red blood-cells. It is now known, however, that 15 per cent or so of total bile-pigment does not depend on this mechanism but is derived from haemoproteins in the bone-marrow, liver, or kidney. This

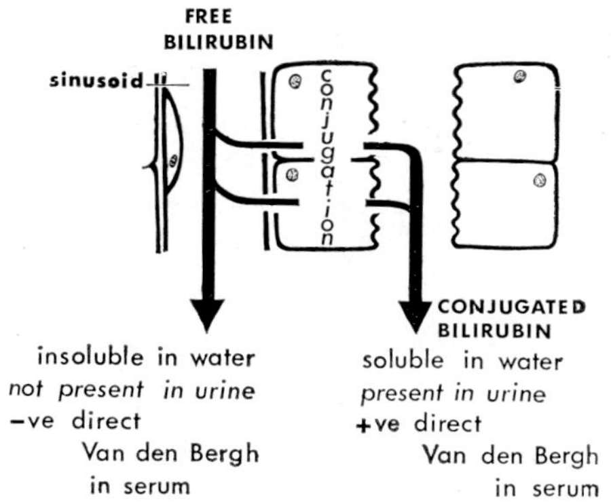

Fig. 26. Characteristics of free and conjugated bilirubin.

fraction of the bile-pigments is therefore not dependent on red-cell destruction. The pigment, loosely bound to serum albumin, is transported to the liver cell which they enter. They are probably accepted by two Y and Z acceptor proteins, and they undergo conjugation with glucuronic acid by enzymes in the smooth endoplasmic reticulum of the liver cell. Transport of conjugated pigment across the cell and secretion into the bilary canaliculi by an active process then takes place. There is apparently a continuous process of deconjugation and reconjugation operating in the obstructed liver which depends on the presence of hepatic β-glucuronidase. Staining techniques demonstrate that in obstructive jaundice some of the retained pigment is unconjugated.

OBSTRUCTIVE JAUNDICE

Obstruction to the outflow of bile from the biliary tract leads to retention of bile-pigment, largely conjugated bilirubin in the blood (*Fig. 26*). As this is water-soluble, bile is found in the urine.

AETIOLOGY
(*Fig. 27*)

Obstruction inside the Liver (Intrahepatic—Lesions affecting Biliary Canaliculi or Cholangioles)

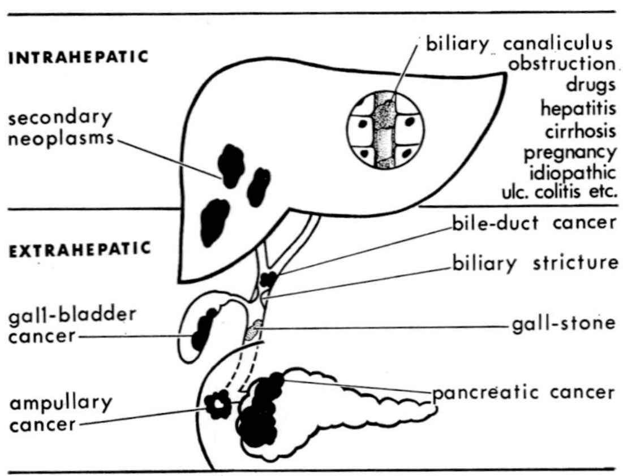

Fig. 27. Causes of obstructive jaundice.

1. *Acute*

 a. Drugs: chlorpromazine; arsphenamine; norethandrolone; methyl testosterone; chlorpropamide, oral contraceptives, etc.
 b. Viral hepatitis, 'cholangiolitic hepatitis'.
 c. In pregnancy (last three months).
 d. Intrahepatic neoplasms and reticulosis, e.g., Hodgkin's disease.

2. *Chronic*

 a. 'Primary' biliary cirrhosis and some cases of non-biliary cirrhosis.
 b. Some cases of drug jaundice, particularly arsphenamine; chlorpromazine.
 c. In infancy—congenital obliteration of the bile-ducts.
 d. Of unknown cause (often recurrent)—recurrent idiopathic cholestasis.
 e. In ulcerative colitis.

Obstruction outside the Liver (Extrahepatic—Lesions affecting the Common Bile-duct or both Hepatic Ducts)

a. Neoplasm
- Ampulla of Vater
- Head of pancreas or neoplastic spread from neighbouring organs
- Bile-ducts and gall-bladder.

b. Gall-stones in common bile-duct.

c. Stricture in common bile-duct.

d. Rarely, chronic pancreatitis, parasites.

PATHOLOGY

In intrahepatic obstruction the lesions responsible for obstruction of the biliary canaliculi are probably several, depending on the cause. Electron microscopy has established that some forms of intrahepatic obstruction are associated with an abnormality of the small processes, 'microvilli', which line the biliary canaliculi and which presumably have important secretory functions such as the passage of bile-pigment into the bile-duct system.

Changes in the villi may, however, be the result rather than the cause, and recently interest has centred on the possibility that certain irritant bile-acids could cause this type of lesion. Certainly lithocholic acid—a monohydroxy bile-acid—produces damage to bile-ducts and gall-stone formation experimentally and biliary obstruction results. Schaffner and Popper (1969) postulate that liver damage of various types could result in altered bile-salt production resulting in increased hepatic monohydroxy bile-salt concentrations.

In *extrahepatic* biliary obstruction the whole of the biliary tract behind the obstruction is dilated, the liver enlarging as a result. In *intrahepatic* obstruction the biliary tract is collapsed so that at first hepatomegaly is less pronounced. The spleen may be enlarged, particularly if obstructive jaundice is of some duration. *Histologically*, in intrahepatic obstruction there may be few changes except centrilobular bile-retention and bile-ducts may be inconspicuous. In extrahepatic obstruction, bile-duct proliferation, biliary necroses—'bile lakes'—and polymorph infiltration of portal tracts are all common. In some cases, however, histological distinction between intrahepatic and extrahepatic biliary obstruction may be difficult.

CLINICAL PICTURE

Jaundice varies in intensity according to the degree of the obstruction, and if deep is of a greenish hue. It is usually of slow onset so that the maximal degree of jaundice is not reached for some days. On clinical examination the liver is invariably enlarged and, except in cases due to neoplastic involvement, the surface is smooth. Tenderness suggests ascending cholangitis but may also occur with intrahepatic neoplasm. Skin excoriation may accompany pruritus, which is probably due to fixation of bile-salts in the skin. Bile-salt levels in the blood are raised, but there is no precise relationship between the degree of elevation and the presence of pruritus. Splenomegaly may be present in chronic cases. The urine is dark because bile-pigment (conjugated) is present in the urine (positive Fouchet or ictotest). There is no urobilin in the urine (negative Ehrlich test) if biliary obstruction is complete. The stools are pale because they contain no bile-pigment and much fat.

Accompaniments and Complications

The associated features depend on the cause. Loss of weight, palpable enlargement of the gall-bladder (Courvoisier's sign), back or shoulder pain, and intermittent glycosuria suggest a neoplasm of the head of the pancreas. Faecal occult blood-tests are positive when pancreatic neoplasms invade the duodenal loop or with growths of the ampulla of Vater. Biliary colic, fever with rigors, and hepatic tenderness may occur when gall-stones are impacted in the common bile-duct. In this condition the gall-bladder is rarely palpable, for the inflammatory fibrosis of its wall caused by calculus cholecystitis prevents dilatation. Bruising of the skin and other haemorrhagic manifestations of prothrombin deficiency may occur if obstruction is complete or of long standing. If it has lasted for some months, as in primary biliary cirrhosis, common duct stricture, or a slowly growing neoplasm of the bile-ducts, other complications may occur, such as osteomalacia, causing bone pain and spontaneous fractures due to malabsorption of calcium and vitamin D. Osteoporosis due to protein deficiency may also occur. Melanin pigmentation of the skin makes the jaundice appear much deeper. Xanthelasma and later xanthomata in the palmar creases and over pressure-points are caused by high serum lipid values. Similar deposits may be seen in the bones and in peripheral nerves. In this latter situation they may be associated with peripheral neuropathy.

DIAGNOSIS

Jaundice with pale stools and dark urine accompanied by persistent pruritus suggests obstructive jaundice. Biochemically there is a raised serum bilirubin with a high percentage of conjugated bilirubin, a raised serum alkaline phosphatase (usually greater than 30 K.A. units), and some-times a raised serum cholesterol value. The elevation of the serum lipids seen in obstructive jaundice may be associated with the presence of a specific lipoprotein (lipoprotein X). Though only found in obstructive jaundice it occurs only in some cases. Raised lipoproteins are responsible for the positive Jirgl flocculation test.

The flocculation tests are negative, the transaminases normal or moderately raised, and electrophoresis of serum proteins may show an $alpha_2$-beta globulin increase. In patients with neoplastic disease there may be a reduction in the serum albumin level.

INVESTIGATIONS

1. The history should include details of drugs taken by the patient in the past six months.

2. Liver function tests and serum amylase estimation. The serum amylase may be elevated if there is pancreatic duct obstruction by a neoplasm or in pancreatitis.

3. Tests for occult blood in the faeces, possibly indicating intestinal cancer.

4. Plain films of the abdomen may show gall-stones.

5. Barium-meal studies to exclude an abnormality of the duodenal loop due to a pancreatic or ampullary neoplasm.

6. Percutaneous needle biopsy of the liver may differentiate intrahepatic from extrahepatic biliary obstruction.

7. *Transhepatic Cholangiography.* The dilatation of the biliary tract seen in extrahepatic biliary obstruction makes aspiration of bile from the biliary tract and replacement with radio-opaque material easy. Obstruction of the biliary tract in areas difficult to visualize at operation, such as the hepatic ducts, can then be radiologically detected. Knowledge of the site of obstruction before operation allows the surgeon to plan the operation accordingly. Because biliary soiling of the peritoneum may follow needling of the liver, laparotomy must follow at once. Retrograde cannulation of the bile-duct via a fibreoptic endoscope is a less hazardous recent development.

8. An ACTH or corticosteroid test may help to differentiate intrahepatic obstruction due to hepatitis from other types of intrahepatic and extra-hepatic obstruction (*see Chapter 24*).

9. Scintillography using ^{131}I rose bengal may not only delineate an intrahepatic neoplasm but can be used to detect patency of the biliary tract. Gall-bladder filling and subsequent emptying are detected with the aid of a counter over the abdominal wall in the left iliac fossa and following the stimulus of a fatty meal, or better still an i.v. injection of chole-cystokinin.

10. *Laparotomy.* If undiagnosed obstructive jaundice has lasted for six or more weeks and the patient has been adequately treated with parenteral vitamin K, an exploratory operation is justified. If the surgeon finds no apparent cause for obstruction he should take a needle liver biopsy, explore the common bile-duct, and perform an operative cholangiogram. If needling of the liver at operation reveals dilated bile-ducts (aspiration of green or white bile) he should make an intensive search for high extra-hepatic biliary obstruction.

Medical Management of Chronic Obstructive Jaundice

In those patients with chronic obstructive jaundice which cannot be relieved surgically chronic jaundice may become a medical rather than a surgical problem. This is most classically seen in patients with primary biliary cirrhosis; details are given in Chapter 13.

LIVER CELL JAUNDICE

Damage to liver cells interferes with uptake of bilirubin, its conjugation and excretion into the biliary tract.

AETIOLOGY

1. *Acute*

    a. Viral hepatitis (serum or infective) and that due to certain other viruses (*see* pp. 120, 126).

    b. Drug hepatitis—monoamine oxidase inhibitors, e.g., Nardil. Antituberculous drugs, e.g., PAS, INAH. Antirheumatic drugs, e.g., butazolidine. Anaesthetics, e.g., halothane.

    c. Liver cell poisons—carbon tetrachloride; alcohol.

    d. Spirochaetal: Weil's disease; canicola fever.

    e. Infectious mononucleosis.

2. *Chronic*

    a. Cirrhosis with liver cell failure.

    b. The congenital hyperbilirubinaemias.

PATHOLOGY

Histological findings are dependent upon the cause. The picture is complicated by the rather limited histological response of the liver to these damaging agents. Various degrees of liver cell destruction (swollen liver cells, hyaline change, etc.) may be seen in all acute lesions, but in patients with viral hepatitis the centrilobular areas may show evidence of most damage. In the portal zones in viral hepatitis, infectious mononucleosis, and Weil's disease there is a cellular infiltrate consisting mainly of lymphocytes and monocytes. Mononuclear infiltration of the sinusoids is seen in infectious mononucleosis. Fat is prominent in acute alcoholic disease of the liver and as a result of other liver poisons. Mallory's alcoholic hyaline is found with the fat in alcoholic liver disease but is not specific for this condition and may be found for example in Wilson's disease and 'Indian childhood cirrhosis' (a cirrhosis of unknown cause found in well-nourished Indian children). The histological distinction between drug jaundice and viral hepatitis can in many cases by very difficult, if not impossible.

The liver is usually enlarged in the initial phase of the disorders mentioned, but acute or subacute hepatic necrosis can shrink the liver both in viral hepatitis and drug jaundice. The spleen may be enlarged from congestion and reticulo-endothelial proliferation.

CLINICAL PICTURE

Jaundice can be mild, as in decompensated cirrhosis, or very deep, as in severe hepatitis with hepatic necrosis. When deep, the jaundice is classically of an orange-yellow hue. Jaundice is of relatively sudden onset in the acute lesions, the maximal serum bilirubin level often occurring within one or two days. There is bile in the urine and usually increased amounts of urobilin and urobilinogen. The faeces may be paler than normal but usually they retain some pigment. The liver may be enlarged or smaller than normal, and in the latter case the area of percussion dullness is diminished.

In Weil's disease signs of meningeal irritation, pyrexia, severe muscle pains, and renal manifestations (e.g., albuminuria, oliguria) may be found.

In glandular fever generalized lymphadenopathy and splenomegaly with ulceration of the pharynx and skin rashes may occur. In cirrhosis there may be cutaneous and other stigmata of chronic liver disease.

Accompaniments and Complications

Some forms of acute liver cell disease are likely to be complicated by acute hepatic necrosis with rapid destruction of the liver parenchyma and collapse of the reticulin framework. Deepening jaundice, fluid retention, and neuropsychiatric complications then develop, and renal failure, hypotension, and a haemorrhagic tendency often occur as terminal manifestations.

DIAGNOSIS

Jaundice of any severity with dark urine and some pallor of the faeces, but without persistent pruritus, suggests liver cell disease. The liver function tests show a raised serum bilirubin with elevation of both conjugated and free bilirubin. The serum transaminases and certain other enzyme values are often raised to high levels (SGPT and SGOT in particular may be up to 2000 units per ml.). The serum proteins may be abnormal and with subacute or chronic liver cell disease the serum albumin may be decreased. The globulin level is increased even in acute liver cell disease, the increase being principally due to the gamma and to a lesser extent the beta fraction. Because of these increases, which represent the reaction of the reticulo-endothelial system to liver cell injury, there are positive flocculation tests (zinc sulphate turbidity, thymol turbidity, colloidal gold, etc.).

Bile is excreted in the urine because conjugated bilirubin which is water soluble passes the renal filter. Because liver cells are destroyed the serum levels of iron and vitamin B_{12} which are stored in these cells may be elevated.

In the diagnosis of liver cell jaundice the history and clinical examination are particularly important. The history is not complete unless it includes inquiry about drug consumption, occupational hazards, alcoholism, exposure to hepatitis, and injections and transfusions received up to six months before the onset of jaundice. Even such procedures as dental extraction and tattooing may transmit the virus of hepatitis.

Apart from the history and clinical examination the following procedures may be helpful.

1. *Blood Investigations*

Leucopenia is found in viral hepatitis, but a leucocytosis is found in Weil's disease, alcoholic hepatitis, and hepatic necrosis, whatever the cause. Eosinophilia may complicate drug hepatitis. Serum tests for Weil's disease and infectious mononucleosis may help, and a diminished prothrombin concentration in the serum, if found, is not completely correctable by parenteral vitamin K. Identification of Australia antigen is of diagnostic help in serum hepatitis.

2. *Liver Biopsy*

This is undertaken after adequate precautions have been taken. (The prothrombin time in particular should be normal.)

3. *Vitamin B_{12} and Serum Fe Levels*

These are raised in liver cell disease.

Note on Congenital Hyperbilirubinaemia

Four types have so far been described, and only one form, that of Najjar and Crigler, causes severe jaundice and has a poor prognosis. It is a disease of newborn babies who may die with kernicterus because the high levels of unconjugated fat-soluble bile-pigment damage the brain.

The features of the four known forms are briefly tabulated below (*Table 11*). The Dubin-Johnson syndrome is the only one with an abnormal histological picture. These disorders are often familial, and apart from the infantile type are of no significance. Great care must be taken not to

Table 11. THE CONGENITAL HYPERBILIRUBINAEMIAS

	TYPE			
FEATURE	*Najjar and Crigler*	*Dubin-Johnson*	*Gilbert*	*Rotor*
Familial	—	+	+	+
Severity	+++ (fatal)	+	+	+
Age-group	Infancy	Any	Any	Any
		(usually first noted in childhood)		
Type of bilirubin in serum	Unconjugated	Conjugated	Unconjugated	Conjugated
Bile in urine	No	+	No	+
Histology of liver	Normal	Pigment present ? melanin	Normal	Normal. ? same condition as Dubin-Johnson but *without* pigment
Other abnormalities	Kernicterus	Bromsulphthalein retention ↑ at 2 hours. Non-filling gall-bladder. Alkaline phosphatase ↑	Normal BSP metabolism	Bromsulphthalein retention ↑ at 2 hours. Non-filling gall-bladder. Alkaline phosphatase ↑
Cause	Total glucuronyl transferase deficiency	Defective excretion of conjugated bilirubin	? Impaired uptake of bilirubin (unconjugated) by liver + partial glucuronyl transferase deficiency	As for Dubin-Johnson

diagnose liver disease in subjects with hyperbilirubinaemia. Not infrequently such patients are confined to bed with 'chronic hepatitis' and may occasionally be subject to unnecessary operations on the biliary tract. Treatment other than reassurance may occasionally be necessary where jaundice is deep and persistent. Phenobarbitone and dicophane have been used in Gilbert's disease to reduce raised serum unconjugated bilirubin levels. This they achieve possibly by stimulating (enzyme induction) glucuronyl transferase production in the liver with increased production and excretion of conjugated pigment. Unconjugated neonatal hyperbilirubinaemia may be lessened by treating mothers of 'at-risk' babies (prematernity) with phenobarbitone. Blue light using an ultra-violet light over the cot lessens bilirubin levels but may possibly produce equally dangerous by-products of bilirubin.

Subjects with congenital hyperbilirubinaemia suffer from 'liver cell jaundice', but this probably depends on enzyme deficiency and liver cell function is otherwise unimpaired. Patients with Gilbert's disease certainly show decreased levels of hepatic glucuronyl transferase and also a decreased uptake of bilirubin into the liver. Those with the Dubin-Johnson syndrome show evidence of excretory impairment by the liver cell.

The Gunn strain of rat which has an inborn enzyme defect suffers from jaundice of the Gilbert type, and consequently has been a useful tool in the investigation of bilirubin metabolism.

A similar Gilbert-type hyperbilirubinaemia can occur in humans after the use of drugs such as *Felix mas* (for the treatment of tapeworm) or cholecystographic contrast medium, and the antibiotic rifampicin. These seem to compete with unconjugated bilirubin for entry into the liver cell. The antibiotic novobiocin can also produce an unconjugated hyperbilirubinaemia but here the lesion seems to be one of interference with glucuronyl transferase (and hence conjugation) in the smooth endoplasmic reticulum.

HAEMOLYTIC JAUNDICE

This is due to an overloading of a *normal* liver with excess bilirubin produced by increased red blood-cell destruction. Conjugation and transfer of bile-pigment proceed normally, but the supply of free bilirubin is greater than the liver can manage.

AETIOLOGY

If it is severe enough to cause jaundice there is usually anaemia. The causes of increased haemolysis are:

1. Abnormal haemoglobins (e.g., haemoglobin S in sickle-cell disease).
2. Abnormal red blood-cells (e.g., congenital spherocytosis).
3. The action of drugs and chemicals, either directly, due to hypersensitivity, or because of a red blood-cell enzyme defect (e.g., glucose-6-phosphate dehydrogenase).
4. In some protozoal, bacterial, and virus infections.
5. Associated with an enlarged spleen (e.g., Hodgkin's disease).

6. Due to antibodies in the serum, e.g., rhesus or transfusion incompatibility or due to auto-immune haemolytic disease.

PATHOLOGY

There is no major abnormality in the liver in most forms of haemolytic jaundice, although in sickle-cell disease hepatic scarring due to infarction may be found and for a similar reason there may be splenic atrophy. There are increased deposits of iron in Kupffer cells. The spleen is otherwise commonly enlarged.

CLINICAL PICTURE

Jaundice is never severe even in a haemolytic crisis. If deep icterus and haemolysis coexist it means that some other cause of jaundice is also operating, or that the patient has accompanying liver cell disease. Obstructive jaundice due to pigment stones in the biliary tract may complicate haemolytic jaundice. Liver cell damage and haemolysis may occur together in chronic active hepatitis. Mild jaundice, with normal or dark coloured stools and urine which is also darker than normal, particularly on standing, suggests pure haemolysis. The dark urine is *not* due to bile but to increased amounts of urobilinogen (positive Ehrlich's test). Pruritus does *not* occur, unless perhaps a reticulosis is the cause of haemolysis.

Accompaniments and Complications

If haemolysis is proceeding rapidly enough to produce jaundice there must be anaemia. Complications of chronic haemolytic anaemia caused by the presence of abnormal haemoglobins are leg ulceration, bone abnormalities, and retarded development.

Raised free serum bilirubin levels are neurotoxic, but, except in haemolytic disease of the newborn, the level is never high enough to produce kernicterus.

DIAGNOSIS

A history to exclude the taking of drugs and contact with poisons is important, as in other forms of jaundice. The serum bilirubin is raised

Table 12. CLINICAL PROCEDURE IN THE PRESENCE OF JAUNDICE

Assess its severity
Look for scratch-marks.
Examine the liver—Is it enlarged or small? Smooth or nodular? Tender?
Look for splenomegaly and enlargement of the gall-bladder.
Test for free fluid in the abdomen.
Look for cutaneous stigmata of liver disease—spiders, liver palms, clubbing, etc.
Look for evidence of portal hypertension—splenomegaly, abdominal wall veins, etc.
Examine the rectum.
Examine the urine for bile and urobilin.
Examine the faeces—Are they pale? Is there occult or frank blood present?

(usually less than 5 mg. per cent) and this is nearly all free (unconjugated) bilirubin. The rest of the liver function tests are normal. Raised gamma-globulins may be found in auto-immune haemolytic anaemia. There is an increased excretion of urobilinogen in the urine and stercobilin in the faeces.

Investigations which may help to determine the cause of haemolytic jaundice and anaemia are as follows:

1. A blood examination may show anaemia. Reticulocytes can be demonstrated in the peripheral blood-film, and cellular abnormalities in the red corpuscles such as Heinz bodies may be found in drug-induced lesions. The white blood-count may be raised in acute cases and hapto-globins reduced.

2. A direct Coombs test may detect an antibody globulin coating the patient's red blood-cells.

3. Cellular fragility may be increased particularly in congenital sphero-cytosis.

4. L.E. cells should be looked for.

5. Red-cell enzymes, particularly glucose-6-phosphate dehydrogenase (G6PD), should be measured.

6. Electrophoretic studies will detect abnormal haemoglobins.

7. More complex tests to detect 'warm' and 'cold' reacting haemag-glutinins, to detect decreased levels of glucose-6-phosphate dehydrogenase (glutathione stability), or the Ham test for nocturnal haemoglobinuria are sometimes required.

Tables 12 and *13* and *Fig. 28* summarize the procedure and features of the three types of jaundice.

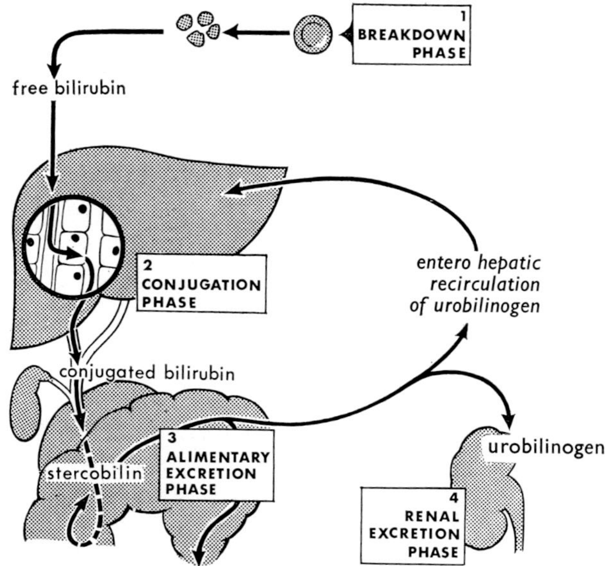

Fig. 28. Metabolism of bile-pigments.

Table 13. SUMMARY OF JAUNDICE

FEATURE	OBSTRUCTIVE	LIVER CELL	HAEMOLYTIC
Colour	Yellow-green	Orange-yellow	Pale yellow
Depth	Mild–deep	Mild–deep	Mild
Pruritus	+ + and persists	+ not persistent	—
Urine colour	Dark (conjugated bilirubin)	Dark (conjugated bilirubin)	Normal. May darken (urobilin)
Faeces colour	Pale { no stercobilin / increased fat	Pale { less stercobilin / increased fat	Normal or dark (increased stercobilin)
Liver size	Increased	Increased, normal, or decreased	Normal
Other important physical signs *sometimes* found	Gall-bladder palpable. Spleen may be enlarged	Spleen +	Spleen +
Positive liver function tests	1. High percentage conjugated bilirubin in blood 2. Raised alkaline phosphatase 3. Raised cholesterol 4. Raised $\alpha_2\beta$ globulins 5. Positive test for lipoprotein X	1. Raised conjugated and free bilirubin 2. Raised transaminases 3. Positive flocculation tests	1. High unconjugated bilirubin
Negative liver function tests	Flocculation tests	Alkaline phosphatase (but sometimes raised)	Flocculation tests. Alkaline phosphatase
Relevant 'special' tests	1. Occult blood in faeces 2. Barium meal 3. Liver biopsy 4. ? ACTH test 5. Cholangiography 6. Laparotomy	1. ? Liver biopsy 2. Blood picture 3. { Vitamin B_{12} / Serum Fe / levels	1. Coombs test 2. Saline fragility 3. Tests for 'warm' and 'cold' agglutinins 4. Haptoglobins 5. L.E. cells 6. Electrophoresis of haemoglobin, etc.

A NOTE ON JAUNDICE AND LIVER DISEASE IN CHILDHOOD AND INFANCY
(*Table 14*)

In childhood, acute viral hepatitis is a common cause of liver cell jaundice though obstructive jaundice is rare. Amongst the causes of obstruction one should remember the possibility of *choledochal cyst*. Certain types of cirrhosis are seen in childhood, notably the '*juvenile*' variety, that accompanying *Kinnier-Wilson* disease and *fibrocystic disease of the pancreas*, and the rare *Fanconi syndrome*.

Portal hypertension, which is often secondary to portal vein thrombosis, is commonly extrahepatic at this age. Intrahepatic causes include both cirrhosis and *congenital hepatic fibrosis*, a disorder characterized by alimentary bleeding and a dense fibrosis of the liver which causes occlusion of the finer portal venules; as it is a form of polycystic disease a similar renal abnormality may coexist (*see* p. 199).

In infancy and the neonatal period certain other hepatic lesions occur. In the newborn, jaundice is often physiological because the immaturity of the liver leads to relative deficiency of the glucuronyl transferase which

Table 14. JAUNDICE IN INFANCY AND CHILDHOOD

	HAEMOLYTIC (*Common*)	LIVER CELL (*Rare*)	OBSTRUCTIVE (*Common*)
Neonate and infant	Physiological Rhesus incompatibility————————→ | (Low glucose-6-phosphate dehydrogenase) may increase severity	Sepsis Galactosaemia→	Neonatal hepatitis 'Inspissated bile syndrome' Obstructive syn-drome Bile-duct atresia
	(*Rare*)	(*Common*)	(*Rare*)
Child	Haemolytic anaemia, e.g., spherocytosis	Viral hepatitis └————————→	Choledochal cyst Parasites 'Cholangiolitic' hepatitis

conjugates free bilirubin with glucuronic acid. Jaundice caused by excessive red-cell destruction is of the 'haemolytic' type, and the unconjugated bilirubin is neurotoxic. In premature babies physiological jaundice of this type sometimes causes kernicterus (damage to the basal ganglia of the brain by bilirubin). The severest types of haemolytic jaundice are, however, associated with rhesus incompatibility. Destruction of foetal red cells is due to the presence of maternal antibodies to foetal red cells (iso-immuni-zation). The baby may have anaemia, oedema, and hepatosplenomegaly as well as jaundice. The jaundice is present at or before birth so that the symptoms of kernicterus—feeding difficulty, muscle rigidity, and respira-tory difficulty—are part of the clinical picture. Replacement of blood is required in those infants whose serum bilirubin is over 20 mg. per cent. Vitamin K in excessive doses increases the likelihood of kernicterus by increasing the concentration of unconjugated bilirubin in the serum. Sometimes, plugging of bile-ductules with inspissated bile causes an obstructive phase known as the 'inspissated bile syndrome'. Steroids found in maternal serum and milk may also prolong neonatal jaundice because they inhibit bilirubin conjugation. Pregnane-3α-20β-diol is a possible cause of jaundice associated with breast feeding in one rare form of neonatal hyperbilirubinaemia, whilst in another an unidentified serum factor produces a similar but familial unconjugated hyperbilirubinaemia not related to breast feeding (Lucey-Driscoll syndrome).

Liver cell jaundice in the newborn is either due to neonatal viral hepatitis due to *rubella* or to *cytomegalic inclusion disease*. Histologically the liver shows rather prominent multinucleated liver cells and hence the name '*giant cell hepatitis*' is sometimes used. This is thought by some observers to be not a true inflammatory disease and the possibility of the disorder being genetically determined is favoured by those who have noted the occurrence of the disease in sibs. A recent finding is of diminished serum levels of an α_1 globulin (α_1 antitrypsin) in some of these cases. This abnormality is known in adults to be associated with pulmonary emphysema and there seems to be some relation too to this and possibly other varieties of chronic liver disease. Another difficulty is that there are biochemical signs of obstructive rather than liver cell jaundice, so that the disorder can be indistinguishable from that produced by a failure of development of the biliary tree, *atresia of the bile-ducts*. In both these disorders jaundice develops a week or more after birth, gradually deepens, and is obstructive in type. A restricted laparotomy with surgical biopsy and cholangiography may be the only way to distinguish them, and as certain types of biliary atresia which affect the extrahepatic ducts are operable the distinction is of importance. Surgical correction, though difficult, can best be done when the child is a few months older, Otherwise, biliary cirrhosis develops and causes death in a year or two.

Infections of the liver by septicaemia, umbilical infection, and syphilis produce a more classic liver cell type of jaundice, while galactosaemia may cause both liver cell and obstructive jaundice.

FURTHER READING

Bile-pigment Metabolism
BILLING, B. H., and LATHE, G. H. (1958), 'Bilirubin Metabolism in Jaundice', *Am. J. Med.*, **24**, 111.

Jaundice in Pregnancy
THORLING, L. (1955), 'Jaundice in Pregnancy: a Clinical Study', *Acta med. scand.* suppl. 302, **151**, 1.

The Congenital Hyperbilirubinaemias
SCHIFF, L., and BILLING, B. H. (1959), 'Congenital Defects in Bilirubin Metabolism as seen in the Adult', *Gastroenterology*, **37**, 595.

General
SHERLOCK, S. (1962), 'Jaundice', *Br. med. J.*, **1**, 1359.

Cholestasis
SCHAFFNER, F., and POPPER, H. (1969), 'Cholestasis is the Result of Hypoactive Hypertrophic Smooth Endoplasmic Reticulum in the Hepatocyte', *Lancet*, **2**, 355.

Congenital Hyperbilirubinaemia
BILLING, B. H., WILLIAMS, R., and RICHARDS, T. G. (1964), 'Defects in Hepatic Transport of Bilirubin in Congenital Hyperbilirubinaemia: an Analysis of Plasma Bilirubin Disappearance Curves', *Clin. Sci.*, **27**, 245.
DUBIN, I. N., and JOHNSON, F. B. (1954), 'Chronic Idiopathic Jaundice: A Review of 50 Cases', *Am. J. Med.*, **24**, 268.
ISRAELS, L. G., SUDERMAN, H. J., and RITZMANN, S. E. (1959), 'Hyperbilirubinaemia due to an Alternate Path of Bilirubin Production', *Ibid.*, **27**, 693.
POWELL, L. W., HEMINGWAY, E., BILLING, B. H., and SHERLOCK, S. (1967), 'Idiopathic Unconjugated Hyperbilirubinaemia (Gilbert's Syndrome): A Study of 42 Families', *New Engl. J. Med.*, **277**, 1108.

Acute Diseases of the Liver

A. INFECTIONS

ACUTE INFECTIONS of the liver may be due to viruses, protozoa, spirochaetes, or bacteria.

1. Viral — Virus hepatitis — Infective hepatitis / Serum (syringe hepatitis)
   Infectious mononucleosis (in some cases), Cytomegalovirus, Rubella, Coxsackie B, Echo, etc.
2. Spirochaetal — Weil's disease / Canicola fever / Relapsing fever } Leptospira
3. Protozoal — Amoebic hepatitis and amoebic abscess
4. Bacterial — Liver abscess / Cholangitis / Portal bacteriaemia } Pyogenic bacteria

1. VIRAL DISEASES

AETIOLOGY

1. Though numerous viruses have been isolated from patients with viral hepatitis none has been found consistently and some of those which have been isolated may be 'associated' viruses. Recent interest centres on the finding in the acute phase of serum hepatitis of an antigen 'Australia antigen', which is in some way related to the virus itself. It is better named 'Hepatitis Associated Antigen' (HAA). Apart from syringe hepatitis this antigen is seen in some patients with chronic hepatitis and in some (about 30 per cent) of children with Down's syndrome. Australia antibody is also sometimes identifiable but does not protect against HAA-induced hepatitis.

HAA, which is usually identified by an immunological reaction, has been recently characterized by electron microscopy in the acute phase in serum of carriers of the disease as well as in some with progressive liver disease.

2. The epidemic form of hepatitis is particularly liable to affect armies in the field, was well known in ancient times, and large civil outbreaks, such as the one that occurred in Delhi in 1955 (100,000 cases), are well recorded. There are two theories of infection, the one involving faecal contamination, the virus being excreted in the faeces during the active stage, and the other, and less likely, incriminating droplet infection. Occasional sources of infection are food, such as shellfish, and water. People of all ages may contract the disease, but schoolchildren and young adults are the most susceptible. Epidemics may vary in intensity because

they are caused by viruses, which though of the same group are perhaps of differing virulence.

PATHOLOGY
(*Fig. 29*)

There are generalized changes throughout the liver. Classically, centri-lobular areas show most cell destruction, but there is scattered damage throughout all zones of the lobule. Except where steroids have been used

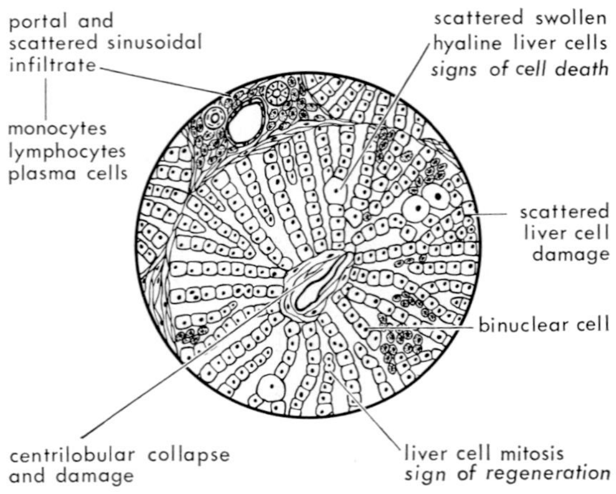

Fig. 29. Pathology of acute hepatitis.

therapeutically, cellular infiltration of the portal zone consisting mainly of mononuclear cells and lymphocytes is seen. As the disease regresses scarring of no prognostic importance occurs in this area. A different histological picture occurs in 'obstructive' hepatitis, where there may be minimal evidence of liver cell necrosis and portal infiltrate, but where there is marked retention of bile in the form of bile-plugs in centrilobular zones and bile in Kupffer cells. When acute hepatic necrosis complicates hepatitis large numbers of liver cells may be destroyed, the reticulum collapses, and the liver shrinks. It is also appreciated that in the acute stage other organs may show evidence of microscopical damage. This is noted in the small bowel (villus shortening) and in the kidney where inflammatory changes are present in the glomeruli.

CLINICAL PICTURE
(*Fig. 30*)

The onset is usually acute. After an incubation period of 2–6 weeks there is an *initial illness* lasting several days, when alimentary symptoms such as anorexia, nausea, vomiting, and upper abdominal pain occur. Pyrexia is usual and a distaste for smoking may develop. In other patients there may be no initial illness or the symptoms may be those of 'flu with headaches and generalized aching of the limbs. There follows in most patients an *icteric phase*, the severity of which is very variable, but which is usually accompanied by transient pruritus, dark urine, and pale faeces. With the onset of jaundice the patient's condition may improve and after

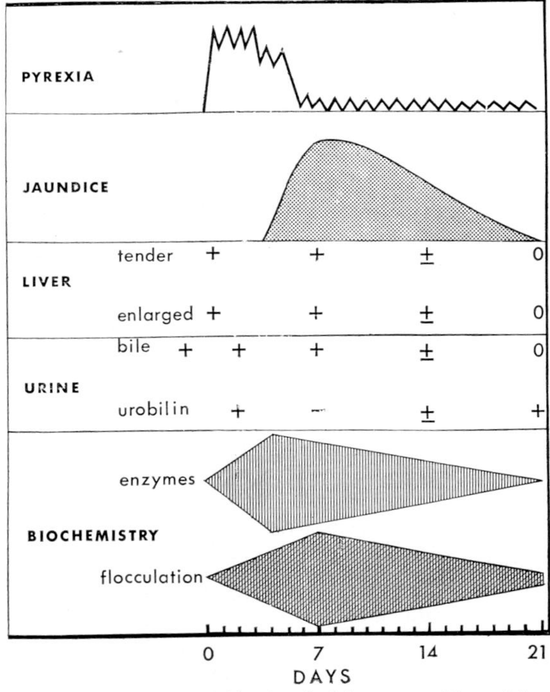

Fig. 30. Clinical and biochemical features of hepatitis.

a variable period lasting from a few days to several weeks the jaundice begins to fade. Other clinical manifestations include skin rashes, arthralgia, and meningeal symptoms, but these are not common.

During the initial illness pyrexia and liver tenderness are the only signs that can be elicited, but the urine may contain bile so that its detection is of importance at this stage. In the icteric phase jaundice is accompanied by moderate hepatomegaly. The liver is tender on firm palpation, and in about a quarter of all cases the spleen is palpable. Some enlargement of the right supraclavicular lymph-nodes may be found.

Accompaniments and Complications (Fig. 31)

1. RELAPSE

In the vast majority of patients the jaundice fades, the liver recedes, and health returns. Adequate convalescence and abstinence from alcohol for three to six months are necessary to avoid the possibility of relapse, in which jaundice and constitutional upset may be worse than in the original disease.

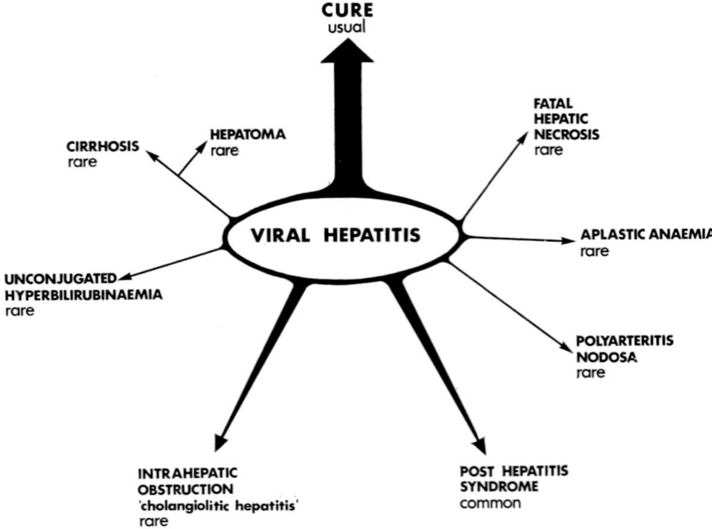

Fig. 31. The outcome of virus hepatitis.

2. HEPATIC NECROSIS

Persistence of vomiting and deterioration in general condition, deepening
jaundice, and the development of neuropsychiatric complications (mental
confusion, hepatic 'flap', and hepatic foetor in the patient's breath) may
herald the onset of acute hepatic necrosis. If this progresses the patient
passes into coma and bleeds profusely into the skin and mucous membranes. The liver shrinks so that it is no longer palpable and even the liver
dullness disappears.

Hyponatraemia, hypotension, and oliguric renal failure are terminal
manifestations of this condition. Hepatic necrosis may develop with the
onset of hepatitis or may develop later after a variable duration of jaundice. It carries a high mortality—80–90 per cent.

3. SUBACUTE AND CHRONIC HEPATITIS

If jaundice is prolonged for more than six weeks it is possible that permanent damage to the liver may occur. The onset of ascites, the development of skin stigmata of chronic liver disease, and increasing enlargement
of the spleen are also suggestive of continuing activity of the disease
process. This may lead eventually to the development of a coarse or
macronodular type of cirrhosis. The liver function tests remain abnormal
in these patients and a needle biopsy may show progressive changes with
increasing fibrosis and early cirrhotic changes. This type of progression is
known as 'chronic aggressive hepatitis'—lesser changes without the onset
of cirrhosis and with changes confined to the portal zones which eventually
regress constitute 'chronic persistent hepatitis'.

4. 'OBSTRUCTIVE' HEPATITIS

Some observers feel that this is a phase in the course of classic viral hepatitis and others that it is caused either by a different strain of virus or by a variation in host response. The patient, after the initial illness and onset of jaundice, develops persistent pruritus, pale stools, and prolonged jaundice. The biochemical tests show obstructive features rather than those of liver cell damage (alkaline phosphatase more than 30 K.A. units, high percentage of conjugated bilirubin, negative flocculation tests). Biopsy specimens show bile retention in centrilobular areas. Jaundice may last for as long as six months. A steroid test (*see* p. 420) may be helpful in the elucidation of the cause of the disease as the serum bilirubin falls dramatically with corticosteroid therapy.

5. THE 'POST-HEPATITIS' SYNDROME

It is common for patients to complain of fatigue and incomplete restoration of health after hepatitis. Others comment on intolerance for fatty food, flatulence, and tenderness over the liver. These complaints, usually considered to be of functional origin, are not helped by the remarks of friends or relatives whose morbid curiosity leads them to see a fancied sallowness of the skin or yellowness of the eyes.

6. 'ANICTERIC' HEPATITIS

Hepatitis may sometimes be so mild that no jaundice occurs. Detection depends on the results of liver function tests, notably the transaminase and other enzyme levels.

7. HYPOPLASTIC ANAEMIA, ETC.

Recently reports have been published of the development of pancytopenia following hepatitis. This is a serious and often fatal complication which is fortunately rare. It presumably represents the effects of viral involvement and damage to the bone-marrow. There is a possibility that foetal damage may occur in the pregnant patient who contracts hepatitis, and a viral myocarditis may be a further complication. Some patients after an attack of viral hepatitis may show for a period of time an elevated unconjugated serum bilirubin level.

DIAGNOSIS

The diagnosis is easy when an epidemic is in progress, but a sporadic case should be considered in any acute gastro-intestinal upset. Drug jaundice of the liver cell type is the most difficult diagnostic problem and therefore an inquiry about drug taking *must* be part of the history. Hepatitis due to infectious mononucleosis and Weil's disease can usually be distinguished. Serum (syringe) hepatitis is a similar illness in most respects, but it is important to detect those cases due to the therapeutic administration of blood or blood products. A history of recent transfusions in a patient with viral hepatitis will lead to the identification of carriers and their further exclusion as blood donors. The presence of HAA is of help in identification of serum hepatitis.

Notes on Serum (Syringe) Hepatitis (SH)

The following are the usual points quoted as differentiating the two forms of viral hepatitis:

1. Different viruses are known to be involved.

2. Serum hepatitis is transmitted by the introduction of contaminated blood or blood products into the patient's tissues and possibly to a small extent by the faecal oral route.

3. The incubation period of serum hepatitis is longer (6 weeks to 6 months) than that of infective hepatitis (2–6 weeks).

4. The onset of serum hepatitis may be more insidious.

5. The illness may be more serious, particularly as the condition may, because of its mode of transmission, affect patients who have already had a previous illness or operation. A mortality-rate of 10–20 per cent may be seen in the debilitated, particularly in those with cancer. Polyarteritis, glomerular nephritis, arthralgia, and urticaria are possible accompaniments and complications related to vascular damage by antigen–antibody complexes.

6. If serum hepatitis is diagnosed and blood or plasma infusions are at fault then it is vital to inform the blood transfusion service. Detection of Australia antigen now has a place in the discovery of 'carrier' blood donors. The incidence of serum hepatitis in this country is low (risk 1 : 1000 units of blood), whilst in the U.S.A. and Japan it is higher. The disease is common in dialysis units where perhaps because of altered immunological tolerance patients on dialysis programmes may harbour the virus without apparent ill effects though fatal hepatitis may result in other patients and nursing and medical staff.

The investigations of use in the diagnosis of infective hepatitis are:

1. A blood-count which shows a leucopenia.

2. The urine contains bile often before jaundice is apparent. At the height of jaundice urobilin may disappear from the urine. Its reappearance is a sign of recovery.

3. The liver function tests show a raised serum bilirubin value (except in anicteric cases), the flocculation tests, notably zinc sulphate turbidity, are positive at an early stage, and the serum proteins show an increase in the beta- and gamma-globulins. Serum albumin is normal in uncomplicated cases. The alkaline phosphatase may be raised but not usually to levels greater than 30 K.A. units. Liver cell enzymes such as transaminases, isocitric dehydrogenase, etc., appear in the serum in high concentration. S.G.P.T. may be elevated to 2000 units per ml.

4. Liver biopsy is unnecessary unless there is diagnostic difficulty and it may be dangerous.

5. HAA detection in serum (immunological or electron microscopy techniques) for virus B cases.

TREATMENT

All cases should be treated by rest in bed during the phase of maximal jaundice. Provided that the serum bilirubin is falling and the patient feels well enough he can be allowed to get up to use the toilet. An appetizing high-protein diet is provided, and it is customary, though of unproven value, to give a high-carbohydrate–low-fat intake as well. In fact, fat produces nausea in many patients so that a low fat diet is just common sense. In the initial phase fruit drinks with glucose are the only form of nutrition which may be acceptable. Most patients show a return to good health after 1–3 weeks' jaundice and can be sent for a holiday before return to work or school.

If the jaundice persists, corticosteroids hasten its disappearance. The reason for this effect is not fully known, though it is possible that bile-pigment precursors are disposed of through alternative metabolic pathways. The fall in the transaminases and return of serum proteins to normal suggest that there must be a beneficial effect on the liver cell. Prednisone, 20–40 mg. a day in divided doses, reducing after the serum bilirubin has started to fall to 10 mg. a day, is a reasonable dose. Corticosteroid drugs should be continued until jaundice has gone, and as they are tailed off a careful watch should be kept for signs of a relapse. Relapse seems more common in patients given corticosteroids than in those treated without and persistence of HAA may be a hazard in serum hepatitis.

Patients who have *obstructive hepatitis* are expected to respond to corticosteroid drugs and if the ACTH (or other corticosteroid) test is positive (*see Chapter 25*) they are so treated. An unnecessary laparotomy in a patient with obstructive hepatitis can precipitate liver failure.

Hepatic necrosis is often fatal. The usual therapeutic régime for hepatic coma is employed with administration of intravenous and intragastric glucose solution (20 per cent) with adequate potassium supplements, and protein exclusion, neomycin 1 g. 6-hourly, aperients, and corticosteroids. Although part of this treatment is aimed at preventing bacterial decomposition of protein in the gut, this is a relatively unimportant factor when there is gross liver cell failure. Bleeding manifestations must be treated with vitamin K and small fresh blood transfusions. Exchange blood transfusion has been used and results though occasionally dramatic have not resulted in a significant change in mortality. Demands on the blood-transfusion service are high particularly if exchanges involving 5 litres of blood are repeated several times. Pig liver perfusion has similarly not resulted in many permanent cures. Survival is unusual, but if it occurs because of the regeneration of liver cells, cirrhosis does not necessarily follow.

Prevention of Hepatitis

The importance of personal hygiene is obvious if the occurrence of fresh cases is to be prevented. The virus of infective hepatitis is found in the faeces of the patient during the active phase and the patient and nursing attendants must be very careful to wash their hands. Gamma-globulin has been shown to have a protective effect and can be administered in an epidemic to reduce the severity of the disease or to protect certain patients. Gamma-globulin should be given to a doctor or nurse who accidentally pricks his or her finger with a needle used to collect blood from a hepatitis patient. Dose required 0·06 ml. per kg. of a 16 per cent solution. A high titre antibody containing serum is available for serum hepatitis exposure cases.

Infectious Mononucleosis (Glandular Fever)

In this disorder involvement of the liver can occur. This may be clinically silent or there may be jaundice from liver cell dysfunction. The disease is characterized normally by pyrexia, pharyngitis, splenomegaly, generalized lymphadenopathy, and skin rashes. Jaundice is usually mild, but abnormal liver function tests include positive flocculation tests and raised gamma-globulin and transaminase levels. The serum alkaline phosphatase is usually abnormal, the rise occurring in anicteric cases or mildly jaundiced patients. The histological changes in the liver include infiltration in the portal tracts and sinusoids with many atypical mononuclear cells. Scattered foci of liver cell damage also occur.

DIAGNOSIS

This is based on the clinical picture, supported by the presence of abnormal mononuclear cells in the peripheral blood-film and a positive Paul-Bunnell reaction (heterophil antibody test), the titre not being altered by absorption with guinea-pig kidney. In patients with glandular fever and a negative Paul-Bunnell test the possibility of cytomegalovirus infection and toxoplasmosis must be remembered (*vide infra*).

TREATMENT

Treatment is symptomatic unless antibiotics are required for severe pharyngitis.

PROGNOSIS

The prognosis is excellent and the hepatic changes are never progressive.

Cytomegalovirus Hepatitis

Cytomegalovirus infection may be responsible for some examples of neonatal hepatitis and in adult life (apart from Paul-Bunnell negative glandular fever) hepatitis may result. Jaundice may be prolonged and is often associated with evidence of both liver cell disease and cholestasis. Patients who have had massive blood transfusion—open-heart surgery—or who have malignant disease or who are on immunosuppressive drugs are particularly at risk. Diagnosis is aided by detection of urinary excretion of the virus and evidence of a rising antibody titre against the virus.

2. SPIROCHAETAL DISEASES

Weil's Disease (Leptospirosis) (*Fig. 32*)

AETIOLOGY

This disease is caused by a spirochaete (*Leptospira icterohaemorrhagiae*), but other leptospirae which are pathogenic to man may also cause jaundice, though less often. Rats are the reservoir of infection, excreting the organisms in their urine. Contact with material or water contaminated by this

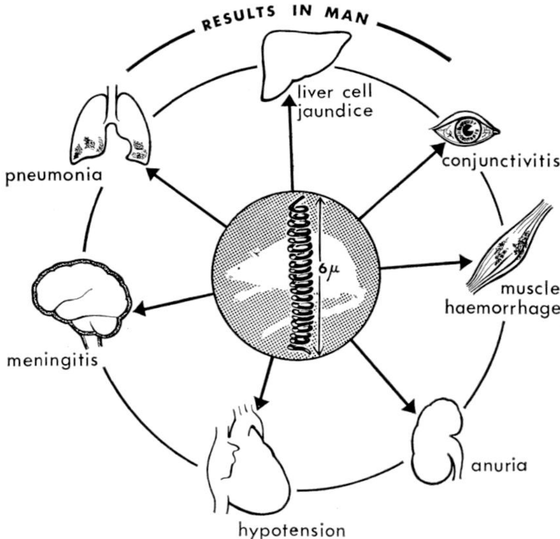

Fig. 32. Weil's disease.

accounts for the special disease-risk noted in farm workers, sewage men, fish cleaners, and knackers. The disease may also be contracted while bathing in stagnant pools, the leptospira penetrating the skin through minute abrasions. *L. canicola,* an organism which causes a severe illness in its vector—the dog—is also capable of infecting humans.

PATHOLOGY

The liver shows rather minimal evidence of liver cell damage with active regeneration in areas of scattered necrosis. There is an accompanying portal cell infiltration of mononuclear cells. The kidneys are swollen and show degenerative changes in the tubules with interstitial inflammatory changes. Histological changes in the muscles are necrosis of muscle-fibres and small blood-vessels. Petechial haemorrhages occur in the meninges where there is a meningeal reaction.

CLINICAL PICTURE

The disease is of sudden onset after an incubation period of 7–13 days. The initial symptoms are due to the presence of the spirochaete in the blood-stream. Fever, severe aching pains in the back and limb muscles, toxaemia with headache, and signs of meningeal irritation occur. Conjunctivitis is almost invariable and herpes labialis is often haemorrhagic. Other haemorrhagic skin lesions may occur.

After a few days signs of liver and kidney involvement occur, the former indicated by jaundice, hepatic tenderness and enlargement, and the latter by albuminuria, oliguria, and nitrogen retention.

Accompaniments and Complications

Meningeal irritation occurs in most patients and lumbar puncture may show an increased number of cells and raised protein in the cerebrospinal fluid which can be icteric.

Most severe cases have some renal damage and this may progress to oliguric failure because of tubular necrosis. It is the combination of icterus, hypotension, and spirochaetal infection of the kidney which causes this serious complication.

Cardiovascular complications are hypotension, tachycardia, arrhythmias, and electrocardiograph abnormalities. Patchy pneumonia and bronchial infection also occur in ill patients.

DIAGNOSIS

The history of occupational risk is important. Other helpful tests are:

1. The blood-count may show a high white count and a polymorph leucocytosis (cf. leucopenia of viral hepatitis).

2. A lumbar puncture will confirm meningeal involvement.

3. The urine volume is reduced, and the urine contains protein and casts. The blood-urea may be raised.

4. The liver function tests show raised serum bilirubin and transaminases, and the flocculation tests may be positive.

5. Leptospirae may be found by dark ground illumination of the blood during the first week and in the urine later. Guinea-pigs inoculated with infected material develop characteristic lesions from which spirochaetes may be isolated.

6. Serology. A rising titre of specific serum agglutinins is significant.

The *differential diagnosis* includes acute viral hepatitis and drug jaundice, but the occupational history, the polymorph leucocytosis, and the renal, meningeal, and ocular involvement are useful pointers to the diagnosis.

TREATMENT

There is no general agreement as to the best therapy, but in view of the severity of the illness it is usual to administer very large doses of penicillin or broad-spectrum antibiotics. Not all patients respond, however. Immune serum can also be used.

In practice, penicillin 10 mega units daily is given as soon as the clinical diagnosis is made and the patient is watched for the onset of oliguric renal failure, which if it develops is treated by a low protein and fluid intake, exchange resins to prevent hyperkalaemia (important in view of the degree of muscle and tissue necrosis), and a high glucose intake. The prognosis varies and in most series the mortality approximates 15 per cent.

Canicola Fever

L. canicola may cause a similar illness, but one that is milder and has a lower incidence of renal and hepatic involvement, so that jaundice only occurs in a fifth of the cases.

Relapsing Fever

This is only seen in tropical and subtropical regions. It is caused by spirochaetes of the species *Borrelia recurrentis* and can be louse- or tick-borne. The illness is severe, with high pyrexia, prostration, muscle pain, and hepatosplenomegaly. Jaundice is unusual except in severe cases. Relapses occur after apparent clinical improvement and hypotensive bouts are also seen. The spirochaete is found in the blood during the acute febrile phase and penicillin is effective.

3. PROTOZOAL INFECTIONS

Entamoeba Histolytica

AETIOLOGY

The incidence of hepatic involvement in amoebic dysentery is variable. The organism gains entrance to the liver by the portal vein from the infected large bowel. The disease is common in tropical countries, but it should be borne in mind as a diagnostic possibility in patients who have been abroad, even many years before, to places where the disease is prevalent. The causative organism exists as a free-living (trophozoite) and as a cystic form (*Fig. 33*). The latter is able to resist adverse environmental conditions and cystic forms have been found in the stools of healthy people in this country. The circumstances which render harmless cystic forms pathogenic are unknown.

PATHOLOGY

The colon may show evidence of surface ulceration. The liver is enlarged, and owing to the ability of the entamoeba to digest hepatic tissue the liver may contain one or occasionally more abscess cavities, usually in the right lobe. The cavity contains thin pink 'anchovy sauce pus' which is sterile on culture. The wall of the cavity consists of normal hepatic tissue in which amoebae can be found. If secondary infection of the cavity occurs, bacterial culture will be positive because of this factor. A true 'hepatitis' without breakdown of liver tissue may occur and this can be arrested by treatment.

CLINICAL PICTURE

The clinical picture may be complicated by the presence of diarrhoea due to amoebic dysentery. Hepatic disease may occur without bowel symptoms and consists usually of upper abdominal pain, pyrexia with rigors, and weakness. On examination at this time the patient is ill and sweating profusely, the liver is enlarged and tender. Swelling of the soft tissue over the right lobe of the liver may be present and it is common to find signs at the right lung base (impaired percussion note and air entry) due to either

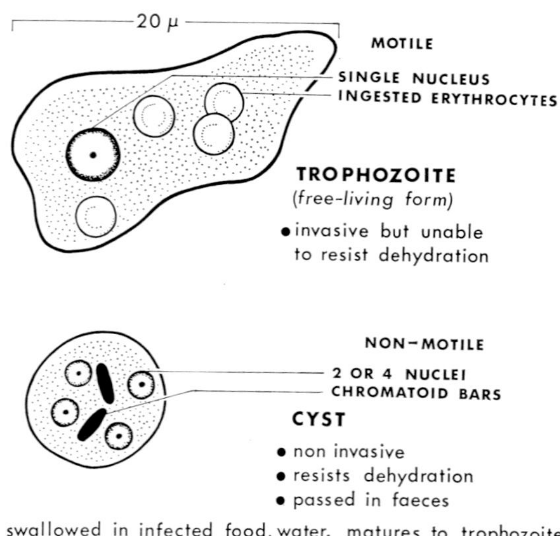

Fig. 33. Amoebiasis.

pulmonary collapse or effusion. The pulmonary collapse is due to enlargement of the right lobe of the liver up into the thoracic cavity. Slight jaundice may occur. In patients without abscess formation the liver may not be much enlarged but it is tender, and 'springing' the right lower ribs causes pain.

Accompaniments and Complications

Patients with hepatic abscess are usually very ill, feverish, and anaemic. *Rupture of an abscess cavity* into the pleural cavity and lung is a serious complication. Rupture into the peritoneal cavity and pericardium is less common, but involvement of the abdominal wall may occur. Investigations show:
1. Anaemia.
2. The white blood-count is raised with a polymorph leucocytosis.

3. Liver function tests may show a slightly raised serum bilirubin and in some patients a raised serum alkaline phosphatase. The serum transaminases are also elevated, but unless the illness becomes chronic the total serum proteins and the flocculation tests are usually normal.

4. Identification is considerably facilitated by isotope scanning of the liver. The abscess cavity appears as a filling defect because of the failure of the destroyed reticulo-endothelial tissue to take up technetium. It may not be possible to decide whether a lesion is an abscess or a tumour without aspiration. Ultrasonic scanning is of particular help in the presence of a fluid (pus)-containing cavity.

5. *Aspiration* of the liver via the intercostal route, if the right lobe is involved, may demonstrate the presence of characteristic pus which is sterile on culture. Biopsy of the abscess wall after aspiration may show the presence of amoebae, but their demonstration in the pus is infrequent. In all cases, whether there is diarrhoea or not, sigmoidoscopy must be performed to look for ulceration in the rectum and colon and to send scrapings and fresh faeces for microscopical examination.

6. A chest radiograph is useful as it shows hepatic enlargement with elevation of the right leaf of the diaphragm, and may show a pleural reaction due to an abscess in the liver or subphrenic space.

TREATMENT

Full amoebicidal therapy is needed and treatment is directed to disease of the colon as well as the liver. Chloroquine (Aralen) is non-toxic, highly active against the amoeba, and is specifically concentrated in the hepatic parenchyma. Oral administration of 1 g. in divided doses (250 mg. 6-hourly) for 2 days, reducing to 250 mg. three times a day, after a few days, brings about an improvement with lowering of the temperature. Emetine hydrochloride 65 mg. by intramuscular injection can accompany this, but not more than 10 daily doses are given because of the risk of damage to the myocardium. Patients on emetine are best kept in bed and the electrocardiograph studied serially.

The alimentary infection is treated with a course of emetine bismuth iodine (E.B.I.) 200 mg. daily for 10 days and with a broad-spectrum antibiotic, e.g., terramycin, tetracycline, or erythromycin. Iodine-containing compounds such as Chiniofon and Diodoquin are nowadays little used, but bismuth glycolylarsanilate (Milibis) is a useful adjunct for treatment of the intestinal disease. Very good results have been obtained with metronidazole (Flagyl). It is active against amoebae in the liver as well as in the bowel and is used in a dosage of 800 mg. three times daily for 10 days. It is also virtually free of side-effects.

Aspiration is indicated when there is good evidence of abscess formation, or if the pyrexia fails to settle with anti-amoebic therapy. When this is done, great care must be taken to ensure a sterile technique. Secondary infection is a serious occurrence in an amoebic abscess cavity. Open operation is usually avoided unless secondary infection or rupture of the abscess has occurred.

4. BACTERIAL INFECTIONS

Routes of Infection

There are four ways in which bacteria can reach the liver:

Route	Possible effects
1. Via the biliary tract	Cholangitis and liver abscess
2. Via the portal vein	Portal pyaemia and multiple abscesses
3. Via a penetrating wound	Liver abscess
4. Via the hepatic artery in septicaemia	Hepatic necrosis; liver abscesses

AETIOLOGY

Obstruction to the outflow of bile as, for example, from a stricture in the common duct, leads to 'ascending' infection of the bile-ducts in the liver. Recently it has been shown that infection does not always 'ascend' the biliary tree but results in many cases from reactivation of a focus of infection in a damaged gall-bladder. In support of this concept 'ascending' cholangitis in patients with neoplastic biliary obstruction is unusual. The ducts are distended with bile-stained pus, and destruction of surrounding liver tissue results in the formation of multiple liver abscesses. Microscopically, there is polymorph infiltration of the bile-ductules in the portal tracts and features of obstructive jaundice.

Multiple abscesses may also arise from infection disseminated by the portal vein from a suppurating appendix, gall-bladder, or, in the neonatal period, from ascending umbilical infection. The pathology is essentially similar to that complicating cholangitis, but the lesion is maximal in the portal venous radicles and is not based on biliary obstruction.

Solitary liver abscess may complicate a penetrating hepatic injury and multiple small abscesses may be found in septicaemias. The common infecting organism in cholangitis and portal pyaemia is *Escherichia coli*.

CLINICAL PICTURE
(See Chapter 15 on Gall-bladder Disease)

The features of cholangitis are described elsewhere. In portal pyaemia the symptoms and signs depend on the initial cause and may be modified by the presence and nature of the causative lesion. The patient is toxic and pyrexial, often having rigors. The liver is usually enlarged and tender and there may be mild jaundice. Deeper jaundice is suggestive of cholangitis rather than portal pyaemia. An abscess in the left lobe may present as an epigastric tumour. A syndrome of chronic portal bacteriaemia has been described in patients with ulcerative colitis in which pyrexia and recurrent bouts of mild jaundice may occur. A solitary liver abscess may cause similar symptoms, but profound malaise with only slight fever and jaundice may be the only clinical signs.

Accompaniments and Complications

Septic thrombosis of the portal venous system may result in portal hypertension with the gradual development of a collateral circulation and bleeding from oesophageal varices. A solitary abscess may rupture into the peritoneal cavity, biliary tract, or subphrenic space.

DIAGNOSIS

In the diagnosis of hepatic sepsis the following tests may be of value:

1. A blood-count will show a polymorph leucocytosis.

2. The liver function tests may show a slightly raised serum bilirubin, raised transaminases, and elevation of the alkaline phosphatase, for the latter is raised in any 'space-occupying lesion' of the liver. Serum vitamin B_{12} levels may be raised due to release of stored protein-bound vitamin B_{12} into the blood.

3. Radiographic examination may confirm the hepatomegaly and show involvement of the subphrenic space (raised immobile diaphragm and pleural reaction). In the detection of deep-seated abscesses tomography may be helpful.

4. Aspiration is indicated if a hepatic abscess is suspected and, using a sterile technique, material is sent for culture and sensitivity studies.

5. The technique of hepatic scintillography, using radioactive technetium or rose bengal, may detect the presence of an abscess, the abscess area failing to take up the labelled material. Similarly, ultrasonic scanning of the liver may confirm one or more filling defects which can be shown to be cystic rather than solid because of their failure to transmit an ultrasonic signal. A recent test which may be helpful consists of the detection in some patients of increased urinary indoxyl sulphate in the urine and impaired vitamin B_{12} absorption. This is because of secondary bacterial colonization of the proximal small bowel from the infected biliary tree.

The other disorders which must be considered when pyrexia and enlargement of the liver occur are amoebic abscess of the liver and primary or secondary neoplasm.

TREATMENT

This must be directed to the primary lesion if one exists. Otherwise, treatment seeks to control the hepatic sepsis. This can be achieved sometimes by aspiration and the use of the appropriate antibiotics. As *Escherichia coli* is commonly the infecting organism tetracycline, chloramphenicol, ampicillin, and kanamycin should be amongst the antibiotics used if no pus can be obtained for diagnostic purposes. If patients fail to respond quickly to aspiration and antibiotics, surgical exposure and drainage may be required. Involvement of the subphrenic space is a further indication for surgical intervention under full antibiotic cover.

B. ACUTE REACTIONS DUE TO DRUGS AND POISONS

In general, drugs and hepatic poisons produce one of two hepatic lesions. These are: (1) Cholestasis. (2) Liver cell injury. (*See Table 15.*) Sometimes the reaction to one drug may be of either variety, e.g., PAS and phenindione.

DRUGS PRODUCING CHOLESTASIS

One group of drugs, such as chlorpromazine (Largactil), arsphenamine, chlorpropamide, etc., produces acute cholestasis in a few patients who are hypersensitive to them. A much larger percentage of patients, when given drugs of the second group, such as methyl testosterone and norethandrolone (Nilevar), develop a milder but similar obstructive lesion which is probably not related to hypersensitivity but is perhaps due to enzyme inhibition in the liver. With prolonged therapy deep jaundice can occur.

In the first group there is often a history similar to that of acute viral hepatitis, the initial illness starting with anorexia, vomiting, and upper abdominal pain followed by jaundice. The jaundice differs from that of ordinary hepatitis in that it is obstructive and accompanied by pruritus, though there may be evidence of accompanying liver cell dysfunction as well. The allergic basis of this type of drug reaction is suggested by the presence of eosinophilia, both in the blood and in the portal cellular infiltrate found in biopsy specimens. Occasionally this type of lesion may be severe and may persist for several months or even years, causing emaciation, and the usual features of chronic obstructive jaundice such as pruritus, skin pigmentation, haemorrhagic manifestations, steatorrhoea, bone thinning, and xanthomata.

The second group of drugs usually causes only mild jaundice, and the alkaline phosphatase may be elevated without icterus. It should be noted that two of the drugs in this group, methyl testosterone and norethandrolone, have been used to relieve the pruritus of chronic obstructive jaundice and although they are effective in doing this, they may also deepen the jaundice. It is probable that some biochemical factor is responsible both for the production of icterus and the relief of pruritus. Both groups cause obstruction to the intrahepatic biliary canaliculi, but the basic pathology is unknown. There is no portal cell infiltrate on obstructive jaundice caused by the second group of drugs.

DRUGS AND POISONS PRODUCING LIVER CELL DAMAGE

There are many drugs and chemicals which can injure liver cells (*Table 15*). With some drugs there is a hypersensitivity factor perhaps best seen with monoamine oxidase inhibitors (Marsilid, etc.), so that the magnitude of the damage is not related to the dose. Notably with industrial poisons there is no allergic factor and damage may be proportional to dosage. The toxicity of alcohol can increase the amount of damage produced by other poisons, and there is often evidence of damage to other organs such as the kidneys.

1. *Example of Drug-induced Liver Cell Jaundice—Mono-amine Oxidase Inhibitors*

The patient may have an illness indistinguishable from infective hepatitis with upper alimentary symptoms followed by jaundice of the liver cell variety. There are only two differences from viral hepatitis. The pyrexia which is usual in hepatitis rarely occurs, and more important still, the prognosis is poor, the mortality being in some series as much as 20 per cent. During an epidemic of hepatitis it may be impossible to distinguish one from the other and because the histology is so similar liver biopsy does not help. Detection of Australia antigen HAA will obviously be helpful in making this distinction in some patients where infection is with virus B. Death is due to hepatic necrosis.

Table 15. HEPATIC LESIONS DUE TO DRUGS AND POISONS

1. Cholestasis
    Chlorpromazine (promazine, etc.)
    Thiouracil
    Methyl testosterone
    Norethandrolone
    Arsphenamine
    PAS
    Chlorpropamide, etc.
    The contraceptive pill

2. Liver Cell
    a. *Drugs*
    Monoamine oxidase inhibitors—phenelzine = Nardil
    Cinchophen
    Sulphonamides
    Butazolidine
    Halothane
    Tridione
    Avertin   { A recent important addition to this list is Paracetamol in massive (suicidal) doses.
    Phenindione
    INAH
    Tetracycline
    Stilbamidine
    Aminopterin, etc.

    b. *Poisons*
    Alcohol
    Carbon tetrachloride and other chlorinated hydrocarbons
    Naphthalene
    Benzene and derivatives, TNT, etc.
    Phosphorus
    DDT
    Certain fungi

2. Example of 'Poison'-induced Liver Cell Jaundice—Carbon Tetrachloride

This is usually seen as a result of carbon tetrachloride fumes being inhaled in a poorly ventilated room. (It is used as a grease solvent in dry-cleaning and in fire extinguishers.) Its toxicity is enhanced by the previous taking of alcohol. The symptoms, which begin a few hours after exposure or immediately if taken orally, are nausea, vomiting, abdominal pain, and, in severe cases, collapse. Evidence of hepatic damage (rapidly deepening jaundice and hepatomegaly) is seen within two days and renal involvement (albuminuria progressing in severe cases to oliguria) occurs a little later. The damaging effects of carbon tetrachloride are sometimes predominantly either hepatic or renal, but usually there is clinical evidence of damage to both organs. In severe cases terminal anuria, pulmonary oedema, and hypotension occur, but in mild cases the patient improves after an illness lasting seven to ten days, though jaundice may persist for three or four weeks. Cirrhosis is a rare but documented possibility following the acute injury.

In the acute phase there is histologically some diffuse fatty degeneration of liver cells with centrilobular necrosis. (*Note*: diffuse fatty change is rare in hepatitis.) In severe cases necrotic changes are seen in the renal tubules. It seems likely that carbon tetrachloride is an indirect rather than a direct hepatic toxin. A metabolic product rather than the carbon tetrachloride itself induces damage to the endoplasmic reticulum with resultant fatty infiltration due to cessation of lipoprotein synthesis. In fact experimentally in the rat the encouragement of carbon tetrachloride metabolism by phenobarbitone administration (enzyme induction) produces a higher incidence of liver damage (and cirrhosis) than carbon tetrachloride alone.

The treatment of liver cell damage due to drugs is mainly supportive, ample glucose being given by gastric tube or intravenously. Corticosteroids may be given if there is hepatic necrosis, and if hypotension and oliguria occur the electrolyte balance and fluid intake must be watched carefully. The usual treatment for hepatic coma may be required.

It cannot be overstressed that as the numbers of new drugs and chemicals increase, so will the incidence of liver disease due to them. An accurate history from the patient, his relatives, his doctor, and his pharmacist becomes vital.

The outlook is favourable when jaundice is mild and evidence of renal impairment minimal, but death from uraemia may occur in severe cases and cirrhosis is a long-term possibility in patients who recover from the acute phase.

FURTHER READING

ACUTE LIVER DISEASE
Australia Antigen
SHULMAN, N. R. (1970), 'Hepatitis Associated Antigen', *Am. J. Med.*, **49**, 669.
Viral Hepatitis
BLUM, A. L., STUTZ, R., HAMMERLI, V. P., SCHMID, P., and GRADY, F. (1969), 'A Fortuitously Controlled Study of Steroid Therapy in Acute Viral Hepatitis', *Ibid.*, **47**, 82 and 93.
HAVENS, W. P. (1962), 'Viral Hepatitis. Clinical Patterns and Diagnosis', *Ibid.*, **32**, 665.
KRUGMAN, S., GILES, J. P., and HAMMOND, J. (1967), 'Evidence for two Distinctive Clinical, Epidemiological and Immunological Types of Infection', *J. Am. Med. Ass.*, **200**, 365.
STOKES, J. (1962), 'The Control of Viral Hepatitis', *Am. J. Med.*, **32**, 729.
Obstructive Hepatitis
DUBIN, I. N., SULLIVAN, B. H., LE GOLVAN, P. C., and MURPHY, L. C. (1960), 'The Cholestatic Form of Viral Hepatitis', *Ibid.*, **29**, 55.
Treatment of Acute Hepatic Failure
JONES, E. A., CLAIN, D., MACGILLIVRAY, M., and SHERLOCK, S. (1967), 'Hepatic Coma due to Acute Hepatic Necrosis treated by Exchange Blood Transfusion', *Lancet*, **2**, 169.
PARBHOO, S. P., KENNEDY, J., JAMES, I. M., CHALSTREY, L. J., AJDUKIEWICZ, A., BROCK, P. J., XANALTOS, C., SAYER, P., and SHERLOCK, S. (1971), 'Extracorporeal Pig-liver Perfusion in Treatment of Hepatic Coma due to Fulminant Hepatitis', *Ibid.*, **1**, 659.
Hepatic Necrosis
LUCKE, B., and MALLORY, T. (1946), 'The Fulminant Form of Epidemic Hepatitis', *Am. J. Path.*, **22**, 867.
TREY, C., LIPWORTH, L., CHALMERS, T. C., DAVIDSON, C. S., GOTTLIEB, L. S., POPPER, H., and SAUNDERS, S. J. (1968), 'Fulminant Hepatic Failure', *New Engl. J. Med.*, **279**, 798.

Infectious Mononucleosis
NELSON, R. S., and DARRAGH, J. H. (1956), 'Infectious Mononucleosis Hepatitis', *Am. J. Med.*, **21**, 26.

Amoebic Hepatitis
LAMONT, N. MCE., and POOLER, N. R. (1958), 'Hepatic Amoebiasis: a Study of 250 Cases', *Q. Jl Med.*, **51**, 389.
WILMOT, A. J. (1962), *Clinical Amoebiasis*. Oxford: Blackwell.

Weil's Disease
DAVIDSON, L. S. P., and SMITH, J. (1936), 'Weil's Disease in Fish Workers', *Q. Jl Med.*, **29**, 263.

DRUGS AND THE LIVER

Cholestasis
GUTMAN, A. B. (1957), 'Drug Reactions characterized by Cholestasis associated with Intrahepatic Biliary Tract Obstruction', *Am. J. Med.*, **23**, 841.
SCHAFFNER, F., and POPPER, H. (1959), 'Morphologic Studies of Cholestasis', *Gastroenterology*, **37**, 565.
———— and CHESROW, E. (1959), 'Cholestasis produced by the Administration of Norethandrolone', *Am. J. Med.*, **26**, 249.

Chronic Chlorpromazine Jaundice
READ, A. E., HARRISON, C. V., and SHERLOCK, S. (1961), 'Chronic Chlorpromazine Jaundice: with Particular Reference to its Relationship to Primary Biliary Cirrhosis', *Ibid.*, **31**, 249.

Drug Jaundice
HOLDSWORTH, C. D., ATKINSON, M., and GOLDIE, W. (1961), 'Hepatitis caused by the Newer Amine Oxidase-inhibiting Drugs', *Lancet*, **2**, 621.
LEADING ARTICLE (1962), 'Hepato-toxicity of Drugs', *Ibid.*, **1**, 1056.
MELROSE, A. G. (1960), 'Drug-induced Jaundice', *Scott. Med. J.*, **5**, 250.
READ, A. E. (1965), 'Drugs and Liver Disease', *Anaesthesia*, **20**, 19.

Halothane Hepatitis
REMMER, H. (1970), 'The Role of the Liver in Drug Metabolism', *Am. J. Med.*, **49**, 617.
SHERLOCK, S. (1971), 'Progress Report Halothane Hepatitis', *Gut*, **12**, 324.

Transplantation
STARYL, T. E., BRETTSCHNEIDER, L., and PUTNAM, C. W. (1970), in *Progress in Liver Diseases* (ed. POPPER, H., and SCHAFFNER, F.), London: Heinemann.

Chapter 11

Chronic Liver Disease

(CHRONIC INFECTIONS; PARASITIC DISEASES; NEOPLASIA)

CHRONIC INFECTIONS

THE IMPORTANT chronic infections of the liver are:
1. Viral hepatitis.
2. Tuberculosis.
3. Brucellosis.
4. Actinomycosis.
5. Hepatic granulomata.

1. Viral Hepatitis

It is possible that the persistence of the viruses responsible for infective and serum hepatitis is the factor which, on rare occasions, leads to chronic liver damage and cirrhosis. Some patients with chronic liver disease have HAA in the blood. Those showing this reaction are, at least in this country, only a small percentage of the total group of cirrhotic patients. Obviously there are considerable differences in the geographical incidence of liver disease associated with HAA, but it is possible that continuing liver damage and even hepatoma could result from such chronic infection.

2. Tuberculosis

The liver is involved in miliary tuberculosis, and granulomatous hepatic lesions can be found by liver biopsy in about 25 per cent of other tuberculous patients. Usually this hepatic lesion, though useful as a means of diagnosis, is merely an incident of haematogenous spread, but, rarely pyrexia, jaundice, and hepatomegaly occur with more massive hepatic involvement.

3. Brucellosis

Granulomatous lesions in the liver are a recognized feature of brucellosis, and some authors feel that occasionally it causes cirrhosis.

4. Actinomycosis

Actinomycosis may spread to the liver from an ileocaecal lesion. The liver may become a honeycomb of abscess cavities separated by fibrous tissue. and sinuses may discharge on to the skin. Examination of the discharge from a sinus may reveal the typical 'sulphur granules' which show under the microscope a branching filamentous structure with clubbed ends. The patient, who is usually very ill, often has evidence of skin involvement over the liver, the chest wall, or the caecal area. Treatment is with massive doses (10 mega units a day) of penicillin.

5. Hepatic Granulomata

A granulomatous lesion in the liver consists of a collection of epithelioid and giant cells surrounded by lymphocytes. The lesions are clearly demarcated from the surrounding liver substance. The presence of hepatic granulomata in a biopsy specimen may indicate one of the following conditions: tuberculosis, sarcoidosis, brucellosis, berylliosis, ascariasis, infectious mononucleosis, *Toxocara canis* infestation, etc. Dogs and cats throughout the world are infested with roundworm. *T. canis* and *T. cati* and ingestion of larvae excreted in the animals' faeces may result in widespread visceral involvement. Larvae form granulomata in various tissues and may be found in liver biopsy material. Certain drugs, e.g., allopurinol, may cause granulomata. If widely disseminated within the liver, granulomata may cause elevation of the serum alkaline phosphatase. Granulomatous lesions of sarcoid may be extensive enough to cause portal hypertension and a syndrome closely resembling primary biliary cirrhosis (*see* p. 190). All hepatic granulomata are structurally similar whatever their cause, and it is only the recognition of tubercle bacilli within the lesions, in the case of tuberculosis, or the results of general clinical and laboratory studies, in the case of other diseases, which can determine the diagnosis.

PARASITIC DISEASES

The following are the important chronic infestations which occur in the liver. Amoebic hepatitis is considered separately (*see* Chapter 10, Acute Diseases of the Liver).

Nematodes (roundworms)	*Ascaris lumbricoides*
Trematodes (liver flukes)	*Clonorchis sinensis. Fasciola hepatica. Schistosoma (S. japonicum, S. mansoni, S. haematobium)*
Cestodes (tape-worms)	*Echinococcus granulosus* (hydatid disease) *Toxocara*

Ascaris Lumbricoides

Involvement of the liver is usually secondary to biliary obstruction. This in turn is associated with the presence of one or many adult worms in the bile-ducts. It is a cause of biliary colic, jaundice, and eosinophilia in areas where infestation is common. Piperazine citrate (Antepar) given by mouth in a dosage of 150 mg. per kg. is effective treatment though the dosage may have to be repeated 1 week later.

Clonorchis Sinensis

This condition is widespread in the Far East. The worm develops from cysts found in uncooked fish. The adult fluke causes irritation of the bile-ducts with adenomatous changes and thickening of the walls. It is the tendency to secondary bacterial infection which probably accounts for the jaundice and cholangitis which may occur.

Neoplastic change in the bile-ducts may follow chronic infestation. Biliary cirrhosis is rare but it may follow secondary infection which in turn may kill the flukes. Eosinophilia accompanying jaundice should make one think of a drug reaction or liver-fluke infestation.

Fasciola Hepatica (Sheep Liver Fluke)

Interest in this condition occurring in man has been recently revived with reports of cases in this country. The infection is acquired by eating contaminated watercress and the fluke enters the liver by penetration of the duodenum. The intermediate host is a fresh-water snail. Jaundice, fever, urticaria (with dermatographism), and right upper abdominal pain are the main symptoms. Eosinophilia is usually found, and the faeces may contain ova after infestation has been present for two or three months. Chloroquine seems to be effective therapy. Malignant change in the bile-ducts, secondary infection, and biliary cirrhosis are possible complications in chronic cases. The most recent epidemic in this country (1970) was reported from Gloucestershire.

Schistosoma

Schistosomiasis (*Fig. 34*), which is endemic in Africa, Asia, and South America, is acquired by contact with infested water. Cercariae penetrate the skin and so enter the lymphatic and blood-streams by which they reach the portal venous system. The adult worms develop here and eggs are laid in the vesical, mesenteric, and intestinal veins. Ova not extruded

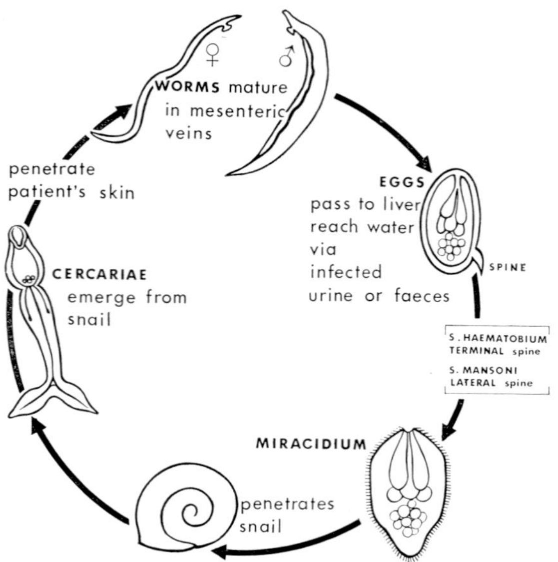

Fig. 34. Schistosomiasis.

into the bowel or bladder are swept back into the liver. A variable histo-logical picture is produced by the ova in the liver. A fibrous tissue reaction results in presinusoidal portal hypertension (pipe-stem fibrosis), and this in turn causes splenomegaly and oesophageal varices. There is a difference of opinion as to whether the portal hypertension is due to the schistoso-miasis and the immunological reaction to it, or on rare occasions to a complicating cirrhosis. An initial urticarial rash, followed several weeks later by diarrhoea with blood in the stools and eosinophilia, may be found. The urinary form (*S. haematobium*) does not usually affect the liver. Symptoms of lung involvement and, later, right-sided heart failure also occur, caused by a fibrotic lesion around ova in the lungs. Diagnosis of intestinal schistosomiasis is confirmed by sigmoidoscopy which reveals ulceration and inflammation of the rectal mucosa. Ova with a lateral spine can be demonstrated in a rectal 'snip' or in the faeces. Snips of rectal mucosa are best examined pressed out between two microscope slides. With liver involvement ova may be found on liver biopsy and tests of liver function may be abnormal. Oriental schistosomiasis, *S. japonicum*, pro-duces a similar but more intense inflammatory lesion in the gut and is diagnosed in a similar way.

Treatment for active infestation is with sodium or potassium antimony tartrate, given intravenously slowly and carefully. Dosage increases from 40 to 120 mg. on alternate days, a total of 2 g. being given in a course. Toxic reactions are common with circulatory collapse, neuritis, vomiting, and epigastric and chest discomfort. For this reason there is a tendency to avoid the use of sodium or potassium antimony tartrate in favour of niridazole (Ambilhar). This drug is given orally (dose 25 mg. per kg. body-weight daily in divided doses) for 7–10 days. The drug is effective in urinary and intestinal disease and apart from mild neuropsychiatric disturbances usually without side-effects.

Echinococcus Granulosus (Hydatid Disease)

AETIOLOGY AND PATHOLOGY
(*Fig. 35*)

The cystic stage of the dog tape-worm is sometimes found in man. Dogs become infested by eating sheep viscera which contain hydatid cysts. Contact with dogs can lead to swallowing of ova which adhere to the dogs' coats, or from consumption of vegetables contaminated with dogs' faeces. After the chitinous envelope has been dissolved by gastric juice, ova burrow through the intestinal wall into the liver; an adult cyst or cysts results. This consists of an outer fibrous coat derived from the liver and an intermediate coat lined by an inner germinal epithelium. The germinal epithelium gives rise to brood capsules containing scolices which form embryo adult worms. The right lobe of the liver is usually affected. The disease is sporadic in sheep-raising areas of England but is less rare in Wales.

8

CLINICAL PICTURE

Unless there are complications the only sign is a rounded abdominal swelling which moves with the liver on respiration. This may be obviously cystic and there may be a fluid thrill.

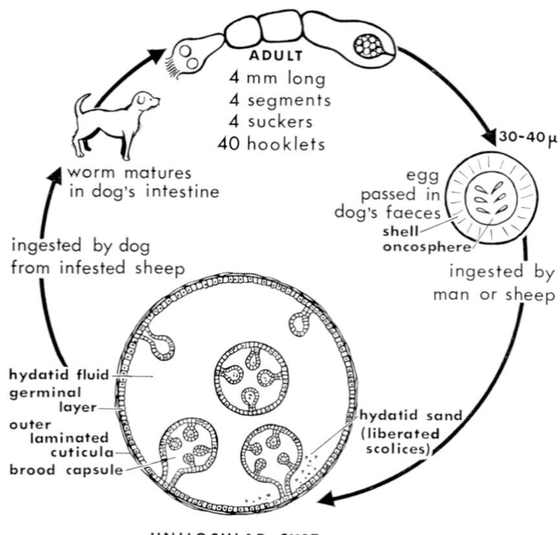

Fig. 35. Echinococcus granulosus.

ACCOMPANIMENTS AND COMPLICATIONS

1. *Rupture,* usually into the peritoneal, intestinal, biliary, or pleural cavities, may occur at any time.

2. *Allergic* phenomena, including urticaria or severe anaphylactic shock due to hypersensitivity to cyst protein, may follow rupture of the cyst.

3. *Secondary infection* from the biliary tract into which the cyst ruptures.

Cysts, sometimes multiple, in the lungs, kidney, spleen, brain, etc., may accompany the hepatic lesion.

DIAGNOSIS

Diagnosis is aided first by having a high index of suspicion concerning cystic swellings in the liver and by the use of the following tests:

1. A radiograph may show calcification in the cyst wall and tomography may show cavitation.

2. A blood-count may show eosinophilia.

3. The Casoni intradermal test (using sterile hydatid fluid) may show a positive immediate response followed by induration of the injected area after twelve hours. A complement-fixation test may also be positive.

TREATMENT

Surgical treatment of hydatid cyst in the liver is necessary because of the risk of rupture, and to avoid this during laparotomy great care is necessary, while the injection of 2 per cent formalin into the cyst before handling it is an important precaution. Rupture may cause multiple recurrent cysts in the peritoneal cavity.

NEOPLASIA

Tumours of the liver may be benign or malignant, primary or secondary.

PRIMARY TUMOURS OF THE LIVER

1. *Simple.* Adenoma. Fibroma. Haemangioma.
2. *Malignant.* Haemangio-endothelioma. Hepatoma (liver cell). Cholangioma (bile-duct cell).

Simple tumours of the liver are of little importance as they rarely grow to any size. They are usually an incidental surgical finding, but sometimes a haemangioma may reach massive proportions.

Primary Malignant Tumours

Of the three primary malignant liver tumours the haemangio-endothelioma is the rarest. It is a primitive and highly malignant tumour of endothelial cells which develop into blood-filled spaces. It usually occurs in children and young adults.

Primary hepatic cancer is usually a hepatoma, a tumour derived from liver cells or a cholangioma derived from bile-duct cells. Sometimes the growth shows both elements histologically. As there is little clinical difference between these types they will not be separately described.

AETIOLOGY

Two important facts are known about the aetiology of hepatic cancer. First, there is a strong association between cirrhosis and hepatoma, and secondly, there is a marked geographical variation in the percentage of livers, both normal and cirrhotic, which develop cancerous change. Incidence is particularly high in the South African Bantu, the Malay, and the Chinese. Reasons for this difference are probably many, but dietary factors may be of importance. Experimentally an extract of the mould *Aspergillus flavus* called Aflatoxin can produce hepatic tumours in rodents, poultry, and trout. The effect seems to be due to a direct interference of this substance with cellular protein synthesis. The mould is commonly found on cereal crops which are being stored and it seems possible that this together with changes in cellular activity in the liver associated with malnutrition could explain the high incidence of hepatoma in some parts of the world such as the Far East and tropical Africa. The relationship with cirrhosis is more easily understood because of the proliferative activity in the damaged liver. The formation of regeneration nodules may lead to autonomous growth resulting in a cancer. Any type of cirrhosis may be complicated in this way, but it is perhaps commonest in the macronodular type and in that complicating haemochromatosis. The association of a hepatoma with cirrhosis and a positive serum reaction for HAA is also being reported from overseas, a further indication of the possible importance of preceding infection with viral hepatitis.

It should be remembered, too, that patients who received thorium as an angiographic contrast material in the early days of this form of radiology also run a risk of tumour formation in the liver and other parts of the reticulo-endothelial system where the material is deposited indefinitely. Both hepatoma and haemangio-endothelioma may later result from use of this substance though this has long since been abandoned.

PATHOLOGY

There may be one large tumour or multiple small lesions. The right lobe is most frequently involved. Where there are multiple malignant lesions it is arguable whether they represent multiple foci of neoplasia or the results of intrahepatic spread from a single lesion. The portal venous radicles are frequently infiltrated, but metastases outside the liver are not common.

Histology

Histologically a hepatoma consists of columns of cells resembling those of the hepatic parenchyma, but the size and nuclear configuration are variable. Cholangiomata derived from bile-duct epithelium have a tubular arrangement.

CLINICAL PICTURE

1. In association with cirrhosis:

The development of the following lesions in a patient with established cirrhosis should make one suspicious of hepatic cancer:

a. Pain and tenderness of the liver which are not usual features of cirrhosis (unless due to haemochromatosis).

b. A hepatic tumour may cause ascites when the serum albumin level has not altered much and the fluid may be blood-stained or of high protein content (3 g. per cent or more).

c. Increasing size and nodularity of the liver.

d. General decline in health, loss of weight, and pyrexia together with jaundice. Glands may be present in the right supraclavicular fossa.

e. Owing to the tendency of hepatomata to grow into and obstruct the portal venous radicles, haematemesis due to portal hypertension may occur. A fatal intraperitoneal haemorrhage from the tumour itself may be the first indication of a hepatoma.

2. Without cirrhosis:

Patients with hepatomata usually have massive hepatomegaly, jaundice, and ascites which is often haemorrhagic. They complain of pain, anorexia, and wasting. The liver is hard on palpation, irregular, and tender. The abdomen is swollen and the overlying venous pattern is prominent.

DIAGNOSIS

A hepatoma should always be remembered as a cause of rapid downhill progression in a cirrhotic. It tends to be forgotten as a possibility when not associated with cirrhosis.

Helpful diagnostic tests include:

1. A raised leucocyte count, contrasting with the leucopenia of most cirrhotics, and a raised E.S.R. are non-specific but helpful clues.

2. Raised serum alkaline phosphatase values are of value in non-cirrhotics but are of little value in patients with cirrhosis where abnormal values are common. An $\alpha_2\beta$-globulin increase may be of diagnostic importance in those without cirrhosis. Abnormal protein bands simulating those found in myeloma may also occur and raised lipoproteins may be found.

3. Radiographic features include changes at the right lung base and diaphragm (collapse, effusion) and the features of portal hypertension (oesophageal varices) in cirrhotics. Portal venography is of some value in the demonstration of hepatic tumours. An avascular area in the liver, together with compression of surrounding vessels, is evidence of an intra-hepatic space-occupying lesion. Pneumoperitoneum may outline the surface of the liver and detect irregularity due to neoplasm. Hepatic scinti-scanning may be helpful if it shows one or more areas where there is no uptake of radioactive material. Most helpful of all may be coeliac axis angiography when an abnormal tumour circulation arising from the hepatic artery can be detected.

4. Liver biopsy may provide a histological answer. Material should be obtained from the site of maximal hepatic tenderness and nodularity.

5. Vitamin B_{12} levels may be raised but do not differentiate between primary and secondary hepatic neoplasms. Rarely, with massive tumours there is hypoglycaemia. Abnormal endocrine activity may also result in *hypercalcaemia* (stupor, anorexia, thirst, constipation, etc.) which may, if there are profound neurological symptoms, need differentiation from hepatic encephalopathy, and *hyponatraemia* also with mental changes when there is an inappropriate production and secretion of ADH (antidiuretic hormone). *Polycythaemia*, though difficult to demonstrate because many cirrhotics are already anaemic, may represent the effects of erythropoietin secretion by the tumour.

6. Recently a further diagnostic test has been used following the observation that 60 per cent of Ugandan patients with hepatoma showed the presence in the serum of an abnormal protein—α-fetoglobin. Though produced normally by the foetus this protein disappears soon after birth and its reappearance is due to its production by the more primitive tumour cells. Its detection by immunophoresis is not difficult, but the incidence of this abnormality is less than 50 per cent in Caucasians with hepatoma.

It must be remembered that secondary hepatic growths are thirty times as common as primary ones and a careful examination of the patient is necessary to exclude the more likely cause of intrahepatic malignancy. Diagnostic laporatomy is necessary in many cases.

TREATMENT

Removal of the right or left hepatic lobe is now a well-established surgical procedure and as a hepatic growth may remain restricted to one lobe for some time, rapid diagnosis may lead to curative, though major, hepatic surgery.

Other treatment, such as radiotherapy and alloxan, which had a short-lived vogue in the treatment of hepatomata, are now of secondary therapeutic importance, but regional use of cytotoxic drugs may be of increasing usefulness and this may be combined with hepatic artery ligation. This therapy is useful where there is severe pain.

Secondary Hepatic Neoplasms

There can be few sites of primary neoplasia which have not caused secondary tumour in the liver, which can be involved by direct spread from neighbouring organs, e.g., stomach, blood spread, by the portal vein from organs such as the rectum and colon, and by the hepatic artery from the bronchus and skin (melanoma).

The common sites of the primary tumour are:

Gastro-intestinal tract	Stomach and oesophagus
	Large bowel and rectum
	Pancreas
Respiratory tract	Bronchus
Skin and eye	Melanoma
Reproductive organs	Breast
Endocrine	Thyroid
	Adrenal
Renal tract	Kidney

PATHOLOGY

There may be one small secondary deposit in the liver or massive involvement so that there is little normal tissue left. It may weigh ten times more than normal, but weights of 5 or 6 kg. are quite common.

Secondary deposits often show umbilication at the centre due to necrosis. The deposits other than melanomata are usually grey-white. Histologically, it is not usually possible to identify the primary source of the tumour unless there is distinctive cytology, e.g., oat-cell tumour of bronchus. Mucus-containing deposits suggest that the origin is in the intestinal tract. Apart from discrete tumour masses, the hepatic sinusoids are often infiltrated by malignant cells, while the portal tracts may contain inflammatory cells.

CLINICAL PICTURE

Patients with secondary neoplasia are usually ill with cachexia, anorexia, and anaemia; fever may occur.

The patient's past history may be of importance and the clinical and histological features of lesions found at previous operations should be checked. Melanomata previously considered not frankly malignant should be reviewed when a patient presents with a liver full of secondary deposits. Pelvic examination and radiographs of the chest and alimentary tract may show up the primary lesion, and tests for faecal occult blood can help. The breasts should always be palpated. In many patients, tests which are of little practical value once the presence of secondary disease in the liver has been confirmed may not be justified.

As the liver is often grossly enlarged, palpation should start in the right iliac fossa. The surface may be nodular and central umbilication of deposits can be felt. Tenderness, pain in the right upper abdomen on breathing, or a dull continuous ache may be complained of. A palpable and audible friction rub over the liver is said to be pathognomonic of neoplasia. Enlarged axillary and right cervical lymph-nodes may be palpable. Occasionally because of the marked vascular supply of the tumour—from the hepatic artery—a bruit may be heard over the liver.

Ascites and jaundice are common, the latter usually being obstructive.

DIAGNOSIS

Secondary neoplastic disease may be difficult to distinguish from cirrhosis and the hepatomegaly of obstructive jaundice. The reticuloses may also involve the liver, in which case splenomegaly and enlargement of lymphatic glands may be found. Biopsy of lymph-glands or liver will differentiate between reticulosis and secondary carcinoma. The distinction is of importance because of the response of reticulosis to radiotherapy and cytotoxic drugs.

ASSESSMENT AND TREATMENT

There is no therapy of use in the treatment of secondary carcinoma of the liver unless the primary growth is hormone-dependent. Regional perfusion of the liver with cytotoxic drugs may relieve pain, and occasionally a solitary deposit may be removed by partial hepatectomy. It is also possible that hepatic artery ligation combined with perfusion of cytotoxic drugs via a cannula in the distal hepatic artery or portal vein will be helpful in the relief of pain and in the production of tumour shrinkage. It is important to remember, too, the relatively good prognosis in the carcinoid syndrome. This may be improved by local resection of liver metastases or by cytotoxic perfusion. Serotonin antagonists may alleviate diarrhoea (*see* p. 292).

FURTHER READING

Schistosomiasis
HAMILTON, P. K., HUTCHISON, H. S., JAMISON, P. W., and JONES, H. L. (1959), 'The Pathology and Pathogenesis of the Hepatosplenic Disease associated with Schistosomiasis', *Am. J. clin. Path.*, **32**, 18.

Primary Hepatic Cancer
ALPERT, M., URIEL, J., and DE NECHAND, B. (1968), 'Alpha fetoglobulin in the Diagnosis of Human Hepatoma', *New Engl. J. Med.*, **278**, 984.
CRUICKSHANK, A. H. (1961), 'The Pathology of 111 Cases of Primary Hepatic Malignancy collected in the Liverpool Region', *J. clin. Path.*, **14**, 120.
DAVIES, J. N. P. (1957), 'Incidence of Primary Liver Carcinoma in Kampala', *Acta Un. Int. Cancr.*, **13**, 606.
TIEN-YU LIN (1970), 'Primary Cancer of the Liver. Quadrennial Review', Proceedings of the 4th World Congress of Gastro-enterology, *Scand. J. Gastro-enterology*, **5**, Suppl. 6, 223.

Secondary Hepatic Cancer
CONN, H. O., and YESNER, R. (1963), 'A Revaluation of Needle Biopsy of the Liver in the Diagnosis of Metastatic Cancer of the Liver', *Ann. intern. Med.*, **59**, 53.
FENSTER, L. F., and KLATSKIN, G. (1961), 'Manifestations of Metastatic Tumours of the Liver', *Am. J. Med.*, **31**, 238.

Chapter 12

Chronic Liver Disease

(VASCULAR DISEASE AND THE LIVER; THE LIVER IN GENERAL DISORDERS)

VASCULAR DISEASE AND THE LIVER
(*Fig. 36*)

LESIONS OF THE HEPATIC VEINS

Obstruction (Budd-Chiari Syndrome)

THE DISORDER produced by obstruction of venous drainage of the liver produces a fairly characteristic pathological and clinical picture.

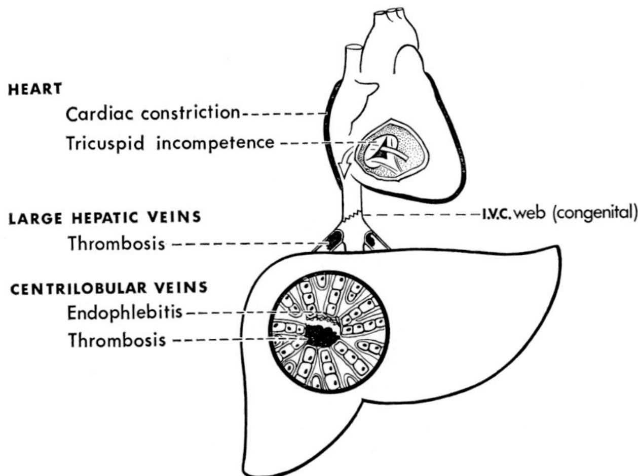

Fig. 36. Causes of increased hepatic venous pressure.

AETIOLOGY

It can be due to lesions of the large hepatic veins or to the central hepatic veins of the individual lobules. The causes of the clinical picture are:

1. Obstruction of large hepatic veins:
   a. Thrombosis, e.g., in polycythaemia and, rarely, after trauma and subphrenic sepsis. Cases are reported complicating the use of the contraceptive pill.

   b. Neoplastic invasion particularly by a hypernephroma, or retroperitoneal sarcoma, and sometimes as part of the thrombophlebitis complicating distant neoplasia.

   c. As a rare congenital disorder due to a membranous web across the inferior vena cava blocking the hepatic veins.

   2. Obstruction of small lobular veins:

      Due to toxins such as *Senecio* (veno-occlusive disease) and, rarely, drugs, such as urethane and possibly other cytotoxic agents, e.g., Busulphan.

PATHOLOGY

The liver is enlarged and tense, the edges rounded. Obvious thrombus may be seen in the larger hepatic veins. There is a gross 'nutmeg' pattern of the freshly cut surface which is due to central congestion of lobules and surrounding fatty change.

Microscopically, the areas around centrilobular veins show congestion and frank haemorrhage with liver cell necroses. Intracellular fat 'cysts' may occupy the rest of the lobules. Large hepatic veins may be obstructed.

CLINICAL PICTURE

The clinical picture varies with the primary lesion; for instance, a hypernephroma may cause haematuria, pyrexia, and a loin tumour, and polycythaemia will be accompanied by splenomegaly, cyanosis, and other thromboses. The onset of hepatic venous obstruction is indicated by pain, hepatic enlargement, vomiting, and ascites. On examination the liver is tender and signs of ascites are present. A useful sign is said to be the failure of the jugular veins to fill when the liver is pressed.

Accompaniments and Complications

Thrombosis of the major venous channels such as the portal vein will cause abdominal pain, ascites, and bloody diarrhoea, while blockage of the inferior vena cava may lead to albuminuria, prominent veins in the loins, and, rarely, a nephrotic syndrome. In acute cases severe liver cell failure with neuropsychiatric complications can develop and bleeding from oesophageal varices may occur.

DIAGNOSIS

In acute cases the sudden onset of pain and ascites should be helpful, particularly if a condition causative of thrombosis is present. In chronic cases the differentiation from cirrhosis, cardiac cirrhosis, and neoplastic disease may be difficult. The following tests are helpful:

   1. The ascitic fluid is usually of high protein content and may be frankly blood-stained. Protein usually 3 g. per cent or more.

   2. Liver function tests, though usually abnormal (positive flocculation tests, raised transaminases, and serum bilirubin), are non-specific.

Three tests are of diagnostic value:

3. Liver biopsy, the specimen showing characteristic congestive changes in centrilobular zones.

4. Catheterization of the inferior vena cava and injection of radio-opaque dye during a Valsalva manœuvre may show venous obstruction. The hepatic veins fail to fill or there is no 'streaming' of the opacified vena cava by blood flowing from the liver. The patency of the inferior vena cava can be verified at the same time.

5. Hepatic scintiscanning may show an increased amount of activity around the midline of the hepatic scan. This may be due to relative sparing of the caudate lobe.

TREATMENT

The treatment is that of the primary lesion and of the ascites. This latter may be refractory to medical therapy which should be intensive. In refractory cases repeated tapping may be required and consideration should be given to performing a portacaval anastomosis operation to by-pass the block. Surgical therapy may also be required for inferior vena caval stricture. Anticoagulant drugs should be given in diseases such as polycythaemia.

Veno-occlusive Disease (Obstruction of Centrilobular Veins)

AETIOLOGY

This is a disease of the West Indies, but sporadic cases of a similar condition are seen in other countries, such as Egypt, India, America, and Great Britain. It is thought to be due to certain toxins of plant and vegetable origin which cause an endophlebitis and thrombosis of central hepatic veins. In the West Indies the toxins are in 'bush teas' made from infusions of various plant leaves used medicinally after childbirth and for sick children. The toxins are contained in *Senecio* and *Crotolaria* extracts, both of which can produce experimental veno-occlusive disease in animals.

PATHOLOGY

The gross appearances are identical with those previously described. Histologically there is swelling of the subintima of the centrilobular veins and surrounding hepatic cell necrosis, congestion, and fatty change. In subacute cases centrilobular collapse leads to fibrosis and disorganization of the lobule so that cirrhosis results.

CLINICAL PICTURE

The disease is commonest in children aged 1 to 10 years. An acute phase with abdominal pain, hepatomegaly, and ascites may follow a respiratory infection. The disease can be fatal at this stage, but if a subacute phase is reached, though hepatosplenomegaly and ascites are present, the general health improves and abdominal pain goes. In the chronic phase which may follow, hepatic cirrhosis develops and the general health then deteriorates rapidly.

DIAGNOSIS

Diagnosis is helped by the dietary history and the typical clinical course.
Special tests of value are:
1. Liver biopsy.
2. Hepatic vein–inferior vena cava catheterization, as previously described, which will help to exclude obstruction of large hepatic veins.
3. Liver function tests. These are non-specific, but mirror the changes of liver cell function. A falling serum albumin level is a bad prognostic sign.

TREATMENT

This is largely symptomatic and is concerned with the control of ascites. In chronic disease bleeding from oesophageal varices may require standard treatment. Abstinence from bush teas is essential. The prognosis is reasonable, about 50 per cent of patients showing complete recovery, but the remainder develop cirrhosis.

The Syndrome of Prolonged Raised Hepatic Venous Pressure

In cardiac failure hepatic enlargement is common, and the enlarged liver is often tender.

Microscopically, the liver shows congestion, liver cell damage, and sometimes frank haemorrhage at the centre of the lobules, presumably because the oxygen tension in the cells is lower at this point.

Jaundice is due to impaired liver cell function and to absorption of bile-pigment from the pulmonary infarcts which are common. The serum bilirubin is rarely greater than 8 mg. per cent. Bromsulphthalein retention (*see* p. 418) is almost always increased, but the alkaline phosphatase is less commonly elevated. The serum transaminase may occasionally rise to 1000 units per ml. or more in acute cardiac failure, if it is severe. Changes in the serum proteins, such as low albumin and raised globulin, may occur, but rarely is the latter altered enough to give rise to positive flocculation tests.

Cardiac 'Cirrhosis'

AETIOLOGY

Permanent damage to the liver because of severe or persistent elevation of central venous pressure may occur in:
1. *Chronic cardiac failure*, particularly that complicating mitral stenosis with tricuspid incompetence. In certain tropical countries endomyocardial fibrosis of the right side of the heart is a common cause.
2. *Cardiac constrictive syndromes* due to pericarditis or myocarditis.

PATHOLOGY

The lesion is a progression of that in cardiac failure. Centrilobular congestion and liver cell damage lead to condensation of fibrous tissue and linking up of adjacent central veins. This 'pseudolobular' pattern of fibrosis is typical of cardiac failure and rarely leads on to a true cirrhosis with nodular regeneration and disorganization of portal tracts. The liver has a uniformly nodular surface with a thickened or 'sugar icing' capsule.

CLINICAL PICTURE

Chronic heart failure causes cachexia and certain hepatic features, such as mild jaundice and ascites, which are often refractory to medical treatment. The liver, which is enlarged and firm, usually pulsates. The jugular venous pulse may show systolic pulsation if there is tricuspid incompetence or a sharp 'y' descent in constrictive heart disease. If there is extensive fibrosis of the liver pulsation may disappear. Congestive splenomegaly is often found and oesophageal varices may arise because of portal hypertension. The heart is usually enlarged and murmurs are present, but in constrictive heart disease the cardiac size may be normal and there may be none.

Helpful diagnostic tests are of two types: (1) those which may help to diagnose the cardiac condition, e.g., electrocardiogram, radiograph of the chest, cardiac catheterization, and angiography, and (2) tests that show up the hepatic damage.

1. The liver function tests tend to show mild jaundice, reversal of the albumin-globulin ratio, a low serum albumin, and increased bromsulphthalein retention. The serum transaminase levels are slightly raised, but after an exacerbation of cardiac failure brought on by a respiratory infection they may rise steeply.

2. A liver biopsy will reveal the degree of liver damage.

ASSESSMENT AND TREATMENT

It is important to detect cases of constrictive pericarditis, for these respond to pericardectomy. Otherwise the prognosis is poor. The presence of intractable ascites leading to multiple abdominal paracenteses accentuates the gross wasting and cachexia.

LESIONS OF THE HEPATIC ARTERY

Normally about 25 per cent of the hepatic blood-flow is derived from the hepatic artery and in cirrhosis a larger percentage may come from this source. Occlusion of the hepatic artery may occur as the result of surgical trauma or embolization, e.g., in subacute bacterial endocarditis. The result of hepatic arterial occlusion is infarction, and clinically this is accompanied by right upper abdominal pain, jaundice, hypotension, and hepatic coma. It is a surprisingly rare condition. Ligation of the hepatic artery was once practised as a means of controlling portal hypertension in cirrhosis. In view of the important contribution of arterial blood to nutrition of the liver in cirrhosis, it is not surprising that the operation carried a high mortality. However, there has been a recent tendency to use hepatic artery ligation in the treatment of hepatic tumours, particularly vascular haemangiomata, primary hepatoma, and some cases of hepatic secondaries.

THE LIVER IN OTHER VASCULAR DISEASES

Cirrhosis occasionally complicates hereditary telangiectasia, and in polyarteritis nodosa, hepatic arterioles may be affected. Thus liver biopsy can be a helpful method of making a diagnosis of this disease. In liver biopsies from patients with Osler's disease abnormal blood-vessels are seen in a cirrhotic liver, but liver biopsy is not to be considered a means of diagnosing the disease.

THE LIVER IN GENERAL DISORDERS

Type of lesion	*Disease*
I. Metabolic	A. Diabetes
	B. Amyloidosis
	C. Galactosaemia (childhood)
	D. Glycogen storage disease (childhood)
	E. Gargoylism
	F. Porphyria
	G. Lipoidoses
II. Nutritional	A. Fatty liver
	B. ? Cirrhosis
	C. Hepatoma
III. Tropical	A. Malaria
	B. Kala-azar
IV. Pregnancy	A. Serum and infective hepatitis
	B. Intrahepatic cholestasis
	C. Gall-stones
	D. Eclampsia
	E. Fatty liver
	F. Drugs
V. Neoplastic	A. Reticuloses
	B. Myeloproliferative diseases

1. METABOLIC DISORDERS AND THE LIVER

A. Diabetes Mellitus

The liver is the main source of glucose which is in turn produced by the breakdown of hepatic glycogen. In diabetes hepatomegaly is common, and in diabetic ketosis severe upper abdominal pains are usually attributed to distension of the hepatic capsule by a swollen liver.

In thin diabetic patients who need insulin hepatomegaly may occur. The reason for the hepatomegaly is sometimes fatty infiltration and sometimes increased glycogen stores. Hepatomegaly is particularly common where there is poor diabetic control, but with improvement the liver may return to normal size. In the obese, mild, and usually elderly diabetic not requiring insulin, hepatomegaly is due to fatty infiltration. Fatty degeneration of the liver is common in subjects who are obese but not diabetic, so that this lesion may be as much an indication of obesity as of diabetes. Cirrhosis of the liver seems to be somewhat commoner in diabetics than non-diabetics. It must be remembered too that in haemochromatosis diabetes and cirrhosis are found together, but also that in 30 per cent of cirrhotic patients diabetes—usually mild—can be demonstrated.

B. Amyloidosis

Amyloid is the name given to the waxy appearance of organs infiltrated by fibrillar protein material in a mucopolysaccharide ground substance. The fibrils are produced by reticulo-endothelial cells and the material has an affinity for metachromic dyes, e.g., Congo red.

Two types have been recognized, and the previous classification was into:

1. Primary amyloid which was not related to previous sepsis and was found particularly in mesodermal structures, e.g., myocardium, tongue, skin, and in relation to blood-vessels, and

2. Secondary amyloid which was sometimes related to chronic suppuration, such as chronic osteomyelitis and empyema, and was found particularly in the liver, spleen, and kidneys.

The present-day classification which stresses site of deposition is into:

1. *Pericollagenous* (primary) where deposition is in connective tissue and where there is no causative disease. The amyloid of myelomatosis, familial Mediterranean fever, and an idiopathic form are examples of this type.

2. *Perireticular* (secondary)—here deposition is particularly related to small blood-vessels, and diseases which were of aetiological importance, e.g., pulmonary tuberculosis and empyema, have been replaced by rheumatoid arthritis, and to a lesser extent ulcerative colitis, Crohn's disease, and certain reticuloses.

CLINICAL PICTURE

This varies with the distribution of the amyloid and the associated conditions.

When there is hepatic involvement the liver is enlarged and firm and spleen and kidneys are often palpable. There may be jaundice and ascites, together with symptoms or signs in the tongue, heart, peripheral infiltration nerves, and intestine. Renal involvement is indicated by proteinuria which may on occasion be so pronounced as to cause a nephrotic syndrome. Since amyloidosis is an incomplete diagnosis, an intensive search for a possible cause should include a careful history and examination to exclude suppurative and general diseases.

Accompaniments and Complications

These are largely dependent on the cause of the amyloid and its distribution in other organs. Tests which are helpful in the diagnosis of amyloid disease are:

The *Congo red* test, which depends on the affinity of amyloid material for this dye and therefore its more complete disappearance from the serum in patients with amyloidosis than in normals. It should be noted that the Congo red test is only positive where there are large amyloid deposits, so that a positive result is only to be expected if there is hepatomegaly. A limited amyloid infiltration is thus unlikely to be detected (*see Chapter 24*).

Biopsy

A variety of tissues may be examined, but biopsy of the liver, small bowel, rectum, or kidneys may give a positive result if these organs are involved.

From whatever site obtained, it is important that stains should be used which are capable of detecting amyloid.

Except for the bromsulphthalein retention test and the alkaline phosphatase, liver function tests are rarely helpful. The serum albumin may be low for a variety of reasons.

TREATMENT

If a cause is found for amyloidosis, such as chronic osteomyelitis, this must be treated vigorously. In many cases there can be no treatment. Cortisone should not be given because of its possible aggravating effect.

C. Galactosaemia

This is an inborn error of metabolism in which there is a specific defect of galactose metabolism so that there is defective formation of glucose from it.

AETIOLOGY

This disorder is inherited as an autosomal recessive and is due to deficiency of the enzyme galactose-1-phosphate uridyl transferase which converts galactose-1-phosphate to glucose-1-phosphate:

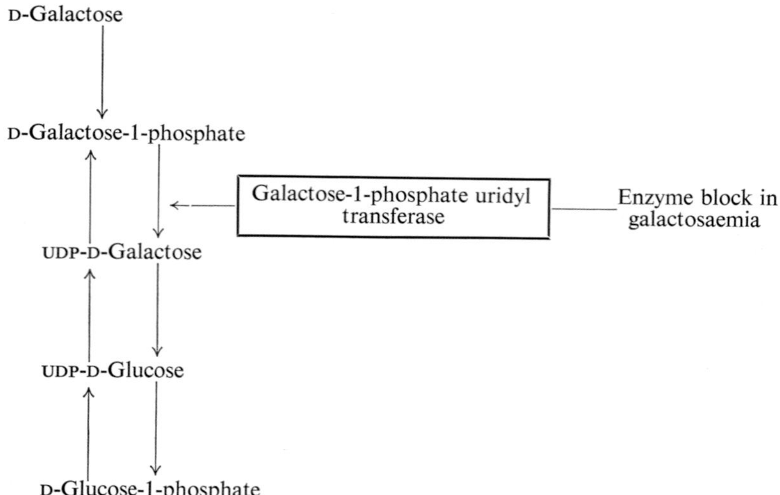

The deficiency of the enzyme can be detected in various tissues such as the red cells.

PATHOLOGY

The principal abnormality is found in the liver where there is fatty change proceeding to a portal cirrhosis. Jaundiced cases have histological signs of bile retention.

CLINICAL PICTURE

The diagnosis is suggested by any of the following clinical syndromes occurring in infancy:

1. Jaundice, vomiting, and loss of weight in the neonatal period. The liver and spleen may be enlarged and ascites may develop. There is failure to thrive.

2. Failure of normal development, feeding difficulties several months after birth, when physical examination may reveal hepatomegaly and cataracts.

3. Mild cases may show disturbance of growth, mental retardation, or other nervous disorders.

In all these situations the diagnosis is confirmed by the finding of a reducing substance in the urine which does not give a positive clinistix or testape reaction.

Accompaniments and Complications

Cataract is due to the toxic effect of galactose on the lens. Proteinuria and amino-aciduria are presumably due to a similar effect on the renal tubular epithelium. Mental deficiency, which may develop in untreated or un-recognized cases, is possibly caused by persistent hypoglycaemia brought about by hyperinsulinism stimulated by elevated blood-galactose levels.

DIAGNOSIS

The presence of a reducing substance in the urine in infancy must be followed by its biochemical identification. A negative clinistix test can be supplemented by urine chromatography. Other helpful tests include:

1. Elevated levels of serum galactose and reduced glucose levels.

2. Deficiency of galactose-1-phosphate uridyl transferase can be demonstrated in red blood-cells, and abnormal accumulation of galactose-1-phosphate can be demonstrated in galactosaemic red cells incubated with galactose *in vitro*. The first test is sensitive and rapid whilst the latter is a more lengthy procedure.

3. The galactose tolerance test is of value in children over the age of 2 years if the urinary galactose excretion is not high enough for diagnosis, but in infants the test is risky because of hypoglycaemia.

4. Liver function tests may show a raised serum bilirubin and alkaline phosphatase with a prolonged prothrombin time. Liver biopsy may reveal evidence of liver cell damage with fatty infiltration and, later on, cirrhosis.

5. Urine may show the presence of protein and generalized amino-aciduria.

ASSESSMENT AND TREATMENT

Treatment is dependent on the complete exclusion of all milk, lactose, and galactose from the diet. Special lactose-free feeds have been devised to this end, and they are given with vitamin supplements. The rigid régime is maintained for several years and clinical improvement occurs. In clinically normal patients with an abnormal galactose tolerance small quantities of milk may be allowed, but even these patients are improved if it is excluded.

D. Glycogen Storage Disease

In the commonest variety of this disorder there is excessive accumulation of glycogen in the tissue, particularly the liver, heart, kidneys, and muscles.

AETIOLOGY

The common form of this disease is inherited as a Mendelian recessive and is caused by a deficiency of glucose-6-phosphatase, an enzyme which is required for the normal production of glucose from glycogen. The block leads to the accumulation of glycogen in the tissues. At least five other types of glycogen storage disease which are dependent on other metabolic deficiencies, such as abnormality of the 'brancher' enzyme which determines glycogen molecular size, have been recognized. It is important to remember that Types I (glucose-6-phosphatase deficiency) and III (amylo-1,6-glucosidase deficiency) are the most important as regards identification, as surgical treatment (*vide infra*) may be possible.

PATHOLOGY

The liver is enlarged, pale, and glassy. The hepatic cells are enlarged and contain excess glycogen. A perilobular fibrosis may be found in chronic cases. Tissue must be taken into alcohol to stain for glycogen.

CLINICAL PICTURE

There is a general failure of health and development with mental retardation. The liver is enlarged and smooth and as a result the portal venous pressure may be elevated. Attacks of hypoglycaemia, related to reduction of glucose output by the liver, are common. In contrast to the failure of physical development mental development is normal. Jaundice and splenomegaly are not found.

In the presence of the above clinical features help may be obtained from the following tests:

1. The liver function tests are helpful in that they are normal.

2. There is a low serum glucose level which fails to rise 30 min. after the injection subcutaneously of 0·75 ml. of 1 : 1000 adrenaline, or after glucagon.

3. Aspiration biopsy of the liver shows increased deposits of glycogen, and histochemical techniques can be used to demonstrate deficiency of glucose-6-phosphatase or other enzymes.

TREATMENT AND ASSESSMENT

This disease was invariably fatal but now certain types are amenable to surgery using the operation of portacaval transposition. At this operation portal venous blood containing normal amounts of glucose is shunted directly into the inferior vena cava (systemic circulation). The distal part of this vessel is connected to the portal vein, the net effect being that glucose can by-pass the liver, and venous drainage from the lower extremity passes to the liver. The operation is only possible where the basic defect is confined to the liver (Types I and IIIb). At least two successful operative results are documented and though the operation may be technically difficult in a young patient with gross hepatomegaly the results are encouraging. Increased growth and mental development can occur.

E. Gargoylism

This inherited disorder is characterized by widespread deposition of mucopolysaccharide. It is clinically associated with dwarfism, coarse facial features, mental retardation, congenital heart disease, and hepatosplenomegaly. The diagnosis is aided by liver biopsy, where the vacuolated appearance of the liver and Kupffer cells and the biochemical findings are specific.

F. Porphyria

These are a group of inborn metabolic disorders of unknown aetiology, in which there is an abnormal metabolism of porphyrins associated with increased porphyrin excretion in urine and faeces.

Porphyrins are normally biochemical stages in the formation of haemoglobin and normally only coproporphyrin is excreted, as a result of normal red-cell destruction. Porphyria is usually classified as follows:

1. Congenital (or erythropoietic)

An extremely rare childhood disease characterized by:

a. Severe photosensitivity with consequent mutilating injuries from exposure to light.

b. Pigmentation and fluorescence of teeth and bone (due to uroporphyrin).

c. Anaemia, probably related to marrow porphyrin deposition. Liver normal.

Urine contains uroporphyrin, and is red; no porphobilinogen.

2. Porphyria cutanea tarda or (hepatic)

A disease of middle age often related to excess alcohol intake:

a. Mild photosensitivity of exposed areas.

b. Pigmentation.

c. Disturbed liver function or frank alcoholic cirrhosis may be present. Oestrogen therapy may aggravate.

A group of young patients with intermittent evidence of liver cell disease and jaundice, who have a similar type of porphyria, give no history of alcoholism. (Deterioration of liver function produces relapse.)

Urine contains uroporphyrin, and may be red; no porphobilinogen.

3. Acute intermittent   A disorder seen in young adults with:
   (or hepatic)
                              a. Abdominal colic of great severity, sometimes with oliguria and constipation.
                              b. Coma, mental confusion, and paralysis which may give rise to fatal respiratory paralysis. Later, psychotic changes occur.

Attacks are precipitated by barbiturates and sedatives as well as alcohol. This is the result of enzyme (ALA-synthetase) induction in the liver with increased synthesis of porphyrin precursors (δ-ALA-amino-laevulinic acid and porphobilinogen).
Urine contains uroporphyrin *and* porphobilinogen and may be red.

The commonest type is the acute intermittent type. The test for porphobilinogen is the same as Ehrlich's aldehyde test for urobilinogen, except that chloroform is added. Urobilinogen is soluble in chloroform and therefore forms a pink colour in the lower (chloroform) layer. The pink colour due to uroporphyrin stays in the aqueous phase.

Otherwise, the diagnosis of porphyria rests on the spectroscopic or chemical detection of these substances.

G. The Lipoidoses (*Fig. 37*)

There are three well-recognized forms of lipoid storage disease, the type of fatty material deposited varying in each case; all involve the liver.

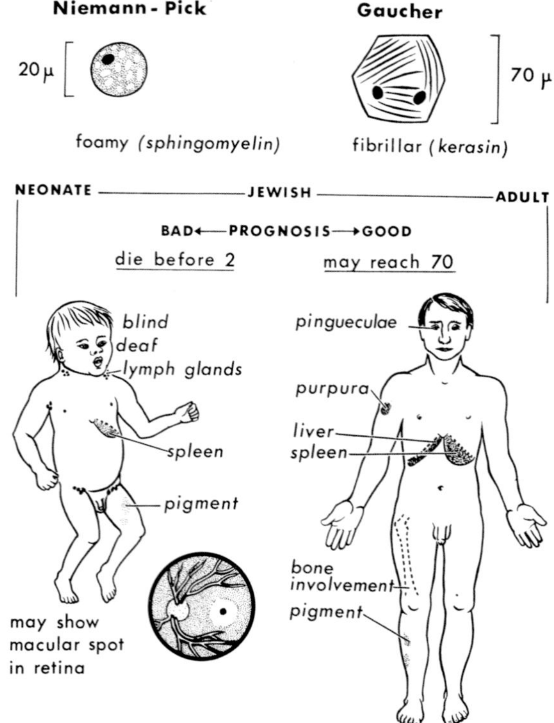

Fig. 37. The lipoidoses.

1. Gaucher's disease, associated with kerasin deposition.
2. Niemann-Pick disease, associated with sphingomyelin deposition.
3. Hand-Schüller-Christian disease, associated with cholesterol deposition, is probably not a true lipoidosis but a histiocytosis.

In all varieties the cells of the reticulo-endothelial system are particularly involved.

Features of Gaucher's Disease

In adults there is:
1. Hepatomegaly and gross splenomegaly with hypersplenism.
2. Skin pigmentation, particularly of the legs.
3. Pingueculae in the eyes.
4. Radiological changes in the bones, such as expansion of the lower ends of the femora ('hock bottle femora').

It is common in Jews. Diagnosis is assisted by a positive family history and can be confirmed by the finding of typical Gaucher cells containing kerasin in the marrow or liver. There is an acute fatal infantile form.

Features of Niemann-Pick Disease

This is a fatal disease seen in babies and children under the age of 2 years. The features of the disorder, which are almost always confined to Jewish children, are:
1. Failure to thrive, with hepatosplenomegaly.
2. Pigmentation of the skin and oral mucosa.
3. Deafness, blindness, and mental deterioration. Blindness is accompanied by retinal degeneration giving a 'cherry-red' spot on the macula.

Diagnosis may be aided by the finding of lipoid-laden cells in biopsy tissue from liver, spleen, bone-marrow, or lymph-glands. The 'foam' cell of Niemann-Pick disease contains many refractile vacuoles of lipid.

Features of Hand-Schüller-Christian Disease

The liver may be involved if cholesterol is deposited there. The clinical features include:
1. A tendency to occur in Jewish families.
2. Bony defects starting in the second or third year of life.
3. Hepatosplenomegaly and skin discoloration.
4. Exophthalmos and diabetes insipidus due to bony involvement of the skull and pituitary fossa.

Biopsy of affected tissue shows foam cells similar to those of Niemann-Pick disease, but the lipoid is cholesterol or its esters. The disease is chronic; complications, such as diabetes insipidus, can be treated, while corticosteroids and radiotherapy may bring about healing of bone lesions.

II. NUTRITIONAL LIVER DISEASE

There is considerable controversy regarding the part played by malnutrition in the pathogenesis of liver disease and in particular cirrhosis. There is good experimental evidence which shows that in the rat amino-acid deficiency can produce both fatty infiltration and hepatic necrosis. Further, the experimental fatty infiltration may proceed to a true cirrhosis. Clinicians have unfortunately been too ready to subscribe to the view that human cirrhosis is commonly of nutritional origin.

Kwashiorkor is undoubtedly one hepatic lesion which is caused by protein deficiency. The liver is heavily infiltrated with fat, but it seems unlikely that this is directly due to deficiency of choline or methionine, for the distribution of fat is different from that in the choline-deficient rat. The relation of this fatty infiltrate to the development of cirrhosis is uncertain and no one has produced conclusive evidence that this change commonly occurs. Investigation is surrounded by difficulties, for wherever there are malnourished people diseases such as malaria and infective hepatitis are also common; and the effects of various hepatotoxic agents contained in or contaminating food must be considered. Cirrhosis in such a community may be the result of many aetiological factors. There are also forms of juvenile cirrhosis in tropical countries in which it is recognized that the lesion does not develop from fatty infiltration. Of a particular interest is childhood cirrhosis in India which seems to have a familial incidence without there being evidence of malnutrition. A 'toxic' cause seems likely.

Primary liver cancer, both that occurring in the cirrhotic and in the patient with a normal liver, is common in some parts of the world, e.g., Africa and Malaya, where the diet is poor. In such cases the effect of multiple aetiological factors must again be considered. It is, however, possible that the alternation of periods of relative starvation and plenty which frequently occur in those parts of the globe might induce abnormal proliferative activity in the liver, particularly in the presence of contaminating substances such as Aflatoxin (*see* p. 143).

III. THE LIVER IN TROPICAL DISEASES

A. Malaria

The endogenous or human phase of the malarial cycle begins with the injection of sporozoites from the infected mosquito. They disappear from the blood-stream and develop in the liver parenchymal cells. In relapsing malaria (*Plasmodium vivax* and *P. malariae*) exo-erythrocytic parasites persist in liver cells and, after a latent period, merozoites are formed which may produce the erythrocytic phase of clinical symptoms.

In chronic malaria the liver may be enlarged because of reticulo-endothelial proliferation. The reticulo-endothelial proliferation is accompanied by foci of liver cell damage and sometimes by granuloma formation. The Kupffer cells contain pigment from destroyed red cells and occasional parasites. In severe malaria, such as blackwater fever and other types of falciparum infection, extensive centrilobular necrosis may occur as a result of a low blood-pressure and obstruction of the sinusoids by degenerating red cells. After repeated attacks of malaria coupled with other factors such as malnutrition, periportal scarring and fibrosis may follow. A true cirrhosis does not result from malaria. Giant splenomegaly seen so often in the tropics is sometimes associated with portal hypertension.

This may be an example of an excessive immunological reaction to the malarial parasite. Other types of idiopathic tropical splenomegaly probably have other as yet unknown causes.

B. Kala-azar

This disease, which is caused by a protozoa, *Leishmania donovani*, is characterized by pyrexia, hepatosplenomegaly, anorexia, leucopenia, and hyperglobulinaemia. *Leishmania* bodies present in the blood-stream are ingested by the vector (various species of a sand-fly, *Phlebotomus*), where after development into flagellate forms they are extruded by the infected fly.

The disease causes widespread reticulo-endothelial proliferation due to protozoal proliferation. The spleen is usually greatly enlarged and there is replacement of the splenic tissue by parasitized cells with fibrosis in chronic cases. The liver is less enlarged, but again there is Kupffer cell proliferation. The proliferation may cause damage to liver cells with cloudy swelling and fatty change. Cirrhosis does not result.

IV. THE LIVER IN PREGNANCY
(*Fig. 38*)

A. Serum and Infective Hepatitis

The pregnant patient may be susceptible to syringe hepatitis because of the investigations required during pregnancy, whilst close contact with

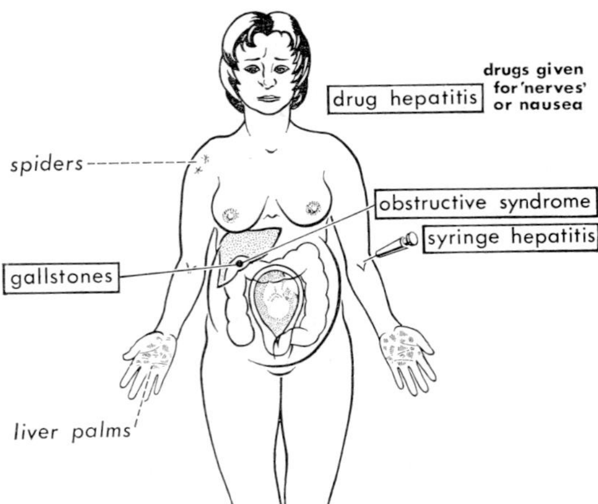

Fig. 38. The liver in pregnancy.

other young children always renders the mother susceptible to infective hepatitis. In most pregnant patients infective or serum hepatitis is of normal severity, but some observers feel that the combination of pregnancy and hepatitis is a bad one, with a high incidence of fatal hepatic necrosis. This is particularly likely to be so in tropical countries. Abortion and premature labour are further hazards for the foetus.

B. Intrahepatic Cholestasis

A syndrome of mild obstructive jaundice with pruritus and a raised alkaline phosphatase is recognized in the last trimester of pregnancy. This may represent a further stage of the common pruritus of pregnancy. The disorder occurs in the similar group of patients who manifest obstructive jaundice related to the administration of the contraceptive pill. It varies as does pill jaundice in its geographical distribution, being commonest in the Scandinavian countries and in Chile. In Britain it is much less common.

The jaundice is of little clinical significance as it disappears with parturition, but is likely to return with subsequent pregnancies. The importance of this lesion lies in the diagnostic problem which may arise from failure to recognize it, and also the danger to the baby, which may be stillborn or premature.

C. Gall-stones

Gall-stones tend to form during and after pregnancy.

D. The Hepatic Lesion of Eclampsia

The liver may be damaged by the widespread vasculitis in this disorder. Haemorrhages occur around the portal zones causing focal necrosis of liver cells. There are usually no clinical signs.

E. Fatty Liver in Pregnancy

A fatty infiltration of the liver from the fat mobilization which accompanies hyperemesis does not cause jaundice. Intravenous tetracycline in high dosage may cause both jaundice and fatty liver. At term, an acute fatty liver accompanied by deep jaundice is both rare and of unknown aetiology. It carries a high mortality (50 per cent) and there is a rather characteristic fine fatty infiltration of hepatocytes. Hypoglycaemia is common and must be energetically treated.

F. Drugs

Drugs such as sedatives, tranquillizers, and anti-emetics are an important cause of jaundice in pregnancy. Ergometrine in the presence of existing liver disease may produce peripheral gangrene and renal failure due to inadequate metabolic turnover.

V. THE LIVER IN NEOPLASTIC DISEASES

A. The Reticuloses

1. *In Hodgkin's Disease*

This commonly involves the liver. The hepatic lesion usually consists of small foci of Hodgkin's tissue in the parenchyma or portal zones. In the latter the growth of tissue may produce obstructive jaundice owing to compression of intrahepatic bile-ducts. Hepatomegaly is common in advanced Hodgkin's disease and the liver may provide diagnostic biopsy material at any stage of the disease. Fever, abdominal pain, pruritus, loss of weight, and anaemia are some of the clinical features of this disorder and examination may reveal enlargement of lymph-glands, pigmentation, wasting, and hepatosplenomegaly. Liver function tests may show a raised serum bilirubin (due to haemolysis or hepatic involvement), a low serum albumin, raised globulins, and an elevated alkaline phosphatase. The last finding is particularly suggestive of hepatic involvement even when there is no jaundice. Biopsy of the liver may show cellular foci containing lymphocytes, eosinophils, plasma cells, endothelial cells, and giant cells, thus showing the typical pleomorphism of Hodgkin's disease.

2. *In Lymphosarcoma*

Large necrotic foci which simulate the appearance of secondary carcinoma or multiple infiltrative lesions may occur. In myeloma there may be plasma cell infiltration. In all reticuloses, flocculation tests may be positive because there are abnormal concentrations of proteins in the serum.

B. Myeloproliferative Diseases

1. *In Chronic Leukaemia*

Whether myeloid or lymphatic, the liver may be infiltrated by primitive white cells. In the chronic lymphatic variety the portal tracts are swollen and distorted, but the sinusoids are not infiltrated. In chronic myeloid leukaemia the reverse tends to be true. Liver biopsy plays no part in the diagnosis of chronic leukaemia and because of the haemorrhagic tendency it may be dangerous. The use of cytotoxic therapy in patients with leukaemia and severe psoriasis may result in liver cell damage and even cirrhosis. Deteriorating liver function must not then be ascribed to progression of the initial disease.

2. *Myeloid Metaplasia*

The replacement of the blood-forming marrow of the adult by processes such as carcinomatosis, myelosclerosis, and marble-bone disease leads to the resumption of erythropoiesis in the liver. Myelofibrosis, either primary or secondary to polycythaemia, is probably the best example of myeloid metaplasia in the liver. Liver biopsy, which demonstrates blood-formation in the liver, is a helpful way of confirming such a diagnosis. The clinical picture of anaemia, giant splenomegaly, and hepatomegaly is very characteristic, and the peripheral blood-film shows a leuco-erythroblastic anaemia. Marrow trephine biopsy confirms the fibrosis of the marrow cavity. The bone radiographs may show increased radiological density. The histological picture in the liver is of hepatic sinusoids distended with red and white precursor cells, myeloblasts, myelocytes, erythroblasts, and normoblasts. The biggest and most conspicuous cells are the platelet-forming megakaryocytes. The facility of the liver to undertake extra-medullary erythropoiesis is increased after splenectomy when there may be further hepatic enlargement. Portal hypertension is occasionally found. This is due to a combination of increased splenic blood-flow (enlarged spleen) and increased hepatic presinusoidal resistance to blood-flow due to hepatic cellular infiltration. An exactly similar haemodynamic abnormality is seen in certain reticuloses with hepatic infiltration, sarcoidosis, and the condition of giant tropical splenomegaly which results from chronic malaria (*see* p. 163).

3. *Polycythaemia*

In polycythaemia and myelofibrosis giant splenomegaly may be associated with portal hypertension and oesophageal varices. Thrombosis of the portal or hepatic veins may also occur.

FURTHER READING

Veno-occlusive Disease
STUART, K. L., and BRAS, G. (1957), 'Veno-occlusive Disease of the Liver', *Q. Jl Med.*, **50**, 291.

Cardiac Failure
WHITE, T. J., LEEVY, C. M., BRUSCA, A. M., and GNASSI, A. M. (1955), 'The Liver in Congestive Heart Failure', *Am. Heart J.*, **49**, 250.

Budd-Chiari Syndrome
CLAIN, D., FRESTON, J., KREEL, L., and SHERLOCK, S. (1967), 'Clinical Diagnosis of the Budd-Chiari Syndrome', *Am. J. Med.*, **43**, 544
THOMPSON, R. B. (1947), 'Thrombosis of the Hepatic Veins. The Budd-Chiari Syndrome', *Archs intern. Med.*, **80**, 602.

Galactosaemia
HOLZEL, A., KOMROWER, G. M., and SCHWARZ, V. (1957), 'Galactosemia', *Am. J. Med.*, **22**, 703.
ISSELBACHER, K. J. (1959), 'Galactose Metabolism and Galactosemia', *Ibid.*, **26**, 715.

Glycogen Storage Disease
RIDDEL, A. G., DAVIES, R. P., and APLEY, J. (1967), 'Portocaval Transposition in the Treatment of Glycogen Storage Disease', in *The Liver*, vol. 19 of the Colston Papers (ed. READ, A. E.), 269. London: Butterworth.
SOKAL, J. E., LOWE, C. U., and SARCIONE, E. J. (1962), 'Liver Glycogen Disease', *Archs intern. Med.*, **109**, 612.

Amyloidosis
COHEN, A. S. (1967), 'Amyloidosis', *New Engl. J. Med.*, **277**, 574 and 628.
LEVINE, R. A. (1962), 'Amyloid Disease of the Liver', *Am. J. Med.*, **33**, 349.

Porphyria
GOLDBERG, A. (1971), 'The Porphyrias', *Seventh Symposium on Advanced Medicine* (ed. BOUCHIER, I. A. D.), p. 210. London: Pitman Medical.
WALDENSTROM, J. (1957), 'The Porphyrias as Inborn Errors of Metabolism', *Am. J. Med.*, **22**, 759.

Gaucher's Disease
REICH, C., SEIF, M., and KESSLER, B. J. (1951), 'Gaucher's Disease, a Review and Discussion of 20 Cases', *Medicine, Baltimore*, **30**, 1.

Niemann-Pick Disease
CROCKER, A. C., and FARBER, S. (1958), 'Niemann-Pick Disease, a Review of 18 Patients' *Ibid.*, **37**, 1.

Nutrition and the Liver
A Symposium. *Am. J. clin. Nutr.*, **23**, 447 and 581.

Nutritional Liver Disease
WATERLOW, J. C., and BRAS, G. (1961), 'Nutritional Liver Disease in Man', in *Modern Trends in Gastroenterology* (ed. CARD, W. I.), vol. 3, p. 158. London: Butterworth.

Hodgkin's Disease
BOURONCLE, B. A., OLD, J. U., and VAZQUES, A. G. (1962), 'Pathogenesis of Jaundice in Hodgkin's Disease', *Archs intern. Med.*, **110**, 872.
LEVITAN, R., DIAMOND, H. D., and CRAVER, L. F. (1961), 'The Liver in Hodgkin's Disease', *Gut*, **2**, 60.

Myelofibrosis
PITCOCK, J. A., REINHARD, E. H., JUSTUS, B. W., and MENDELSOHN, R. S. (1962), 'A Clinical and Pathological Study of 70 Cases of Myelofibrosis', *Ann. intern. Med.*, **57**, 73.

Sarcoidosis
MAUDREY, W. C., JOHNS, C. J., BOITNOTT, J. K., and IBER, F. L. (1970), 'Sarcoidosis and Chronic Hepatic Disease. A Clinical and Pathological Study of 20 Cases', *Medicine, Baltimore*, **49**, 375.

Pregnancy (*Recurrent Idiopathic Jaundice*)
SVANBORG, A., and OHLSSON, S. (1950), 'Recurrent Jaundice of Pregnancy', *Am. J. Med.*, **27**, 40.

Chapter 13

Cirrhosis of the Liver

RENÉ LAËNNEC used the name 'cirrhosis' (from the Greek word for 'tawny') because of the colour he observed in the diseased liver at post-mortem. By definition cirrhosis is a disease in which the following histological features are present:

1. Fibrosis.

2. A loss of normal hepatic architecture due to the formation of regeneration nodules.

3. Evidence of liver cell damage.

Of these three factors the second is the most important. The regeneration nodules arise from the proliferation of parenchymal cells, and the result is an area of liver tissue with abnormal features, size, and arrangement of blood-vessels, and perhaps functional impairment also. Fibrosis is an integral part of cirrhosis, but it can be present without cirrhosis if there is no basic upset of lobular pattern. The factor of liver cell damage is also variable and in well-'compensated' cirrhosis the liver cells may look healthy and liver function may be reasonable.

TYPES OF CIRRHOSIS

Essentially three main types of cirrhosis are recognized.

1. *Micronodular*

This shows fine hobnail appearance of the liver, which is often enlarged and in which histologically there is a formation of fine uniform regeneration nodules of about 5 mm. in size.

2. *Macronodular Cirrhosis*

A coarse, irregular surface is apparent. The liver is often small and regeneration nodules are of varying sizes from 1 cm. to the size of an orange.

3. *Mixed*

The regeneration nodules are of varying size.

Primary biliary cirrhosis is a micronodular type of cirrhosis based on chronic biliary obstruction, and cardiac cirrhosis is a fine cirrhosis also. No close relationship exists between the cause of cirrhosis and the configuration of the regeneration nodules. Alcoholic cirrhosis is often micronodular, but in alcoholics with heavy intermittent drinking habits regeneration nodules may be large. Size of regeneration nodules is probably more closely related to the extent of previous necrosis.

CLINICAL RESULTS OF CIRRHOSIS

These may be classified as those which are *harmful* and those which are possibly *beneficial*. Unfortunately, the former are more frequent than the latter.

1. *Harmful Effects*

a. Liver cell failure	Jaundice	
	Hypoalbuminaemia	
	(Fluid retention)	
b. Portal hypertension	Oesophageal varices (bleeding)	
	Abnormal collateral vessels	
	(Hepatic coma and precoma)	
	(*Escherichia coli* septicaemia)	
	Vascular shunts (cyanosis)	
c. Neoplastic change	Hepatoma	
d. Hormonal imbalance	? cause of skin lesions and spider naevi	
	? cause of amenorrhoea, infertility, etc.	
	? cause of fluid retention	
	(Antidiuretic hormone, aldosterone, oestrogens)	
	Low incidence of atheroma, thrombosis, and hypertension.	

2. *Beneficial*

These are probably related to the effect of increased circulating oestrogens, enhanced fibrinolysis (due to the presence of increased plasminogen activators in the serum), and to abnormally low platelet adhesiveness. There may also be decreased sensitivity to pressor substances such as angiotensin or increased destruction of it.

CLINICAL VARIETIES OF CIRRHOSIS
(*Fig. 39; Table 16*)

1. Alcoholic Cirrhosis (Laennec's Cirrhosis)

AETIOLOGY

This disease is common where there is a high incidence of alcoholism. It is the common type of cirrhosis seen in the U.S.A. and in some European countries such as France. It is not rare in the British Isles and perhaps 30 per cent of cirrhotics have an alcoholic history. The patients with this disease in Great Britain are mainly 'well-to-do' or work in the catering trade or as publicans and commercial travellers.

The precise reason why alcoholic cirrhosis develops is unknown. Some people drink heavily and do not develop cirrhosis. It has been shown that alcohol can produce a fatty liver with fat droplets in all liver cells, but there is little knowledge concerning the reason why some patients go on to develop cirrhosis. Perhaps nutritional factors are important in this transformation, but other workers have suggested that constitutional and familial factors may be important. The classic story that the alcoholic buys alcohol and starves himself of protein is often true, but alcoholic cirrhosis can develop in those who drink and eat well. The disease is more common in males than in females.

PATHOLOGY

The liver is often enlarged and an even micronodular type of cirrhosis may be present. The liver often looks greasy and this feature is well demonstrated in histological preparations which show fatty change in the liver cells. Fatty infiltration is indicative of recent drinking, and when drinking stops the fat disappears. Liver cell damage is variable, but following a bout

Table 16. CLINICAL VARIETIES OF CIRRHOSIS

ALCOHOLIC CIRRHOSIS	CRYPTOGENIC CIRRHOSIS
More common in males	More common in females
Jaundice + +	Jaundice ±
Liver large	Liver small
Spleen ±	Spleen + +
Ascites +	Ascites + +
Bleeding varices +	Bleeding varices + +
Hepatic coma +	Hepatic coma + +
Special features	*Special features*
Delirium tremens	May be no preceding history
Peripheral neuritis	of hepatitis
Enlarged parotid glands	
Dupuytren's contractures	
Also pancreatitis, gastritis, and	
duodenal ulcer	

of hard drinking it can be severe with areas of liver cell necrosis and polymorph infiltration. Histologically one other feature is often seen and this is a peculiar hyaline degeneration of the perinuclear cytoplasm in damaged liver cells—'Mallory's alcoholic hyaline'. This is not, however, a feature specific to alcoholic liver disease. It may occur, for example, in the liver in Wilson's disease or Indian childhood cirrhosis. It seems that alcohol itself is the direct cause of the fatty infiltration which only rarely progresses to cirrhosis. Cirrhosis seems particularly likely in those with attacks of severe liver cell dysfunction and jaundice where spotty necrosis is a histological feature, i.e., 'alcoholic hepatitis'.

CLINICAL PICTURE

After heavy drinking bouts the patient may be jaundiced, with anorexia and vomiting, upper abdominal pain, and hepatomegaly. The diagnosis from acute viral hepatitis in these circumstances may be difficult. When cirrhosis develops the signs of liver cell failure (oedema, including ascites and jaundice), together with those of portal hypertension (bleeding varices, neuropsychiatric complications), are similar to those in other varieties of cirrhosis. Certain features other than the history of heavy drinking, which can be difficult to elicit in some cases, may be present. Peripheral neuropathy may be present and a careful examination of the nervous system must take note of calf tenderness, sensory loss, and abnormal tendon-reflexes. The presence of jaundice, if it is of the liver cell variety, must make the clinician think of alcoholic cirrhosis. An association between parotid gland enlargement and contraction of the palmar fascia (Dupuytren's contracture) has been shown to exist in the alcoholic.

Accompaniments and Complications

A coarse alcoholic tremor or frank delirium tremens may occur in alcoholics, particularly when alcohol is withdrawn. Wernicke's encephalopathy, with paralysis of intrinsic and extrinsic ocular muscles, is caused by vitamin B deficiency and may be accompanied by glossitis. Irritation of the skin, 'wine itch', is a complaint of some alcoholics.

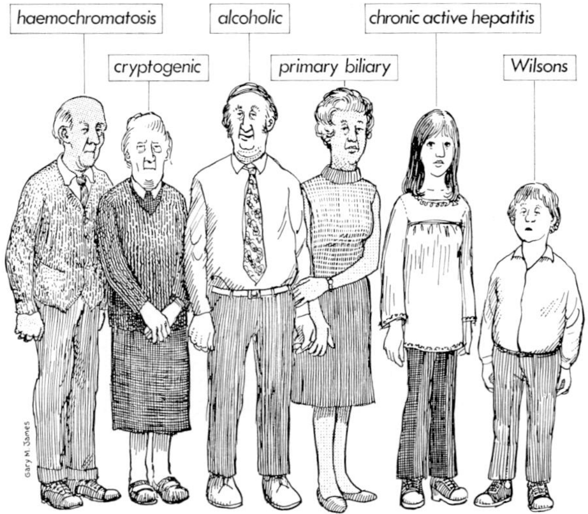

Fig. 39. The cirrhosis family.

In severe cases death is caused by liver cell failure (deep jaundice, hepatic coma, ascites) or bleeding from oesophageal varices may occur. Sudden death, perhaps due to the discharge of fat emboli from the liver, has been described.

There may be difficulty in deciding whether confusion is due to the effects of alcohol on the brain, 'delirium tremens', or to the effects of hepatic precoma, but the patient with delirium tremens is alert, frightened, and agitated unlike the drowsy, confused, inattentive patient with precoma.

Chronic pancreatitis sometimes coexists in alcoholics with liver disease, and tuberculosis, both pulmonary and peritoneal, is common.

Zieve has described a condition of hyperlipaemia and haemolysis of red blood-cells associated with abnormal red-cell shape (acanthocytosis) which occurs in the alcoholic (Zieve's syndrome) though it is doubtful if this is a clear-cut entity.

DIAGNOSIS

There are no tests of liver function which are specific for alcoholic cirrhosis as opposed to other types of cirrhosis, so that if a correct diagnosis is to be made it is most important to extract the history of alcoholism from the patient or his relatives. Jaundice and moderately elevated serum transaminases may occur after acute bouts.

The liver biopsy which shows the features previously described can be of importance in making the diagnosis. The serum protein abnormalities are those seen in any variety of cirrhosis. Estimation of serum lipids may be helpful.

TREATMENT AND MANAGEMENT

This is based upon: (1) The elimination of alcohol from the patient's daily life. (2) The treatment of complications such as fluid retention, bleeding from varices, hepatic coma, etc.

When a patient is admitted to hospital with alcoholic cirrhosis alcohol must be withdrawn, and its removal is most easily effected if large doses of a phenothiazine drug, such as chlorpromazine, are given to prevent the onset of delirium tremens. The patient should be placed on an appetizing and nutritious diet with adequate vitamin supplements particularly of the B group. Magnesium supplements are important, too, and in acute cases there may be a dramatic improvement of neuropsychiatric states following their administration. Stern explanation of the patient's illness is required in order to ensure that he abstains from alcohol when his condition improves. It is not enough to tell the patient that alcohol consumption should be cut down—it must be stopped. The patient's friends and relatives (providing they are not alcoholics) should be encouraged to help him and the help of societies such as 'Alcoholics Anonymous' may be required. An attempt must, of course, be made to find out *why* the patient is an alcoholic, and publicans and commercial travellers should be advised to find another job.

On the whole, the results of trying to make the patient abstain are poor, but patients are often driven to abstinence when they hear the gloomy story of possible complications or read their own liver biopsy report. This latter we find as effective as anything!

It is most important that the patient should be seen regularly at a clinic after the diagnosis has been made. Patients who are not drinking attend regularly, but those who have slipped back to the bottle do not, so that non-attendances should be investigated by the Welfare Department.

Great improvement can occur once alcohol is withdrawn. Oedema and evidence of malnutrition rapidly diminish, while liver function and histology improve. It has been shown quite conclusively that cessation of drinking is associated with an improved mortality and morbidity so that it is a target worth aiming for.

2. Cryptogenic Cirrhosis

AETIOLOGY

This is the commonest type of cirrhosis seen in Britain and is particularly common in middle-aged or elderly females. About half the patients who develop this type of cirrhosis have a past history of viral hepatitis. In many of these patients the attack is not particularly severe as judged by the length of the clinical history. The patient may appear to be in good health for many years before the symptoms of cirrhosis or one of its complications, such as bleeding from oesophageal varices, occur. In others the progression from hepatitis is more obvious.

Presumably this lesion follows patchy necrosis of liver tissue, but the nature and timing of the initial illness are in many cases difficult to elucidate. Presumably viral hepatitis is the all-important cause, but exposure to drugs and poisons and the possible role of auto-immunity must be considered.

PATHOLOGY

The liver is often smaller than normal with a coarse, uneven nodularity of its surface (macronodular cirrhosis). The nodules are of varying size, usually 1–3 cm. in diameter; they are surrounded by coarse bands of fibrous tissue. The histological changes found in portal hypertension often accompany the hepatic lesion. There is a variable cellular infiltration and evidence of liver cell damage.

CLINICAL PICTURE

The patient usually presents in one of the following ways:

1. Because of bleeding from oesophageal varices.

2. Because of ascites or peripheral oedema.

3. Because of confusion or personality change associated with hepatic precoma.

4. The diagnosis is not uncommonly made at laparotomy done for some unrelated reason, e.g., gall-stones.

5. Because of splenomegaly.

6. Because the patient has some abnormality, discovered on routine testing, such as:

a. Urobilin in excess in the urine.

b. A raised serum bilirubin, or globulins, the latter causing a raised E.S.R. A raised serum alkaline phosphatase or transaminases.

c. A low white-cell count or reduced platelets due to hypersplenism.

The patient is more likely to be female than male (3 : 1). There may be cutaneous stigmata of liver disease and finger-clubbing. The liver is in some patients larger, but in others smaller, than normal. The spleen is usually found to be enlarged if the patient is properly examined. Peripheral oedema and/or ascites may be present. The features of portal hypertension with bleeding varices and prominent abdominal collateral veins may be seen together with those of hepatic precoma. Occasionally, patients with chronic liver disease of this type may develop cardiac complications such

9

as a high cardiac output, ejection systolic murmurs, and even cardiomegaly and cardiac failure.

The endocrine changes of chronic liver disease may also be seen, but in elderly female patients they may be limited to absence of body hair. Jaundice is usually non-existent or mild but may develop after a particular insult to the liver, such as alimentary bleeding.

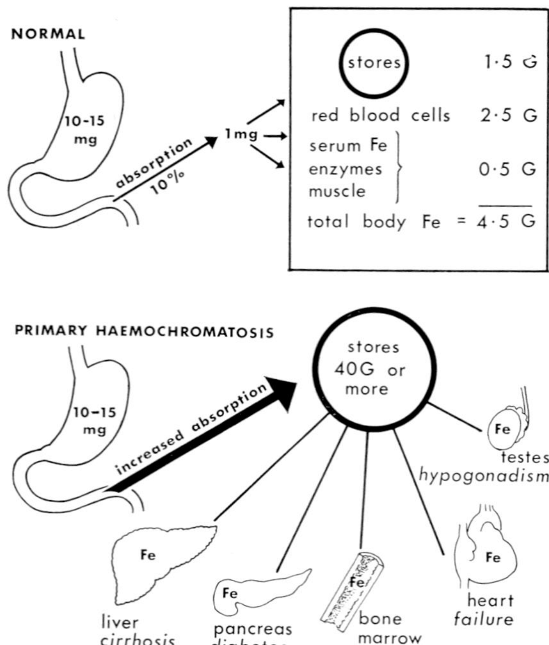

Fig. 40. Normal and abnormal iron metabolism.

DIAGNOSIS

The presentation of cryptogenic cirrhosis can be very variable because of the complications which may occur. In the vast majority of cases the liver function tests are abnormal and helpful information can be obtained from:

1. Tests indicating the production of abnormal proteins, i.e., flocculation tests and the electrophoretic strip. The transaminases may also be moderately raised.

The albumin may be reduced, particularly if there is fluid retention, and the prothrombin index is prolonged.

2. Bromsulphthalein test (*see* Special Tests, Chapter 25) shows abnormal retention.

3. A barium swallow to demonstrate varices.

4. A blood-count may show leucopenia and thrombocytopenia due to 'hypersplenism'. In these circumstances the spleen is usually clinically palpable.

5. Liver biopsy demonstrates cirrhosis, but in view of the size of the regeneration nodules it is not unknown for an apparently 'normal' biopsy to be obtained from the middle of one of them. Usually 90 per cent of cases may be diagnosed in this way whilst collateral evidence may be obtainable by scintiscanning and peritoneoscopy. Diagnostic laparotomy should be avoided if possible.

TREATMENT

No specific treatment is required unless complications have occurred. It is usual to encourage a high protein intake unless this aggravates hepatic encephalopathy. Corticosteroid drugs are not indicated and in the presence of ascites and liver failure may cause infection, severe side-effects, and even increased mortality.

3. Haemochromatosis

AETIOLOGY

This disorder exists in two main forms:

1. A congenital variety (often familial) where there is an inborn error of iron metabolism (*Fig. 40*).

2. An acquired variety due either to therapeutic or dietary iron over-loading or associated with certain rare anaemias, e.g., sideroblastic anaemia, refractory anaemia (*Fig. 41*).

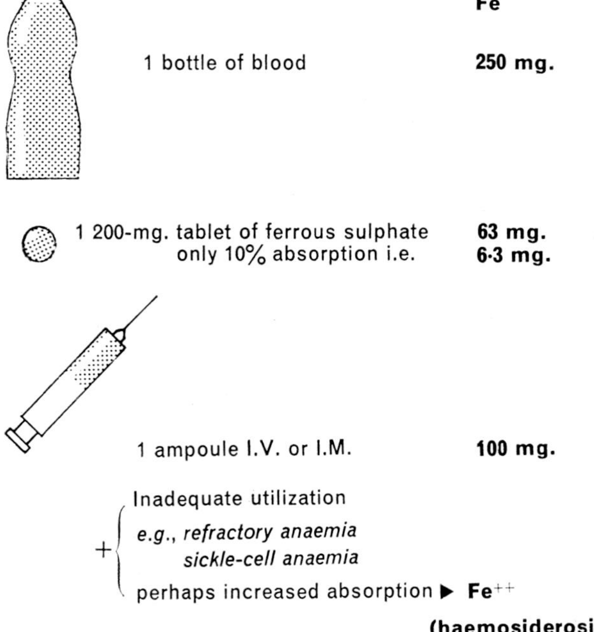

Fig. 41. Haemosiderosis.

It is generally agreed that in the first variety there is an excessive absorption of food iron perhaps because of abnormal avidity of the intestinal mucosa. Recently some evidence has been presented to suggest that an iron-binding protein in gastric juice, 'gastroferrin', may play a significant part in iron absorption. Deficiency of this protein is said to occur in primary haemochromatosis, thus resulting in diminished binding and excess absorption of iron. This work has not been completely confirmed. It has also been pointed out that the *alcoholic* is likely to develop haemochromatosis, and similar findings sometimes develop after portacaval anastomosis. The liver injury itself may therefore be important in determining the degree of 'clinical expression' of the disease, even though the basic defect may be an increased iron absorption. Some observers have shown increased iron absorption in cirrhosis, particularly after portacaval anastomosis, and in alcoholics wine may be an important dietary source of iron.

There has been much argument regarding the differences between the acquired and congenital forms of this disease, but most observers feel that true haemochromatosis can develop from acquired iron overload if the overload is large and continuous in time. Iron overloading without structural damage is called 'haemosiderosis'.

Owing to the safety valve of menstruation and pregnancy, haemochromatosis is largely a disease of middle-aged and elderly males, but elderly women or those who have had a hysterectomy or oophorectomy may suffer. The mode of inheritance is difficult to unravel because minor forms of the disease occur in which the only abnormality is increased iron in the liver, and this can only be detected by biopsy.

PATHOLOGY

The liver usually develops a micronodular type of cirrhosis. It is reddish in colour and usually enlarged. Iron, which can be detected by staining with Perls's reagent, is present in the liver and Kupffer cells. A good 'Oxford' blue colour is obtained in sections from well-established cases. Iron is also present in the *pancreas* where there may be destruction and fibrosis of glandular lesions and atrophy of the islets of Langerhans. It is also in excess in the *bone-marrow, heart muscle, skin,* and the *endocrine glands,* particularly the *testes* and *pituitary (Table 17).*

CLINICAL PICTURE

Classically, the picture is that of cirrhosis in a middle-aged male who has generalized slaty pigmentation of the skin. The patient complains of failing sexual drive and has noticed that shaving is less frequently necessary. Abdominal pain, located in the right upper abdomen, is a common complaint which is difficult to explain. The symptom complex of thirst, polyuria, and loss of weight indicates the presence of diabetes secondary to pancreatic destruction. Some studies have, however, suggested that the diabetes of haemochromatosis is not due to simple destruction of the pancreatic islets but that genetic factors may be involved. The spleen may or may not be palpable; cardiac involvement is indicated by the presence of cardiac arrhythmias, cardiomegaly, or even cardiac failure. The testes may be small and the body-hair sparse. The skin is smooth and fine.

Accompaniments and Complications

Neoplastic transformation is fairly common (15 per cent) and the diagnosis of hepatoma must be considered in any patient with haemochromatosis who begins to deteriorate physically. A syndrome of vasomotor collapse, abdominal pain, and muscle guarding, which has been described in this disease, is perhaps due to the release of vasodilator material from the liver. The diabetes is usually controlled by moderate doses of insulin, but ketosis and coma can occur. The complications of cirrhosis such as portal hypertension, fluid retention, and hepatic coma are rare, but depressive psychosis can develop.

Table 17. WHERE TO LOOK FOR INCREASED STORES OF TISSUE IRON

	DIRECT
Needle biopsy	Liver Bone-marrow Testes
Intestinal biopsy	Stomach Jejunum
Skin biopsy	
Urine examination	In centrifuged deposit (intracellular)
	INDIRECT (Organ dysfunction)
Pancreas	Glycosuria Diabetic glucose tolerance curve
Serum	High serum iron (200 μg. per cent or more) Saturated iron binding capacity (90 per cent or more)
Heart	E.C.G. (arrhythmia, inverted T waves, etc.)
Liver	Abnormal liver function tests
Testes	Low 17-ketosteroids in urine

A polyarthritis may also be present involving the small and large joints. On X-ray examination there may be erosions of articular surfaces and calcification of intra-articular cartilage. The joint fluid may contain crystals of calcium pyrophosphate (pseudo-gout).

DIAGNOSIS

In a classic case the diagnosis is obvious, but any male patient with cirrhosis should be suspected of haemochromatosis.

Helpful tests include:

1. A determination of the serum iron and the iron-binding capacity reveals that the serum iron is high and the iron-carrying protein fully saturated. Normal serum iron (male), 120 μg. per 100 ml. Normal iron-binding capacity, 300 μg. per 100 ml. Normal saturation approx. 30 per cent.

9*

2. Examination of the urine for sugar and a series of blood-glucose determinations will reveal overt diabetes. Latent diabetes can be detected by a glucose tolerance test. Thirty per cent of all cirrhotics have a diabetic tendency and many are pigmented. Thus haemochromatosis may be wrongly diagnosed. The diagnosis should never be made without full liver and biopsy studies.

3. The technique of tissue biopsy to detect iron deposits can be applied to the bone-marrow, liver, gastric or intestinal mucosa, and the testes. Skin biopsy is simple and may give a positive result, but in fact the majority of the skin pigmentation is due not to iron but to melanin.

4. The liver function tests are often normal in this disease in spite of a well-developed cirrhosis. The serum bilirubin, flocculation tests, and transaminases may be helpful.

5. Liver biopsy, besides confirming the presence of cirrhosis, is useful for detecting increased iron deposits (Perls's stain).

6. Radiographic studies may reveal the presence of oesophageal varices and, very rarely, the increased iron in the liver causes an opacity in the abdominal plain film, making the hepatic shadow denser than normal.

7. An E.C.G. may reveal evidence of myocardial damage, such as inverted T waves due to iron in the heart muscle.

8. An estimation of the total iron stores can be made by use of a differential ferrioxamine test. Desferrioxamine is a powerful iron-chelating agent. On chelation it changes to ferrioxamine. By giving radioactively labelled ferrioxamine (^{59}Fe) as well as unlabelled desferrioxamine a measurement of the total ferrioxamine produced by chelation can be made. This value correlates well with the clinical condition and differentiates between cirrhosis with haemosiderosis and true haemochromatosis. The change in total chelatable iron is a valuable way of following treatment.

9. Alpha fetoprotein studies may be helpful in suspected hepatoma which complicates 15 per cent of cases.

10. A megaloblastic anaemia due to associated folate deficiency may occur.

MANAGEMENT AND TREATMENT

The treatment of haemochromatosis is based on depleting the patient's stores of iron. The total iron stores may be raised from the normal 5 to 50 g. or more. The most satisfactory method of doing this is by repeated venesections, a pint of blood (250 mg. of iron) being removed every week for eighteen months to two years until the patient's haemoglobin and serum iron begin to fall.

Venesection may then be carried out at less frequent intervals, but a careful watch must be kept for evidence of relapse. Though desferriox-amine has been shown to be an effective chelating agent its effect is trivial compared with venesection. The change in total chelatable iron is a valuable way of following treatment.

Venesection does not usually affect the cirrhosis, and students must remember that it is done for the following reasons:

1. To effect an improvement in general health.

2. To prevent or improve myocardial involvement which is a common cause of death.

3. To improve the diabetes.

Skin pigmentation lessens as does liver size, but arthritis and sexual drive are not improved nor does the risk of hepatoma lessen.

Patients are often loath to attend for a treatment as drastic as weekly venesection. They should be told firmly about the nature of the disease and the reason for the form of treatment. The improvement in general health is usually enough to encourage them to attend, but one further 'bait' is the regular weekly prescription of testosterone to combat lack of energy and sexual drive.

Diabetes is treated in the usual way and insulin is usually required. Advice about alcohol is important. The liver should be re-examined in case a hepatoma develops. Haemochromatosis is a disease which needs prolonged treatment and close surveillance. The preventive aspects are of growing importance, and tests such as the serum iron–iron binding capacity, liver biopsy, and a differential ferrioxamine may be justified with detection of affected members of the family. These patients should then be treated by venesection until the serum and tissue iron are normal. A careful watch must be kept for hepatoma.

4. Primary Biliary Cirrhosis (Hanot's Cirrhosis; Chronic Non-suppurative Destructive Cholangitis)

AETIOLOGY

There is to date no known reason why this disease develops. Essentially, cirrhosis develops in a liver which is the subject of chronic intrahepatic biliary obstruction. The obstruction is at the level of the bile ductules, and amongst the theories forwarded to explain it are increased biliary viscosity, autoimmune damage, and hormonal factors, the latter suggested by the remarkable predilection of the disease for middle-aged females. Raised values for hepatic copper are found, but though these may be greater than those found in Wilson's disease the significance is unknown. The recent demonstration of the presence of mitochondrial antibodies in the serum of over 90 per cent of patients with the disease and the detection of granulomata around affected bile-ductules has strongly suggested an immunological basis for it. The granulomatous reaction is again a feature of the early disease and one of diagnostic importance.

PATHOLOGY

The liver is large, dark green, and finely cirrhotic. Microscopically, the important features are perilobular fibrosis, lack of bile-ducts in the portal tracts, as well as the features of intrahepatic biliary obstruction. It must be noted that early on there may be neither cholestasis nor cirrhosis.

CLINICAL PICTURE

The patient is usually a middle-aged female with mild obstructive jaundice. Pruritus is noticed before icterus and the skin may be covered with scratch marks. The liver is large and firm and the spleen usually palpable. The urine is dark, the faeces pale, and the jaundiced skin is often pigmented. Xanthomata occur on the eyelids and on the feet (*Fig. 42*) and hands,

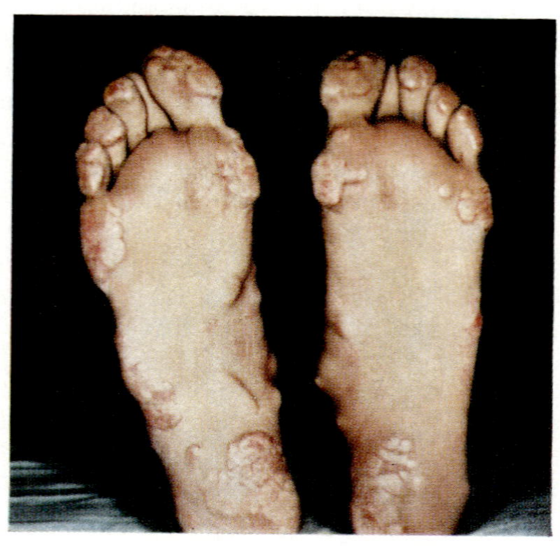

Fig. 42. Xanthomata on feet—primary biliary cirrhosis.

often at sites of pressure, such as under a wedding ring. In gross cases they form in the palmar creases, over bony prominences, on the soles of the feet, and in scars. They also occur in bone and peripheral nerves. Finger-clubbing is common.

Accompaniments and Complications (*Fig. 43*)

Bone pain and bone thinning due to osteoporosis, osteomalacia, and secondary hyperparathyroidism may occur. The osteomalacia is caused by malabsorption of vitamin D associated with the steatorrhoea of bile-salt deficiency. Abdominal pain may be due to peptic ulceration which is a common but unexplained complication of this disease. Bleeding due to prothrombin deficiency may occur. Teeth tend to become carious and dental extraction may be followed by troublesome haemorrhage.

The usual complications of cirrhosis, namely portal hypertension, hepatic coma, and fluid retention, tend to be of late onset, but are usually the cause of death five to ten years after the onset of the disease.

Helpful investigations in a suspected cause of primary biliary cirrhosis include:

1. Liver function tests, which show a serum bilirubin of about 5–10 mg. Most of the bilirubin is conjugated, and there is a raised alkaline

phosphatase greater than 30 K.A. units. The albumin may be normal in early cases and the flocculation tests are positive.

2. A barium meal, which may show varices, peptic ulceration, and flocculation of contrast in the small bowel due to steatorrhoea.

3. Bone radiographs, which show thinning and may show more specific evidence of osteomalacia (pseudo-fractures) and secondary hyperparathyroidism (subperiosteal erosions), best seen in the phalanges of the fingers.

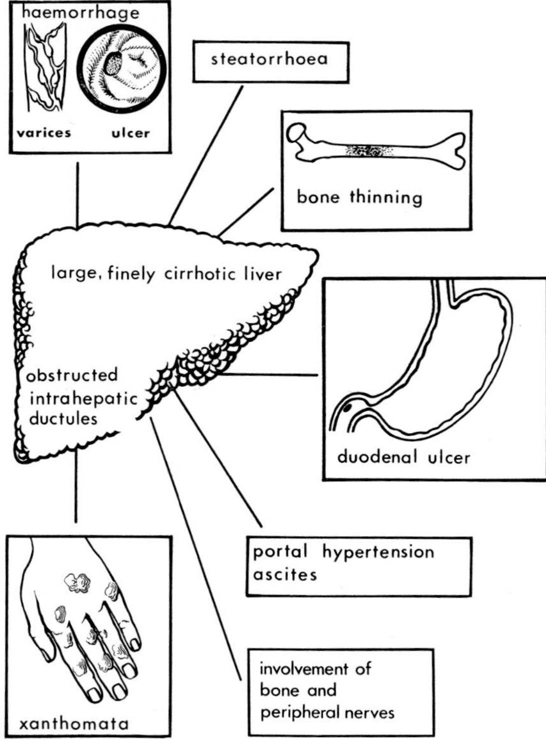

Fig. 43. Accompaniments of primary biliary cirrhosis.

4. Studies of the serum lipids, which show not only a raised total level but also a rise in the individual fractions—phospholipid, cholesterol, cholesterol esters, and neutral fat.

5. The blood contains mitrochondrial antibodies detected by fluorescent studies using mitochondrial preparations derived from rat or human tissue. Though not specific, the fact that over 90 per cent of patients with the disease have a positive test and that it is not found in patients with biliary cirrhosis secondary to extrahepatic obstruction is valuable diagnostically.

It is vital to make sure that the biliary cirrhosis is not secondary to extrahepatic biliary obstruction, and this is why the diagnosis must be firmly established by *laparotomy, liver biopsy,* and an *operative or endoscopic cholangiogram.* Primary biliary cirrhosis is a fatal disease, but secondary biliary cirrhosis may be surgically correctable.

MANAGEMENT AND TREATMENT

There is no cure for this disease and treatment is directed at the prevention of complications.

Pruritus responds to local applications or antihistamines in some cases. Methyl testosterone or the anabolic steroid norethandrolone (Nilevar), which is less androgenic, may be needed if itching is very troublesome. The patient is usually relieved to lose the pruritus, but buys it at the expense of increased jaundice. The use of an oral bile-salt–chelating substance— cholestyramine—may also be effective in the relief of skin irritation, but it is also likely to aggravate steatorrhoea (vitamin D absorption) and may reduce the prothrombin index. It is also unpleasant to take as at least in one form it has a fishy odour and very gritty consistency. It reduces the elevated cholesterol level—dose 6 g. three to four times daily. A more recently obtainable preparation, 'Questran' (Bristol Laboratories), is more pleasant to take. Many of these patients are afraid to go out because of unfavourable comments people make about the jaundice and pigmentation. They need great encouragement, and make-up, if skilfully applied, can restore their morale.

Regular injections of vitamin K, 20 mg., and vitamin D, 100,000 units, are given monthly to prevent bleeding and osteomalacia. Calcium lactate 1 g. three times a day, or calcium-Sandoz, will ensure an adequate calcium intake but may exacerbate the steatorrhoea. The latter, if troublesome, is usually improved by a low-fat, high-protein diet.

The complications of liver cell failure and portal hypertension are treated along the usual lines. The prognosis for life is usually of the order of five to ten years.

5. Chronic 'Active' Hepatitis; 'Juvenile' Cirrhosis (Lupoid Hepatitis, etc.)

AETIOLOGY

This disease is one of early adult life and is more common in females than in males. It is possible that some cases represent the effects of progressive viral hepatitis, and a certain percentage—small in this country—have a positive HAA reaction in the blood. These patients are more commonly males and may be a separate subgroup distinct from the young female sufferers who seem more common here. Because of certain findings, such as positive L.E. cell tests, a tendency to involvement of other organs besides the liver, hypergammaglobulinaemia, and prominent infiltration of the liver with plasma cells and lymphocytes, many observers feel that auto-immune factors play a significant role in the progression of the disease. Though commonest in the young adult the disease can occur at any age. The histology does not always show cirrhosis although a post-necrotic type of cirrhosis is the final end-result. Recently certain drugs, particularly the laxative oxyphenisatin, have been shown to be a further cause.

PATHOLOGY

The liver is enlarged in the early stages and as the disease progresses it shrinks and becomes coarsely cirrhotic. Microscopically, the evidence of liver cell injury is, in the active phase, swollen liver cells with hyaline degeneration. The portal tracts are infiltrated by lymphocytes and plasma cells. Small groups of liver cells are often cut off by advancing fibrous tissue, 'piecemeal necrosis'—so that small rosettes of liver cells are formed.

Fibrosis, starting focally, spreads so that bands of fibrous tissue surround developing regeneration nodules.

CLINICAL PICTURE

The classic picture in this condition is of a young, well-built, icteric female with hepatosplenomegaly and prominent cutaneous stigmata of liver disease. Amenorrhoea is almost invariable. Although attacks of pyrexia with constitutional upset may occur it is a surprising fact that most patients complain but little unless they are deeply jaundiced. If the jaundice is of sudden onset, as it is in about one-third of the cases, it resembles viral hepatitis, but commonly it is insidious. The chronicity of the jaundice (three months to ten years) is variable.

Interest in this disease is heightened by the fact that organs other than the liver are often involved, leading to the following manifestations (*Fig. 44*):

Arthralgia and arthritis
Skin rashes
L.E. cells in blood
Renal disease (nephritis, renal tract infection, glomerular lesions, renal tubular
  acidosis)
Ulcerative colitis
Psychosis
Pneumonia, pleurisy, and pericarditis
Diffuse pulmonary fibrosis—pulmonary hypertension
Haemolytic anaemia with positive Coombs test
Hashimoto's disease
Diabetes
Sjögren's syndrome

The above are usually found during active phases of the disease, but occasionally one of the 'extrahepatic' features precedes the onset of the hepatic disorder.

The disease is chronic and many patients die of liver failure after four or five years. Relapses and remissions occur, the former aggravated by intercurrent infection. Occasionally the disease seems to burn itself out, though the patient may be left with a macronodular cirrhosis.

DIAGNOSIS

Though the diagnosis is essentially clinical, help is given by:

1. *Liver Function Tests.* These show moderate jaundice, raised transaminase, and strongly positive flocculation tests. The serum proteins are grossly abnormal, the albumin is usually more than 3 g., but the globulins are much increased, particularly the gamma-globulin fraction. The fraction may sometimes appear as quite a narrow band on the electrophoretic strip.

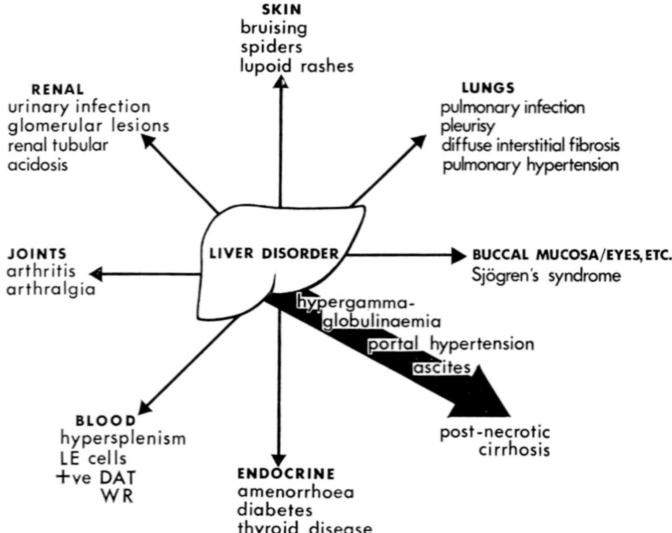

Fig. 44. Associated diseases in 'juvenile' cirrhosis.

2. *Various Serum Reactions.* These give false-positive tests because of the abnormal globulins, including the Wassermann reaction and the differential agglutination test (D.A.T.). Of more diagnostic help is the finding of a positive ANF (antinuclear factor) and rheumatoid factor together with a positive reaction with the patient's serum against smooth muscle (SMA). These patients may also show a positive test for mitochondrial antibodies (30 per cent).

3. The *Coombs test* may be positive and there may be an accompanying haemolytic anaemia.

4. The *blood* may contain L.E. cells. This feature has led some observers to call this condition '*lupoid hepatitis*', and some have believed it to be synonymous with disseminated lupus erythematosus—though in this disease SMA is not present—an important point of distinction.

5. Liver biopsy.

6. Investigation of extrahepatic involvement.

MANAGEMENT AND TREATMENT

If corticosteroids are used there is little doubt that they control 'extra-hepatic' manifestations such as arthritis, ulcerative colitis, and haemolytic anaemia. They also have a beneficial effect on liver cell function, for in most patients bilirubin and transaminase levels fall, and in some patients the globulin levels too. As liver cell function improves menstruation returns. Prednisone is the most convenient corticosteroid drug, and after 30 mg. daily for 7 days a maintenance dose sufficient to control symptoms and prevent the return of icterus is given. It is important to remember that these patients develop side-effects even from small doses, so that a mere 10 mg. a day may be all that can be tolerated. The therapy should be maintained for a year and then withdrawn gradually, but a return of symptoms and jaundice calls for further treatment. Every effort should be made to 'wean' patients from corticosteroids at yearly intervals, for not only are the side-effects troublesome but growth of the young may be impaired. After a lapse of several years and despite normal liver function tests withdrawal of corticosteroids may yet cause a relapse.

Temporary exacerbations caused by intermittent infection must be treated by increased dosage. Sepsis, and especially septicaemia, is a danger, so that careful supervision is necessary.

A trial of immunosuppressive therapy with azathioprine (Imuran), 75–150 mg. daily, has been made in this disease. This therapy may be indicated where the disease appears resistant to corticosteroids or where the side-effects of this treatment are too severe to be tolerated. Azathioprine by itself is generally less effective than corticosteroids but neither seems able to stop the progression to cirrhosis. A low dose of azathioprine (75 mg.) does not usually cause bone-marrow depression and allows use of a smaller dose of prednisone. There has been a recent report of a double-blind trial of corticosteroids in this disease which shows a distinct improvement in mortality as a result of its use compared with a placebo. The mortality in the treated group was about a quarter of that in the untreated.

6. Hepatolenticular Degeneration (Kinnier-Wilson's Disease) (*Fig. 45*)

AETIOLOGY

The basis of this disease is abnormal metabolism of copper. Most authorities conclude that the major abnormality is a deficiency of the protein caeruloplasmin which loosely binds copper in the serum. As a result, copper attaches itself to tissue protein and thus high copper concentration is responsible for the clinical features such as damage to the basal ganglia of the brain, the corneal rings (Kayser-Fleischer rings), hepatic cirrhosis, and probably the renal tubular lesion as well.

The disease is inherited as an autosomal recessive and therefore affected children are sometimes the offspring of cousin marriages.

PATHOLOGY

The liver usually shows a macronodular type of cirrhosis. Excessive deposits of copper can be demonstrated by staining with rubeanic acid. In the basal ganglia of the brain there are degenerative changes and in severe cases frank cavitation.

The disease causes symptoms before the age of 20 years and males are rather more susceptible than females. Siblings may be found who suffer either from asymptomatic or overt forms of the disease and it is important to distinguish them from the unaffected (heterozygotes).

In classic cases the diagnosis is easy. There is a combination of physical signs indicating damage to the central nervous system and the liver. Thus, there may be some mental deterioration, a rather characteristic dysarthria,

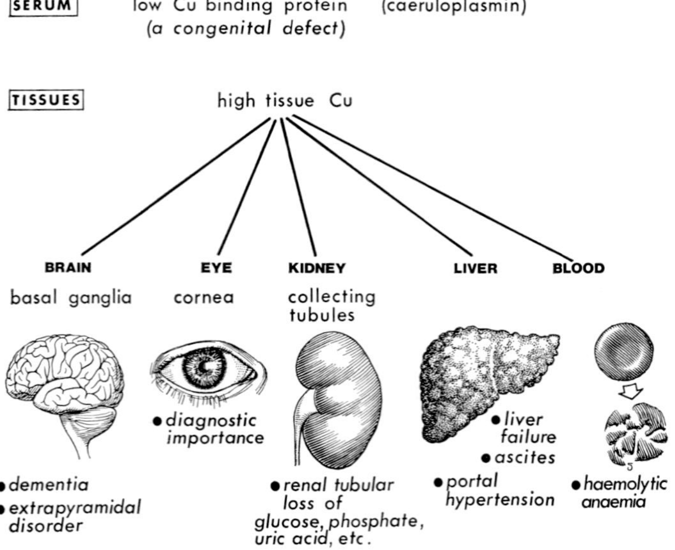

Fig. 45. Kinnier-Wilson's disease.

and involuntary movements. The latter vary from slight intention tremor of the hands to gross spontaneous movements of the limbs and head. The patient smiles vacuously and drools saliva.

The hepatic features of the disease are variable and some patients have had attacks of jaundice. In some cases this is associated with acute haemolysis due to a rapid increase in serum-copper levels sufficient to produce red-cell damage. The increased serum levels are derived from tissue stores. Bleeding from oesophageal varices, ascites, and peripheral oedema are not uncommon. Hepatosplenomegaly may be present.

The physical sign which is always present in chronic adolescent and adult cases, and which clinches the diagnosis, is the corneal ring (Kayser-Fleischer ring) of brownish copper-containing pigment seen just within the corneosclerotic junction (*Fig. 46*). It can usually be discovered with the aid of a torch if the beam of light is directed across the front of the cornea, but in difficult cases a slit lamp may be required. This sign may not be present in young children.

When the main features are hepatic, as in those with portal hypertension or fluid retention, the diagnosis will not be made unless Kayser-Fleischer rings are carefully looked for, and this is especially important in the younger cirrhotic patient. A simple screening test to measure serum copper oxidase (*see below*) is probably justifiable in all such patients. Difficulty can also arise where the symptoms and signs are purely neurological and rapidly progressive.

Accompaniments and Complications

Amino-aciduria is found, and up to 10 g. may be excreted in four hours (normal, less than 1 g.). The amino-aciduria is part of a general renal tubular dysfunction which causes glycosuria and increased excretion of

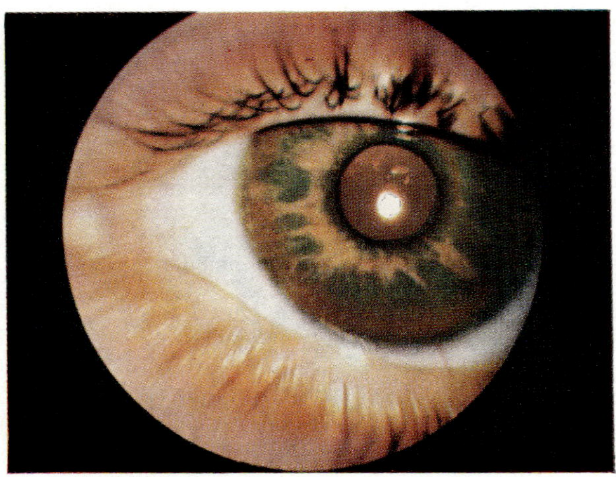

Fig. 46. The Kayser-Fleischer ring.

phosphate and uric acid. Serum levels of phosphate and uric acid therefore drop and, rarely, osteomalacia may occur. Another rare finding is degenerative joint disease. The lunulae of the finger and toe-nails may be coloured blue, perhaps by increased tissue copper.

DIAGNOSIS

Helpful tests are:

1. The estimation in the serum of copper oxidase activity which is proportional to the concentrations of caeruloplasmin. The levels are low (<20 mg. per 100 ml.).

2. Hepatic histology: apart from cirrhosis—fatty change, Mallory's hyaline, and a rather characteristic swelling of liver cell nuclei with glycogen inclusions are seen.

3. Estimation of tissue copper in needle biopsy material from the liver. The fresh tissue must be placed in 1 per cent rubeanic acid in 70 per cent

alcohol if copper is to be demonstrated and another specimen must be stained by conventional methods to demonstrate cirrhosis. Estimation of *total* copper in liver biopsy material is an important way of differentiating the homo- from the heterozygote. The critical level is >25 mg. copper per 100 g. dry weight of liver.

4. Estimation of urinary copper will show increased daily excretion (normal less than 100 μg. per 24 hours). In Wilson's disease excretion is usually 200–1000 μg. per 24 hours.

5. Liver function tests—these may suggest cirrhosis.

6. Urine examination shows amino-aciduria and possibly glycosuria.

7. Radiographic studies of the bones may demonstrate bone thinning and osteoarthritic changes. A barium swallow may reveal oesophageal varices.

In recent years it has been shown that patients with Wilson's disease may have total caeruloplasmin levels which are normal, but fractionation may reveal abnormalities.

MANAGEMENT AND TREATMENT

The basis of treatment is the removal of excess copper from the patient by the use of chelating agents. Until Walshe introduced penicillamine, B.A.L. was used, but has now been abandoned in favour of penicillamine (dimethyl cysteine) which is more effective and can be given by mouth. The dosage is 1–2 g. of D-penicillamine daily in four doses before meals, but allergic skin rashes may occur which can be troublesome enough for desensitization by small doses to be needed. Another alarming feature is the tendency for neurological deterioration to occur during the first few days of treatment. Side-effects also include leucopenia and a nephrotic syndrome, whilst pyridoxine deficiency (associated with an anti-vitamin B_6 action) is a theoretical possibility. The improvement is greatest in the neuropsychiatric condition. Tremor lessens so that the handwriting improves, mental brightening occurs, and the whole outlook of the patient changes. Patients may return to responsible work or school. Kayser-Fleischer rings become less obvious and may disappear.

The prognosis is that of the underlying cirrhosis, and most patients succumb to liver cell failure even if 'decoppering' is effective.

It is customary to administer potassium sulphide 20 mg. three times a day in conjunction with penicillamine, the aim being to prevent copper absorption from the food by precipitating it in the gut as copper sulphide.

The treatment of siblings who do not have the full disease but who have increased hepatic copper is important, for in this way progression of the disorder can be prevented. A careful clinical examination of siblings and serum and liver histology studies is essential. Increased amounts of copper have been found in some patients with familial juvenile cirrhosis. These patients have no other evidence of Wilson's disease, and though the exact significance is unknown, 'decoppering' should be carried out. Others have suggested that similar treatment should be used in patients with primary biliary cirrhosis where liver copper is also high, presumably due to biliary obstruction.

FURTHER READING

Alcoholic Liver Disease
BRUNT, P.W. (1971), 'Alcohol and the Liver', Progress report, *Gut*, **12**, 222.
PHILLIPS, G. B., and DAVIDSON, C. S. (1954), 'Acute, Hepatic Insufficiency in the Chronic Alcoholic; Clinical and Pathological Study', *Archs intern. Med.*, **94**, 585.

Alcoholic Cirrhosis and Cryptogenic Cirrhosis
SUMMERSKILL, W. H., DAVIDSON, C. S., DIBLE, J. H., MALLORY, C. K., SHERLOCK, S., TURNER, M. D., and WOLFE, S. (1960), 'Cirrhosis of the Liver—A Study of Alcoholic and Non-alcoholic Patients in Boston and London', *New Engl. J. Med.*, **262**, 1.

Haemochromatosis
FINCH, S. C., and FINCH, C. A. (1955), 'Idiopathic Haemochromatosis, an Iron Storage Disease', *Medicine, Baltimore*, **34**, 381.
WILLIAMS, R. W., SCHEUER, P. J., and SHERLOCK, S. (1962), 'The Inheritance of Idiopathic Haemochromatosis', *Q. Jl Med.*, **31**, 249.

Primary Biliary Cirrhosis
ATKINSON, M., NORDIN, B. E. C., and SHERLOCK, S. (1956), 'Malabsorption and Bone Disease in Prolonged Obstructive Jaundice', *Ibid.*, **25**, 299.
SHERLOCK, S. (1959), 'Primary Biliary Cirrhosis (Chronic Intrahepatic Obstructive Jaundice)', *Gastroenterology*, **37**, 574.
— — (1968), 'Chronic Cholangitides: Aetiology, Diagnosis, and Treatment', *Br. med. J.*, **3**, 515.

Wilson's Disease
BEARN, A. G. (1957), 'Wilson's Disease. An Inborn Error of Metabolism with Multiple Manifestations', *Am. J. Med.*, **22**, 747.
WALSHE, J. M. (1959), 'Current Views on the Pathogenesis and Treatment of Wilson's Disease', *Archs intern. Med.*, **103**, 155.
— — (1970), 'Wilson's Disease, its Diagnosis and Management', *Br. J. Hosp. Med.*, **4**, 91.
WILSON, S. A. K. (1912), 'Progressive Lenticular Degeneration—A Familiar Nervous Disorder associated with Cirrhosis of the Liver', *Brain*, **34**, 295.

Chronic Active Hepatitis
COOK, G. C., MULLIGAN, R., and SHERLOCK, S. (1971), 'Controlled Prospective Trial of Corticosteroid Therapy in Active Chronic Hepatitis', *Q. Jl Med.*, **40**, 159.
DONIACH, D., WALKER, J. G., ROITT, I. M., and BERG, P. A. (1970), 'Auto-allergic Hepatitis', *New Engl. J. Med.*, **282**, 86.
MACKAY, I. R. (1968), 'Chronic Hepatitis: Effect of Prolonged Suppressive Treatment and Comparison of Azathioprine with Prednisolone', *Q. Jl Med.*, **37**, 379.
READ, A. E., SHERLOCK, S., and HARRISON, C. V. (1963), 'Active "Juvenile" Cirrhosis considered as Part of a Systemic Disease and the Effect of Corticosteroid Therapy', *Gut*, **4**, 378.

General
SCHEUER, P. J. (1970), 'Liver Biopsy in the Diagnosis of Cirrhosis', *Gut*, **11**, 275.

Chapter 14

The Complications of Cirrhosis

Portal Hypertension (*Fig. 47*)

CIRRHOSIS IS NOT the only condition associated with portal hypertension. The following scheme is the usual way in which portal hypertension is classified.

	CAUSE	LESION
1. *Presinusoidal*		
Extrahepatic	1. Portal vein obstruction	Portal vein thrombosis
Intrahepatic	2. Portal venule obstruction	*a.* Hepatic fibrosis, e.g., Schistosomiasis Congenital hepatic fibrosis Tropical splenomegaly (also increased splenic blood-flow) *b.* Hepatic infiltration (reticulosis, sarcoid)
2. *Postsinusoidal*		
Intrahepatic	1. Nodular regeneration	Cirrhosis
Extrahepatic	2. Blocked hepatic veins	Budd-Chiari syndrome
3. *Increased splenic blood-flow*	1. Splenic A.V. shunt	Splenic arteriovenous fistula
	2. Massive splenomegaly (plus/minus hepatic cellular infiltration and portal venous occlusion)	*a.* Tropical splenomegaly *b.* Myelosclerosis

Measurement of Portal Vein Pressure (Fig. 48)

In any variety of portal hypertension proof of the diagnosis can be obtained by measuring the portal venous pressure. Three methods can be used clinically:

1. MEASUREMENT OF THE PRESSURE IN THE PULP OF THE SPLEEN

A needle is inserted into the splenic pulp. The spleen is enlarged so this is usually easy. Pressure can be measured by a simple saline manometer or with a strain gauge. (Normal less than 15 mm. Hg.)

2. MEASUREMENT OF THE 'WEDGED' HEPATIC VEIN PRESSURE

A cardiac catheter is passed into a hepatic vein under radiographic control. By passing the catheter until it 'wedges' in a hepatic venule and by measuring the pressure at that point one *assumes* that this represents portal venous pressure.

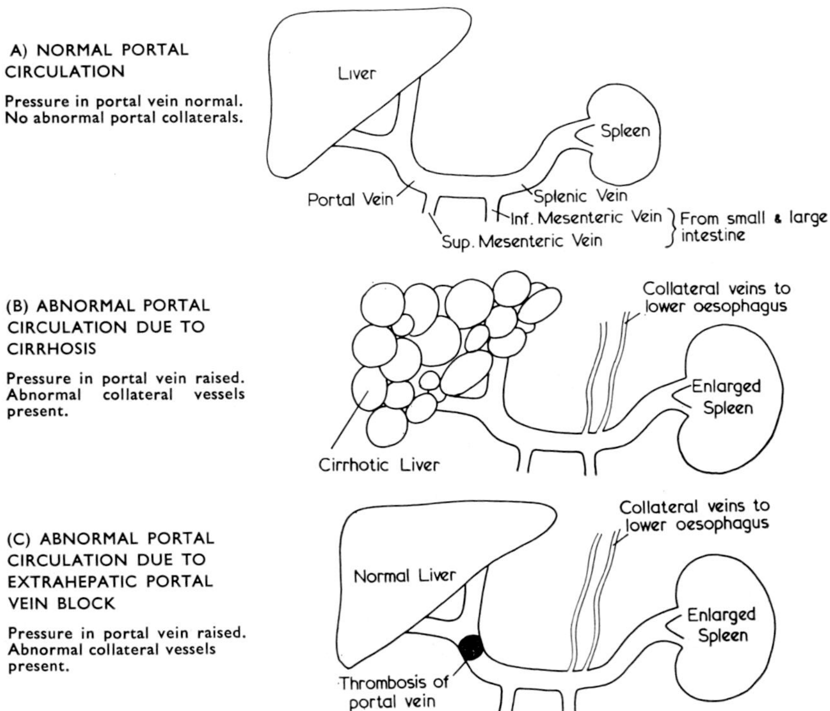

Fig. 47. Portal hypertension.

3. MEASUREMENT OF INTRAHEPATIC PORTAL VENOUS PRESSURE USING A FINE NEEDLE

AETIOLOGY

Cirrhosis is an example (the most important one in England) of portal hypertension due to obstruction of the postsinusoidal type.

Any type of cirrhosis may be complicated by portal hypertension, but perhaps it is most characteristically seen in the macronodular variety.

Portal hypertension occurs because there is distortion of intrahepatic portal and hepatic venous channels by regeneration nodules. An equally important factor is the development of shunts between the hepatic artery and the portal vein in the regeneration nodules so that the portal vasculature is exposed to arterial pressure. Other vascular abnormalities are found in the cirrhotic liver and some of the portal venous blood may be

shunted directly into the systemic circulation by intrahepatic communications. Some observers feel that pressor substances in the portal blood-
stream may increase portal venous pressure and aggravate portal hypertension.

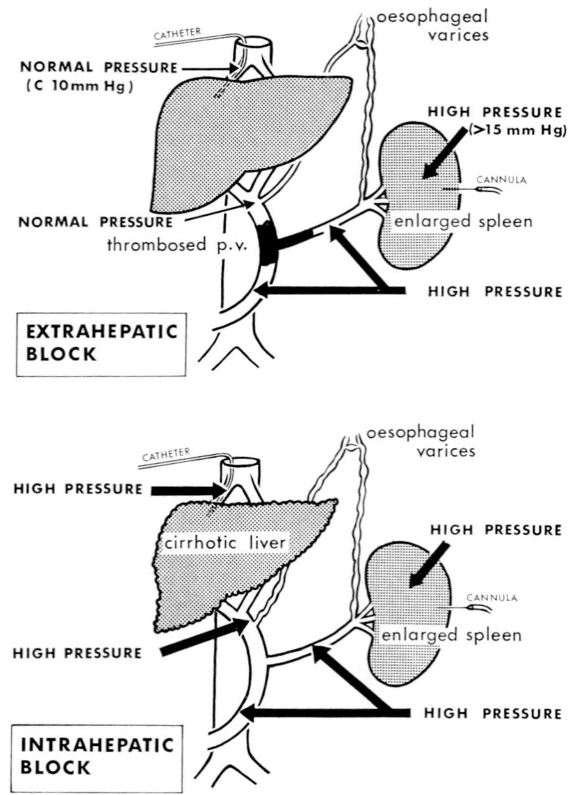

Fig. 48. Portal venous pressure in intra- and extrahepatic obstruction.

PATHOLOGY

The spleen is enlarged from congestion and fibrosis. The capsule is
thickened. The splenic and portal veins are often dilated and may be
thrombosed. Collateral vessels develop, but these are poorly seen at
post-mortem. They are of such importance that a separate description is
indicated.

The Collateral Circulation

Abnormal communications (collateral channels) of clinical importance
develop between the portal vein and the following systemic veins:

1. Veins at the lower end of the oesophagus and gastric fundus (left
gastric and short gastric veins). *These form oesophageal and gastric varices*
which may bleed.

2. Prominent veins are often visible on the abdominal wall and, rarely, they may form a caput medusae around the umbilicus. A murmur may be heard over these collaterals (Cruveilhier-Baumgarten syndrome).

3. Between the inferior mesenteric vessels and the haemorrhoidal veins. *Haemorrhoids* may result from these communications, but students must remember that haemorrhoids in adults are very common and portal hypertension is a rare cause. In babies and young children haemorrhoids usually have an organic cause and portal hypertension is an important one. The inferior mesenteric vein may be considerably enlarged to form systemic communications of its own.

4. Diaphragmatic and retroperitoneal veins with occasional communication with the adrenal, renal, and lumbar veins.

All varieties of collateral vessels carry blood containing nitrogenous products from the alimentary tract directly into the systemic circulation, producing cerebral intoxication and therefore *hepatic encephalopathy*.

Rarely, *cyanosis* develops in patients with portal hypertension because of portopulmonary communications or arteriovenous shunts in the lung. The collateral vessels, by avoiding the filter of the liver, facilitate the development of *E. coli septicaemia*, a not uncommon complication of cirrhosis.

CLINICAL PICTURE

The main clinical manifestation of portal hypertension is alimentary bleeding of variable severity. It can range from severe haematemesis to slow oozing with positive occult blood in the stools. Melaena may occur alone or with haematemesis.

Accompaniments and Complications

Bleeding from varices may be complicated by the following:

1. Jaundice	These are due to further impairment of liver cell function caused by blood-loss and hypotension.
2. Ascites and oedema	
3. Neuropsychiatric deterioration	

DIAGNOSIS

The history may indicate alcoholism, previous hepatitis, haemochromatosis, or Wilson's disease. The possible existence of portal vein obstruction and its principal causes (*Fig. 47*) should not be forgotten. The patient must be examined most carefully for cutaneous evidence of chronic liver disease, hepatomegaly, and splenomegaly. Portal hypertension always causes the spleen to enlarge, and if this is not detected clinically obesity or poor technique may be responsible. If there is doubt the patient should be turned on the right side and examined bimanually.

Hepatic foetor is usually present when collateral vessels link the portal (gut) with the systemic (mouth) circulation. Slight jaundice can best be detected by careful examination of the sclera in a good light.

Helpful tests include the following:

1. A barium meal to verify the presence of varices and to exclude an alternative source of bleeding, e.g., peptic ulcer. Films may also reveal splenomegaly or confirm its clinical presence.

2. A bromsulphthalein (BSP) and other liver function tests. (*See* Special Investigations, Chapter 24.)

3. The blood-count will show anaemia due to haemorrhage, and leucopenia and thrombocytopenia associated with the enlarged spleen (hypersplenism).

4. Endoscopy to show varices if the diagnosis is in doubt.

5. Splenic venography is required to decide whether the bleeding is due to intrahepatic or extrahepatic obstruction of the portal vein. If the spleen has been removed coeliac axis angiography may be used to visualize contrast returning from the spleen via the splenic and portal vein. Otherwise umbilico-portography may be useful though this will require surgical aid.

6. If the Sengstaken compression tube is passed and the bleeding stops, this suggests that oesophageal varices are the cause.

MANAGEMENT AND TREATMENT

The routine treatment of alimentary haemorrhage includes half-hourly pulse and blood-pressure determinations, elevation of the foot of the bed, and blood transfusion where necessary. Sedation, particularly with morphine, must be avoided. If haemorrhage continues, two methods of 'medical' attack are possible:

1. It has been shown that posterior pituitary extract (vasopressin), by means of its constrictive effect on plain muscle in arterioles, reduces the inflow of blood into the portal circulation. Vasopressin, 20 units, is usually given in a 5 per cent dextrose drip over 15–30 minutes. Though it may succeed in stopping haemorrhage it is unpleasant for the patient because it produces abdominal colic, and it is dangerous in patients with coronary artery disease. If successful it can be repeated. The administration of a potent preparation of vasopressin usually produces a bowel movement which can be beneficial in the prevention of hepatic coma. Pitressin by reducing hepatic arterial blood-flow can compromise liver function. Another possible way of stopping variceal haemorrhage is by the use of gastric cooling. The apparatus for this is complicated and the basis of it is that a coolant mixture is circulated through a gastric balloon which is shaped to fit the stomach and is swallowed by the patient.

2. If vasopressin and/or gastric cooling fails and if the patient can be made fit enough for a surgical attack on the bleeding varices it may be justifiable to pass a Sengstaken tube (*Fig. 49*). This triple-lumen tube has two balloons, one spherical, which compresses fundal veins in the stomach, and one tubular, which compresses the oesophageal varices and anchors the apparatus (*Fig. 50*). The apparatus is, in our experience, best passed through the mouth. The gastric balloon is then filled with 10 per cent diodone to indicate its position radiologically. Gentle traction allows the gastric balloon to fit snugly into the fundus. The oesophageal balloon is

distended to 25 or 30 mm. Hg to counteract the elevated portal blood-pressure in the varices. Once the oesophageal balloon has been inflated it is important that (*a*) the nurse never leaves the patient; (*b*) the pharynx must be aspirated frequently by a mechanical sucker, because the patient is unable to swallow.

The hazards of this apparatus must be understood. Because of rupture of the gastric balloon it may ride up the oesophagus to cause *laryngeal obstruction*. If this happens the nurse must first deflate the apparatus by cutting it across with scissors and then rapidly withdraw it.

Respiratory infection is counteracted by physiotherapy, prophylactic antibiotics, and frequent changing of position.

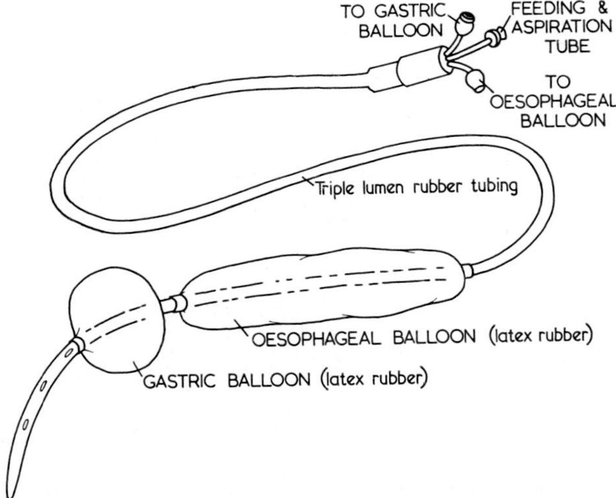

Fig. 49. The Sengstaken oesophageal compression tube.

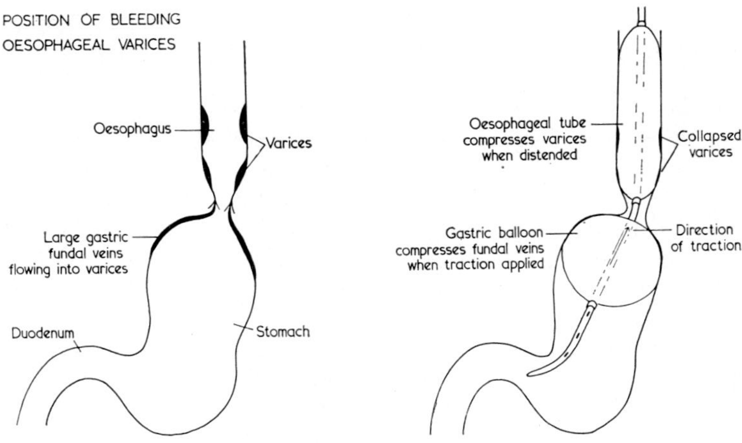

Fig. 50. Mode of action of Sengstaken tube.

Ulceration of the pharynx, lower oesophagus, and fundus of the stomach is prevented by using traction only when absolutely necessary and applying it intermittently.

Regular aspiration of the stomach will detect renewed bleeding.

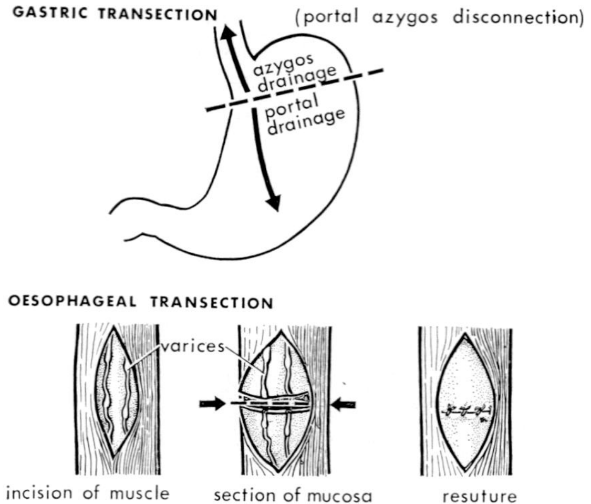

Fig. 51. Gastric and oesophageal transection.

Treatment to prevent or alleviate coma or impaired consciousness is given (*see* p. 208).

The Sengstaken tube is a most uncomfortable and potentially dangerous piece of apparatus. It is unjustifiable to use it if patients with terminal liver disease are bleeding. In these patients injection of sclerosant solutions into the oesophageal varices is the only sort of therapy which can be used, though if haemorrhage can be stopped liver function may improve enough for more radical surgery. A recent suggestion has been that decompression of the portal system by umbilical vein catheterization and/or thoracic duct drainage could be helpful; in fit patients without evidence of liver cell failure, when haemorrhage is not stopped by liberal blood transfusion, vitamin K by injection, and vasopressin, it may be used to prepare the patient for surgery.

The emergency surgical treatment is usually a direct attack on the varices by gastric or oesophageal transection, or more simply a trans-oesophageal ligation of varices without transection (*Fig. 51*), but in some centres an emergency portacaval anastomosis is performed. The mortality of an emergency portacaval anastomosis operation is, however, high (>25 per cent), and careful selection is essential. As opposed to this, oesophageal ligation is a much easier and less hazardous operation.

If the patient recovers from the bleeding, either spontaneously or after emergency treatment, he should be considered for the operation of elective portacaval anastomosis. This reduces the portal pressure by anastomosing the portal vein (high pressure) to the inferior vena cava (low pressure). The operation can be done as an end-to-side or side-to-side operation (*Fig. 52*).

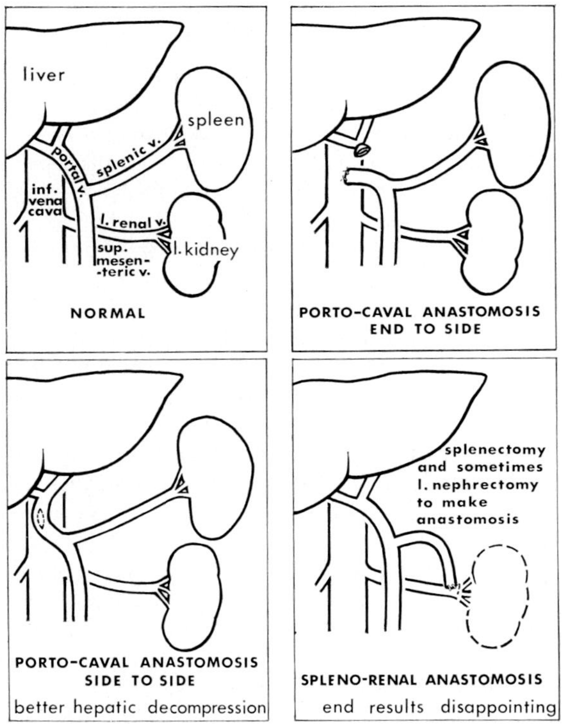

Fig. 52. Shunt operations designed to relieve portal hypertension.

The following are required for a successful anastomosis:

1. There must be a patent portal vein to use.

2. Liver function must be adequate (no jaundice, albumin 3 g. per cent or more, no ascites, no neuropsychiatric episodes).

3. Preferably the patients should be young, as those over 50 years of age are more likely to develop neuropsychiatric complications.

In order to demonstrate a normal portal vein, a splenic venogram is performed. If the spleen has been removed previously a mesenteric venogram is done at laparotomy.

The likelihood of neuropsychiatric deterioration after operation can be assessed preoperatively by observing the patient and his E.E.G. records while he is taking a high protein diet or a diet supplemented with NH_4Cl or methionine. This will simulate the postoperative cerebral intoxication by nitrogenous breakdown products.

If operation is successful the results are as follows:

1. Haemorrhage does not recur.

2. Oesophageal varices shrink and, after a few months, may disappear.

3. Abdominal collateral veins vanish.

4. The spleen diminishes in size—this can start within an hour or so of operation.

5. In some patients there may be further impairment of liver function so that postoperative jaundice and ankle oedema occur.

6. Neuropsychiatric complications may appear in the immediate post-operative period or later, because of the large artificial shunt.

7. Some patients develop a secondary haemochromatosis following a successful shunt operation. This is probably due to increased iron absorption and availability following cessation of alimentary bleeding and also due to continuing liver disease.

Failure to observe these changes means that the shunt has probably not been successful and in these patients ascites and a gross collateral circulation on the abdominal wall develop.

Although this operation can stop the patient from dying of haemorrhage, liver function is likely to be impaired by the deprivation of the portal blood-supply. If an anastomosis cannot be done, resection or transection may be tried, but the results are inferior (*see Fig. 51*).

Because of the small size of the vessels used, splenorenal anastomosis rarely produces a satisfactory drop in portal pressure. It is done only if portacaval anastomosis is impossible because the portal vein is thrombosed or if the patient is not fit for a portacaval shunt. Several series of cases have shown that there is no indication for the operation of prophylactic portacaval anastomosis for patients who have varices but who have not bled. Such operations do not alter the mortality—merely it's causes.

Note on Extrahepatic Portal Vein Obstruction

If the portal or splenic veins are obstructed before the latter enters the liver, extrahepatic portal hypertension develops.

The chief cause of portal blockage outside the liver is sepsis. This may come from any septic lesion in the abdomen. Infection of the umbilical stump after birth and thrombosis following exchange transfusion via the umbilical vein are recognized causes. Septic thrombosis of the portal vein in the adult may result from acute diverticulitis, cholecystitis, or appendicitis and may occasionally occur in the postpartum period. In some cases a cavernomatous malformation of the portal vein is thought not to be congenital, but to be the *result* of portal obstruction. In adults, thrombosis of the portal vein occurs because of pressure from tumours and cysts, and in polycythaemia.

The *similarities* between extrahepatic and intrahepatic (cirrhotic) obstruction of the portal vein are:

1. Haemorrhage from varices and splenomegaly.

2. Hepatic foetor.

The *differences* between extrahepatic and intrahepatic obstruction of the portal vein are as follows:

In extrahepatic obstruction:

1. Patients are usually young.

2. There is a lack of cutaneous stigmata of liver disease.

3. The liver is of normal size, at least initially.

4. Jaundice, ascites, and neuropsychiatric complications after haemorrhage are rare.

5. The liver function tests are normal, apart from abnormal retention of B.S.P. and occasionally raised alkaline phosphatase. Liver function may, however, deteriorate with long-standing occlusion and this may account for odd examples of hepatic failure following intestinal haemorrhage.

6. The histology of the liver is normal.

Proof of extrahepatic portal vein obstruction can be obtained:

1. By catheterization of the hepatic veins and failing to find a raised 'wedged' pressure in the hepatic veins (*see Fig. 48*).

2. By demonstrating a block in the portal vein and an accompanying collateral circulation on a splenic venogram or coeliac axis arteriogram.

MANAGEMENT AND TREATMENT

Though bleeding may be severe, these patients, who have no liver disease, run little risk of liver cell failure, which is the chief cause of mortality in patients with cirrhosis. For this reason, most patients can be managed conservatively. Operations designed to remove the varix-bearing area of the oesophagus and stomach are not a certain cure. The portal vein is rarely obstructed high enough for sufficient tissue to be left to allow portacaval anastomosis, but if it is, patients can be cured surgically. If the portal vein is occluded it may be possible to anastomose the superior mesenteric vein end to side to the I.V.C. which is transected and the distal end ligated (cavo-mesenteric shunt). Splenectomy is often disappointing and may be dangerous because thrombus may spread along the portal vein postoperatively. The high concentration of platelets after this operation may be responsible for this.

The multiplicity of surgical operations devised to prevent bleeding in those with extrahepatic portal hypertension is an index of their unreliability.

Congenital Hepatic Fibrosis

This is a variant of the inherited disorder congenital polycystic disease. The patients may have both renal and hepatic involvement. The hepatic involvement may be due to cyst formation when a massive nodular—and occasionally painful—hepatomegaly is produced or there may be a massive intrahepatic fibrosis without cyst formation. Congenital bile-duct dilatation may also occur (*Table 18*). Congenital hepatic fibrosis causes portal hypertension by obstructing intrahepatic portal vein radicles. The result of this is bleeding from oesophageal varices usually occurring in childhood or early adult life. The family history (of renal failure and hypertension) is often helpful. The liver is enlarged and extremely firm, the kidneys may occasionally be palpable and the liver function tests, apart from the alkaline phosphatase (which is raised), are normal.

The disease is often called 'cirrhosis' and the liver may be so hard that needle biopsy is impossible. A history of one or more unsuccessful attempts at needle liver biopsy in a young patient with 'cirrhosis' and a large liver and spleen should make one suspect such a diagnosis. The portal hypertension is presinusoidal in type and such patients may need a portacaval anastomosis. Wedge biopsy of the liver confirms the diagnosis and shows the normal basic liver architecture and the massive fibrosis and portal venous obliteration.

Though portacaval anastomosis is well tolerated and liver cell function is preserved postoperative renal failure (due to associated renal cystic involvement) is a danger.

Table 18. HEPATIC LESIONS ASSOCIATED WITH POLYCYSTIC DISEASE

LESION	RESULTS
a. Polycystic liver	'Nodular' hepatomegaly Pain
b. Congenital hepatic fibrosis	Hepatosplenomegaly Portal hypertension
c. Congenital dilatation of intrahepatic bile-ducts	Cholangitis Bile-duct stone formation Bile-duct carcinoma

Partial Nodular Transformation of the Liver

This is a rare cause of portal hypertension but a further example of a disorder like extrahepatic portal vein occlusion and congenital hepatic fibrosis where portal hypertension exists with good liver function. The disease is of unknown cause, but there is replacement of much of the liver by a nodular transformation of the parenchyma without much fibrosis and certainly without cirrhosis. It is difficult to diagnose but should be suspected where portal hypertension exists without signs of liver cell failure and where the liver is of normal size. Treatment of bleeding oesophageal varices—the major complication of this disorder—is satisfactorily obtained by portacaval anastomosis. Because of the fact that much of the liver tissue may be normal or even occasionally atrophic the disorder is difficult to diagnose on a random needle biopsy.

ASCITES IN LIVER DISEASE

AETIOLOGY

Hepatic disease is responsible for *fluid retention* because of the following factors:

1. The concentration in the serum of albumin manufactured in the liver is lowered and so depresses colloid osmotic pressure, thus transudation of fluid occurs.

2. Aldosterone excreted in excess increases sodium and fluid retention. Pooling of blood in the splanchnic vessels reduces effective blood-volume and thus may provide the initial stimulus to increased aldosterone secretion.

3. Oestrogens and antidiuretic hormone, which are slowly excreted in liver disease, may accumulate and aggravate fluid retention.

4. Reduction in renal blood-flow and filtration rate may, in some cases, aggravate fluid retention. A more profound upset of renal function can be demonstrated in some patients with liver failure. There appears to be diminution of cortical (glomerular) blood-flow in favour of flow to the medulla, where there is a resultant upset of the counter-current system.

5. A high pressure in the portal circulation acts in two ways by: (*a*) Presinusoidal localizing the fluid retention to the abdominal cavity, giving rise to ascites; (*b*) Postsinusoidal engorging the liver so that excess hepatic lymph is produced.

Students should remember that ascites can develop suddenly if there is deterioration of liver cell function caused by *haemorrhage*, but if bleeding stops the fluid is usually dispersed easily by diuretics.

Chronic ascites is, however, a different problem and may be refractory to diuretic treatment.

CLINICAL PICTURE

Patients complain of abdominal swelling and discomfort. There is anorexia and shortness of breath.

On examination, cutaneous stigmata of liver disease, jaundice, and neuropsychiatric disorders may be found.

The skin over the distended abdomen is tight and shiny from tissue oedema. The distension is greatest in the upper abdomen and flanks, where striae may occur. Portal venous collaterals may appear around the umbilicus and in the epigastrium, while prominent loin veins caused by mechanical pressure on the inferior vena cava are sometimes seen. The patient is wasted, and the thin limbs and sunken face contrast vividly with the distended abdomen. There is a *fluid thrill* if the ascites is tense, and *shifting dullness*. It may not be possible to feel any viscera until ascites disappears.

Complications and Accompaniments (Fig. 53)

1. MECHANICAL

a. The rise of intra-abdominal pressure causes weakness at the *normal abdominal hernia sites* so that umbilical, inguinal, and hiatus herniae may occur. Hydrocele, haemorrhoids, rectal or vaginal prolapse may develop.

b. A rise in central venous pressure causes filling of the jugular veins. Because of this, patients with ascites may be wrongly diagnosed as having heart failure.

c. Pleural effusion is due to a 'leak' of fluid from the abdomen into the chest. This fluid is transferred by diaphragmatic lymphatics and rarely may be transported through an anatomical defect in the diaphragm.

2. DUE TO LIVER CELL FAILURE

In that the ascites of liver disease is a feature of failure of the liver cell, it cannot be overstressed that other evidence of liver cell failure *and* evidence of portal hypertension are usually present. Most cirrhotics have the unfortunate habit of developing neuropsychiatric deterioration at the least provocation.

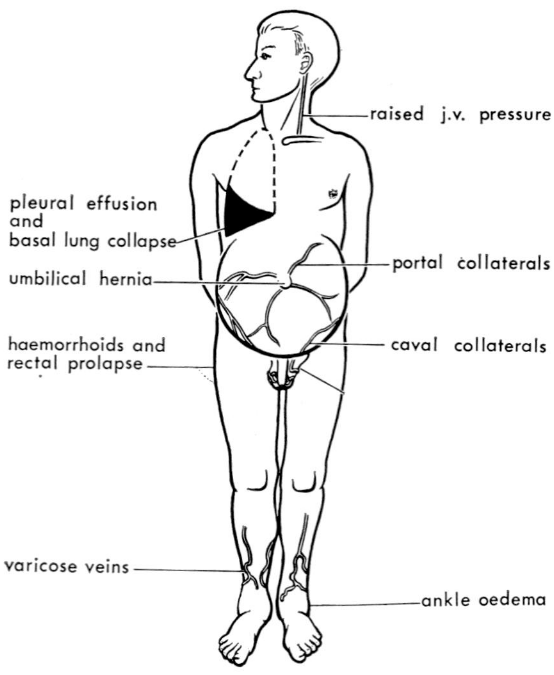

Fig. 53. The mechanical complications of ascites.

The differential diagnosis of ascites is given in Chapter 22. *Investigations* will help, not only to confirm that ascites is due to cirrhosis, but will also help in deciding whether the ascites will clear with drug therapy.

1. *The serum albumin*: The value is usually below 3 g. per cent in cirrhotic patients. Higher values make one think of neoplasia and tuberculosis.

2. *The serum sodium*: A low sodium (less than 132 mEq./l.) is a bad prognostic sign, for hyponatraemia may mean terminal liver failure.

3. *Urinary excretion of sodium*: In patients with ascites from whatever cause sodium retention occurs, and the cirrhotic may show such extreme avidity for sodium that very little is excreted. The amount found in the urine varies little with the intake, but it is conventional to measure the urinary output of sodium when the patient is taking a 22 mEq. sodium diet in each 24 hours. An excretion of less than 1 mEq. per 24 hr. means that ascites will be difficult to control, but higher figures arouse hope.

Confirmatory evidence of cirrhosis comes from results of liver function tests, low protein values in ascitic fluid, and evidence of portal hypertension or liver cell failure.

TREATMENT

(*Fig. 54*)

The following methods, beginning with the simplest and least drastic, and progressing to more complex dietary and drug treatment for refractory cases, are used to control ascites:

1. Rest in bed.

2. Reduction of sodium intake by withdrawal of salt condiments, and the use of salt in cooking.

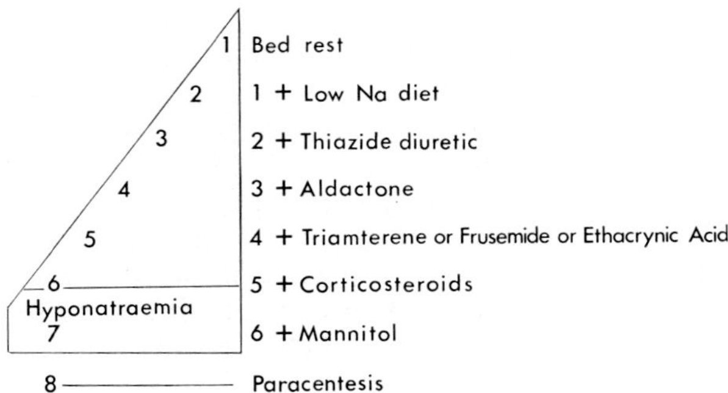

Fig. 54. Ascites in cirrhosis. The therapeutic wedge.

3. Diuretics, usually thiazide derivatives. It is essential that adequate potassium supplements are also given *every day* of the week and not only when diuretics are given, for hypokalaemia may precipitate hepatic coma. If there is no response, treatment is continued with the addition of—

4. Rigid sodium restriction (22 mEq. per day).

5. Diuretics combined with aldosterone antagonists, e.g., spironolactone, 25 mg. q.d.s. Amiloride, 10 mg. q.d.s., and Triamterene, 200 mg. daily, may be helpful as they also increase the diuretic response to thiazide diuretics and in a similar way to spironolactone diminish urinary potassium loss. If these diuretics with spironolactone fail, then the more potent diuretics frusemide and ethacrynic acid can be used though they are both likely to produce a fall of glomerular blood-flow and aggravate nitrogen retention. There has been a recent tendency to use large doses of spironolactone alone before adding other diuretics

6. The previous régime, reinforced by an osmotic diuretic, e.g., mannitol 20 per cent (1–2 litres intravenously). The purpose of mannitol is to increase the sodium flow to the distal renal tubule where aldosterone antagonists operate. If this is not done, aldosterone antagonists may fail because the low glomerular filtration rate allows excessive reabsorption of sodium in the proximal tubule, so that little is left at their site of action in the distal tubule. It is wisest to administer a *trial* dose of mannitol of the

order of 200 ml., a careful watch being made to make sure that the urinary volume is proportionally increased. If this is not done retention of fluid may result in fatal pulmonary oedema or variceal haemorrhage.

Success can be judged by (a) increased urinary volume; (b) a loss of weight (which should be charted daily), and which should not be more than about 2 kg. per day. This is because of the dangers of hepatic encephalopathy when there is too vigorous a diuresis. A vigorous diuresis causes shrinkage of the intravascular fluid compartment and diminishes hepatic blood-flow; (c) a diuresis which is accompanied by loss of sodium and potassium. Fluctuation in the patient's girth may be due to flatulence and so is a less satisfactory way of following a case of ascites.

Ancillary Aids

1. *Infusions* of serum albumin (salt-free) are expensive, and in many cases fail because albumin quickly leaves the vascular compartment to enter the ascites, which becomes worse rather than better. If the albumin is retained in the vascular compartment the serum albumin rises and a diuresis leads to loss of ascites. Albumin infusions can precipitate bleeding from oesophageal varices and acute pulmonary oedema.

2. *Prednisone.* The refractory stage with hyponatraemia can sometimes be remedied by corticosteroids. It is uncertain how these drugs work, but since they cause a diuresis of water rather than sodium, the serum sodium rises enough to promote a diuresis of water and sodium by conventional diuretics.

3. A small '*tap*', by lessening intra-abdominal pressure, may promote a diuresis from ensuing drugs, perhaps by improving renal blood-flow and glomerular filtration rate. Several centres have repopularized the i.v. infusion of ascitic fluid as a way of controlling fluid retention. This can be done if precautions are taken to make sure that both collection and reinfusion can be accomplished in a sterile manner. A diuresis results from an increase in plasma volume in an identical fashion with albumin infusions. A further technique which promises well allows separation of the majority of the ascitic fluid from its concentrated protein. This is done by using a pump and a semipermeable membrane and allows infusion of protein and a smaller amount of fluid.

These measures to control ascites are slow in action and much patience is needed. Ascites is a bad prognostic sign and many patients die within months or a few years of its onset. In those who do not die and in whom a diuresis results in a dramatic improvement in health the long-term effect of the liver disease is unlikely to be affected. Diuretic therapy is also liable to be complicated in nearly three-quarters of all cases by electrolyte abnormalities in the serum and they may precipitate nitrogen retention or frank renal failure. The syndrome of ascites with hypotension and hyponatraemia is a particularly dangerous one.

When treatment is successful patients are amongst the most grateful, for not only does ascites disappear but general health and nutrition are vastly improved.

The Place of Paracentesis Abdominis in the Treatment of Ascites
This method should only be used if:
  1. The patient is uncomfortable and shows respiratory distress.
  2. As a means (via a *small* paracentesis) of promoting a drug diuresis.
  3. In patients refractory to *full medical therapy*.
One unfortunately sees patients who, because of limited facilities (e.g., lack of trained dietitians), have not had the benefit of a full medical 'anti-ascites campaign'. These patients, who are subjected to frequent and unnecessary 'tapping', do not usually survive for long once this method of treatment is employed, but if they do, they are bothered by constant admission to hospital at ever decreasing intervals for this dramatic but dangerous treatment. Over 95 per cent of ascites in cirrhosis is controlled by dietary and diuretic therapy.

Dangers of Paracentesis
  1. *Infection of the Peritoneal Cavity.* This has few diagnostic features in the cirrhotic with ascites, so that pyrexia and the onset of hepatic coma may be the only signs of trouble. In such circumstances culture of ascitic fluid provides the diagnosis.
  2. *Hepatic Coma.* The cause for this occasional hazard is unknown and probably complex. The low blood-pressure, oliguria, haemoconcentration, and biochemical disorders are probably all important.
  3. A *low sodium state* associated with constant oozing from around the paracentesis wound sometimes precedes death. In such patients administration of intravenous sodium almost always precipitates pulmonary oedema.
Portacaval anastomosis has been used in the treatment of refractory ascites. As ascites is evidence of considerable liver cell failure, most patients are not generally fit for operation, but in the few suitable cases side-to-side portal vein–inferior vena cava anastomosis is preferred because this allows adequate decompression of the liver and therefore reduction in hepatic lymph-flow.

HEPATIC DISEASE AND NEUROPSYCHIATRIC COMPLICATIONS

In certain patients liver disease may be complicated by acute bouts of delirium which are known by various names, such as hepatic coma and hepatic precoma, portasystemic encephalopathy, hepatic encephalopathy, etc. Basically, the defect is an alteration of awareness because of the impaired function of certain deep-seated brain structures, probably in the region of the basal ganglia.
  For these changes to occur, one or more of the following are required:
  1. Disease of liver cells—acute or chronic.
  2. Communications between the portal and systemic circulation (either artificial, e.g., after a portacaval anastomosis, or natural, as may complicate portal hypertension).

3. A sensitive brain. Sensitivity probably increases with age, and once neuropsychiatric complications have developed they may be expected to occur more readily on subsequent occasions.

AETIOLOGY

Most workers believe that the changes of hepatic coma are largely due to intoxication of a sensitive brain by breakdown products of protein metabolism produced by bacterial action in the gut. These products are able to by-pass the liver cell because of liver cell disease, and because of abnormal vascular communications in and outside the liver which communicate with the systemic circulation. These nitrogenous products consist of substances other than ammonia, but ammonia, which is itself toxic, offers a convenient marker which can be measured in the blood.

There are other factors which may be of importance. Urea is an important substrate for bacterial and intestinal cellular ureases. These produce ammonia which adds to the ammonia load being dealt with by the already failing liver. Increased bacterial activity in the lower small gut may increase intestinal production of ammonia. *Renal production* of ammonia may be important if hepatic coma follows diuretic therapy, and production or impaired absorption of ammonia by *muscle* may also be a factor.

A *defective synthesis of urea* in the liver due to liver cell disease may mean that higher concentrations of ammonia are present in the blood. The synthesis of urea takes place via an 'ornithine–citrulline–arginine' cycle with the incorporation of ammonia. Defective *removal of ammonia from the blood*, perhaps related to deficient action of alphaketoglutarate or glutamic acid, which acts as ammonia acceptors, may occur.

Abnormal transfer of *ammonia into cells* may occur in response to an alteration in tissue pH.

CLINICAL PICTURE

Hepatic neuropsychiatric changes may occur under the following circumstances. It is important to recognize the different clinical situations under which it occurs, because the treatment and prognosis differ.

1. *Acute*

a. In massive liver necrosis, e.g., following infective hepatitis or drug injury.

b. In established chronic liver disease (cirrhosis) associated with a precipitating factor, such as *surgical trauma; haemorrhage; infection* (e.g., pneumonia, infection of ascites, etc.); *paracentesis abdominis; drugs* (i) diuretics, chlorothiazide, frusemide, ethacrynic acid, NH_4Cl, (ii) sedative drugs, morphine, paraldehyde, etc.; *electrolyte disorders*— hypokalaemia, hyponatraemia.

2. *Chronic*

In established chronic liver disease (cirrhosis) related to permanent poor liver cell function and portal systemic collateral circulation.

Patients in category 1*a* rarely survive because of gross destruction of the liver. Patients in group 1*b* survive the incident of hepatic coma if the precipitating factor can be corrected, and the prognosis is then that of the underlying liver disease. Patients in the chronic category (2) often have other evidence of terminal liver failure.

Patients are often drowsy and may show a disordered sleep rhythm. There may be euphoria as well as confusion, and a gross change in personality. The disorder tends to fluctuate from day to day and even from hour to hour. The speech is often slurred and the face may lack expression. Difficulty with the copying of simple designs may be demonstrated even when other clinical evidence is slight. Handwriting is poor and difficult to read.

Apart from the mental changes the most constant neurological abnormality is the presence of a 'hepatic flap'. This is a coarse tremor which may be seen in any part of the body, e.g., head, limbs, tongue, but which is most easily seen in the hands. The tremor is best demonstrated by asking the patient to hyperextend the wrists and to maintain this position with the fingers spread apart. The flaps take place at the wrist and metacarpophalangeal joints and sometimes there is an added lateral movement. A 'hepatic flap' is not specific for hepatic disease and it may be seen in uraemia and hypercapnoea. It must therefore be related to its clinical context. The patient may also have hepatic 'foetor' when asked to breathe out through the mouth into the clinician's face. The odour defies accurate description but is sweet, not unpleasant, and quite characteristic. Foetor disappears after adequate gut sterilization with neomycin.

Other neurological features, which include muscular rigidity, increased tendon-jerks, and an extensor plantar response, are chiefly found in cases of frank coma. Recently it has been recognized that the syndrome of chronic hepatic encephalopathy produces many disorders caused by widespread damage and dysfunction within the central nervous system. Histological changes with loss of neuronal cells and proliferation of protoplasmic astrocytes are seen in the cerebral cortex, basal ganglia, cerebellum, and spinal cord. The physical signs are therefore extremely variable and consist of signs of cerebral dysfunction as well as ataxia and intention tremor, involuntary movements such as choreo-athetosis, and paraplegia due to spinal cord demyelination. These disorders are particularly likely to occur where there is a large portal–systemic shunt existing over several years. This is most likely after a portacaval anastomosis in a well-chosen subject with good liver function. A correct diagnosis is important as treatment may bring about an improvement.

DIAGNOSIS

The presence of liver damage, either acute or chronic, with the classic triad of confusion, foetor, and flap, makes the diagnosis easy. Wilson's disease is a rare but difficult differential diagnosis and delirium tremens in alcoholics also needs differentiation.

Helpful tests apart from the liver function tests are:

1. *The E.E.G.*

Tracings from patients exhibiting mental and neurological abnormalities are always abnormal. Abnormal records may also be obtained before clinical changes are obvious. The changes which are non-specific consist in a slowing of the normal alpha rhythmic activity of the brain (9–13 c.p.s.) with replacement by *generalized* slow rhythmic activity which in severe cases is in the delta range of less than 4 c.p.s.

2. *Blood-ammonia Levels*

Arterial blood-levels are more reliable than venous because of the part played by muscle in ammonia metabolism. Levels must be determined whilst the patient is fasting. Various techniques are used and the results are not very helpful in determining whether neuropsychiatric abnormalities are due to liver disease or not. For this reason, and the special experience needed, blood-ammonia values are now largely a research procedure.

TREATMENT

It will be obvious from the classification that the treatment of this disorder depends not only on the type of liver disease but on the identification and treatment of precipitating factors. Acute hepatic necrosis may be treated by corticosteroid therapy, possibly the treatments outlined on p. 125, bleeding by transfusion and purgation, morphine reactions by cautious use of nalorphine, etc.

Whatever the cause of the disorder, in each patient a routine 'anticoma' treatment is also applied, consisting of:

1. Removal of all protein from the diet.

2. Ensuring a free action of the bowels with purgatives and wash-outs.

3. The use of non-absorbable antibiotics to prevent the bacterial breakdown of protein in the gut. Neomycin is still probably the most effective way of doing this, given in a dose of 1 g. 4–6-hourly. It is important to check blood levels, particularly where there is renal impairment because of the risk of 8th nerve damage.

4. The provision of large amounts of glucose given either intravenously, 20 per cent into a large vein, or via an intragastric drip.

5. Potassium supplements to correct hypokalaemia and the alkalosis (extracellular) which accompanies it, for both of these factors may potentiate hepatic coma.

6. The use of arginine to encourage incorporation of ammonia into urea, and sodium glutamate which may act as an acceptor of ammonium with the production of non-toxic glutamine, are of unproven value. Other treatments have employed the use of inhibitors of urease and the colonization of the gut with non-ammonia-producing bacteria such as *Lactobacillus casei*. Lactulose, a non-absorbable sugar which is split by colonic bacteria to lactic and acetic acids, produces beneficial diarrhoea and a low

colonic *p*H which encourages the growth of non-ammonia-producing bacteria. It is expensive but may complement oral neomycin.

Serial tests of mental arithmetic, construction of a five-pointed star with matchsticks, a daily handwriting chart, and serial E.E.G.s are ways of checking the patient's progress.

Even those patients whose neuropsychiatric disorder has been precipitated by infection or bleeding will have a reduced protein tolerance, so that after recovery the daily protein intake can be increased in 20-g. steps to determine the level that can be permitted (usually about 40 g. per 24 hours). In chronic cases neomycin may be given continuously but is of decreasing usefulness, since resistant bacteria develop in the alimentary tract.

Colonic by-pass and ileorectal anastomosis, by ensuring free movement of the bowels and short-circuiting the site of most alimentary bacterial activity, have a place in the treatment of chronic cases. It is, however, doubtful whether they do much more than can be achieved with protein restriction and antibiotics and such operations are poorly tolerated in the patient with liver cell failure where there is a high risk of postoperative infection and haemorrhage as well as aggravation of encephalopathy. Certainly the survival of patients with encephalopathy is not increased by this procedure. On the other hand, there are occasional dramatic successes and this treatment may allow a more realistic diet—an important factor for the patient with poor liver function. Levo-dopa has also been claimed to be helpful in chronic cases.

SOME SPECIAL FEATURES OF CIRRHOSIS
(*Fig. 55*)

1. *Changes in the Skin and Nails*

CHANGES IN THE NAILS

Though the reason for this is unknown, cirrhotics may develop finger clubbing or 'white' nails which are opaque and 'frosted' enough to prevent the pink colour of the nail-bed being seen, even when the fingers are clenched. If there is hypoalbuminaemia, transverse bands—'Muehrcke's bands'—across the nails are seen in some patients. Since they occur in any hypoproteinaemic condition they are not pathognomonic of cirrhosis.

SPIDER NAEVI (*see Fig. 55*)

These consist of a central dilated arteriole which is pulsatile, and smaller vessels radiating from it from the 'legs'. The whole 'spider' blanches with pressure on the 'body' with a pin head. Such 'spiders' are often raised above the surface of the skin and can on occasions bleed profusely if injured. They are found either in the skin of the face, neck, arms, hands, or the trunk above the nipple line. Only in young children may they be found on the legs. The distribution is mainly on those parts exposed to the air.

'Spiders' occur in healthy people, for many of us boast one or two which may either persist or fade, to be replaced by others. They should only be considered an indication of liver disease if numerous, large, or developing in crops.

ERYTHEMA OF THE PALMAR SURFACES.

Erythema of the hands and feet is seen not only in some cirrhotic patients, but also in the healthy, the pregnant, and in those with rheumatoid arthritis. The erythema is caused by cutaneous anastomoses. Hormonal factors have again been implicated.

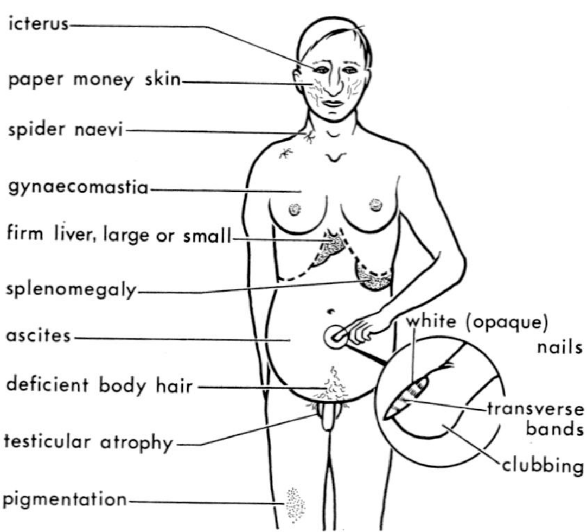

Fig. 55. Physical stigmata of cirrhosis.

STIGMATA OF CIRRHOSIS REVEALED BY SPECIAL TESTS

RADIOLOGICAL
Oesophageal and gastric varices
Presence of portal collateral vessels

CHEMICAL
Raised serum bilirubin
Lowered serum albumin
Raised serum globulin and abnormal flocculation tests
Raised transaminases, 5 nucleotidase L.D.H., etc.
Prolonged bromsulphthalein retention

URINE
Low 17-ketosteroids and 17-hydroxycorticosteroids

HISTOLOGICAL
Liver biopsy usually confirms

SCINTISCANNING
Diminished hepatic uptake
Increased splenic uptake

Cirrhotic patients often have prominent venules on the skin of the face and neck. Some American observers have called it 'paper money skin' because of its likeness to the coloured fabric threads which are present in paper currency.

2. *Hormonal Aspects of Hepatic Cirrhosis*

The vascular abnormalities may be due to disturbances of oestrogen metabolism, and the same may be true for gynaecomastia in male patients. A vasodilator material in the circulation may be the cause of the hyperdynamic circulation sometimes found, and aldosterone, which is often excreted in excess, may potentiate fluid retention. Lack of androgenic hormones may be responsible for the lack of body hair, testicular atrophy, and sterility in male cirrhotics.

The excretion of 17-ketosteroids and 17-hydroxycorticosteroids is low, the latter because there is a failure to break down cortisone to its tetrahydroderivatives. Patients with liver disease are for this reason likely to develop side-effects from modest doses of corticosteroids.

3. *Cirrhosis and Infection*

The patient with hepatic cirrhosis is susceptible to infection. This is probably for a variety of reasons, including poor function of the hepatic bacterial filter due to portosystemic communications and impaired immunological defences, low peripheral white count, splenic enlargement and malfunction, abnormal immunoglobulins, and impaired production of complement. Infection is likely to occur in the lungs (particularly in the alcoholic), in ascitic fluid, in the blood-stream, and in the renal tract where it may be related to an increased incidence of diabetes. Important organisms are the pneumococcus and tubercle bacillus (lungs) and *Escherichia coli* (septicaemia, ascitic and urinary-tract infection). Infection may produce relatively few signs and its presenting symptomatology may be that of hepatic coma. It is essential that clinicians should recognize this fact. Samples of blood and ascitic fluid should be taken for bacterial examination and appropriate antibiotics administered.

FURTHER READING

Portal Hypertension
CONN, H. O., and LINDENMUTH, W. W. (1968), 'Prophylactic Portocaval Anastomosis in Cirrhotic Patients with Esophageal Varices', *New Engl. J. Med.*, **279**, 725.
KERR, D. N. S., HARRISON, C. V., SHERLOCK, S., and WALKER, R. M. (1961), 'Congenital Hepatic Fibrosis', *Q. Jl Med.*, **30**, 91.
READ, A. E., DAWSON, A. M., KERR, D. N. S., TURNER, M. D., and SHERLOCK, S. (1960), 'Bleeding Oesophageal Varices treated by Oesophageal Compression Tube', *Br. med. J.*, **1**, 227.
SHALDON, S., and SHERLOCK, S. (1960), 'The Use of Vasopressin (Pitressin) in the Control of Bleeding from Oesophageal Varices', *Lancet*, **2**, 222.
REYNOLDS, T. B., ITO, S., and IWATSUKI, S. (1970), 'Measurement of Portal Pressure and its Clinical Application', *Am. J. Med.*, **49**, 649.
SHERLOCK, S., FELDMAN, C. A., MORAN, B., and SCHEUR, P. J. (1966), 'Partial Nodular Transformation of the Liver with Portal Hypertension', *Am. J. Med.*, **40**, 195.

WALKER, R. MILNES (1960), 'Transection Operations for Portal Hypertension', *Thorax*, **15**, 218.
— — SHALDON, C., and VOWLES, K. D. J. (1961), 'Late Results of Portocaval Anastomosis', *Lancet*, **2**, 727.

Extrahepatic Portal Vein Obstruction
THOMPSON, E. N., and SHERLOCK, S. (1964), 'The Aetiology of Portal Vein Thrombosis with Particular Reference to the Role of Infection and Exchange Transfusion', *Q. Jl Med.*, **33**, 465.

Ascites
ATKINSON, M., and LOSOWSKY, M. S. (1961), 'The Mechanism of Ascites Formation in Chronic Liver Disease', *Q. Jl Med.*, **30**, 153.
SHALDON, S., MCLAREN, J. R., and SHERLOCK, S. (1960), 'Resistant Ascites treated by combined Diuretic Therapy', *Lancet*, **1**, 609.
SHERLOCK, S., WALKER, J. G., SENEWIRATNE, B., and others (1966), 'The Complications of Diuretic Therapy in Patients with Cirrhosis', *Ann. N.Y. Acad. Sci.*, **139**, 497.

Hepatic Coma
READ, A. E., MCCARTHY, C. F., AJDUKIEWICZ, A. B., and BROWN, G. J. A. (1968), 'Encephalopathy after Portacaval Anastomosis', *Lancet*, **2**, 999.
SHERLOCK, S. (1961), 'Hepatic Coma', *Gastroenterology*, **41**, 1.
— — SUMMERSKILL, W. H. J., WHITE, L. P., and PHEAR, E. A. (1954), 'Portosystemic Encephalopathy', *Lancet*, **2**, 453.

Hepatic Failure
SHERLOCK, S. (1961), 'Liver Failure', in *'The Scientific Basis of Medicine' Annual Reviews*, 1961. British Postgraduate Medical Federation. London: Athlone Press.

Cutaneous Abnormalities
BEAN, W. B. (1953), 'The Arterial Spider and Similar Lesions of the Skin and Mucous Membranes', *Circulation*, **8**, 117.
MUEHRCKE, R. C. (1956), 'The Finger Nails in Chronic Hypoalbuminaemia', *Br. med. J.*, **1**, 1327.

Infection
JONES, E. A., CROWLEY, N., and SHERLOCK, S. (1967), 'Bacteraemia in Association with Hepatocellular and Hepatobiliary Disease', *Post-grad. med. J.*, **43**, March Suppl., p.7.

Chapter 15

Diseases of the Gall-bladder and Bile-ducts

BILIARY PHYSIOLOGY

BILE CONSISTS of a solution of bile-pigments, bile-salts, cholesterol, phospholipids, hormones, and electrolytes, together with mucus. Approximately 1 litre of hepatic bile is produced daily and this is secreted at a pressure of about 20 cm. of water. Gall-bladder bile differs from the hepatic variety in being concentrated ten times or so by the active removal of water and electrolytes by the gall-bladder mucosa. The gall-bladder contracts and discharges its concentrated bile into the duodenum. The contraction is produced by a hormone cholecystokinin which is released from the upper small bowel by contact with food and in particular by fatty foods.

BILE-SALTS

By far the most important solids in the bile (60 per cent of the total) are the bile-salts. There are the *primary* bile-salts—a trihydroxy bile-salt (cholic acid) and a dihydroxy bile-salt (chenodeoxycholic acid) which comprise 80 per cent of the total bile-salts and are present in roughly equal amounts. The precursor substance is cholesterol. Primary bile-salts are broken down by bacteria in the gut. *Secondary* bile-salts are formed, namely a dihydroxy bile acid (deoxycholic acid) from cholic acid and smaller amounts of a monohydroxy bile acid (lithocholic acid) from chenodeoxycholic acid. All of these primary and secondary bile-salts exist in bile as conjugates with taurine and glycine.

The bile-salts play an integral part in fat absorption and in bile are responsible for the formation with phospholipids and cholesterol of polymolecular aggregates called 'micelles' which allow cholesterol to be kept in solution. The bile-salts share a specific active reabsorption site in the ileum and there is an essential recycling process back to the liver—an enterohepatic circulation. The mixed micelles in bile contain bile-salts, phospholipids, and cholesterol—the latter is kept from precipitation by this configuration and both bile-salts and phospholipid (lecithin) help to maintain cholesterol solubility.

GALL-STONES

AETIOLOGY

Gall-stones are found at post-mortem in about one-fifth of all subjects. They steadily increase in incidence from about 30 years of age. Although they are commonest in obese females who have borne children they can occur in both sexes and in any age-group. They can be single or multiple and, though usually found in the gall-bladder, may migrate or be found in other parts of the biliary tree. There is good evidence of increasing incidence of gall-stones in countries which have developed the Western form of civilization. A very high incidence is, however, seen in North American Indians.

Gall-stones are of several varieties.

	COMPOSITION
1. Pure	Bilirubin Cholesterol
2. Mixed (often laminated)	Calcium salts Cholesterol Bilirubin

The present tendency, however, is *not* to distinguish too clearly between the various types. Little is known of the factors leading to the formation of gall-stones.

BILE-SALT METABOLISM AND GALL-STONES

Defective bile-salt metabolism could be associated with gall-stone formation in the following way. In gall-stone disease the *hepatic* bile is known to be abnormal (lithogenic). This means that it is the liver rather than the gall-bladder which is the organ at fault. Further in this lithogenic bile the total concentration of bile-salt is reduced—this factor producing impaired micelle formation and precipitation of cholesterol. The cause for this alteration in bile-salt concentration is unknown, but there is presumably a hepatic biochemical defect, presumably acquired and perhaps related to a diminished total bile-salt pool. This in turn possibly represents diminished hepatic synthesis, but the cause for this is unknown.

A further abnormality of lithogenic bile is its increased concentration of mucus derived from the gall-bladder epithelium. Mucus increases bile viscosity and prevents the evacuation of cholesterol–bilirubin–bile-salt complexes and precipitates them as microspheroliths—miniature gall-stones. It has also been suggested that because of the finding of unconjugated bile-pigment in the centre of mixed gall-stones increased concentrations of (an enzyme) B-glucuronidase may be responsible for the presence of unconjugated bilirubin in bile and this substance may serve in turn as a source of precipitation of complexes of calcium and bilirubin. The situations in which there is an interruption or inefficiency of the enterohepatic circulation—namely ileal disease, chronic liver cell disease, and ileal resection—are situations in which gall-stone formation is found with increased frequency. Great interest also centres around the fact that lithocholic acid which normally is poorly absorbed from the gut and produced only in small amounts gives rise in the experimental animal to bilirubin stones and cholestasis. Increased lithocholic conjugates might be found where bile-salts are exposed excessively to bacteria—such as in the blind-loop syndrome and ulcerative colitis or in ileal disease. In ileal disease or resection there is increased influx of bile-salts into the colon where colonic bacteria produce secondary di- and monohydroxy bile acids in increased amounts.

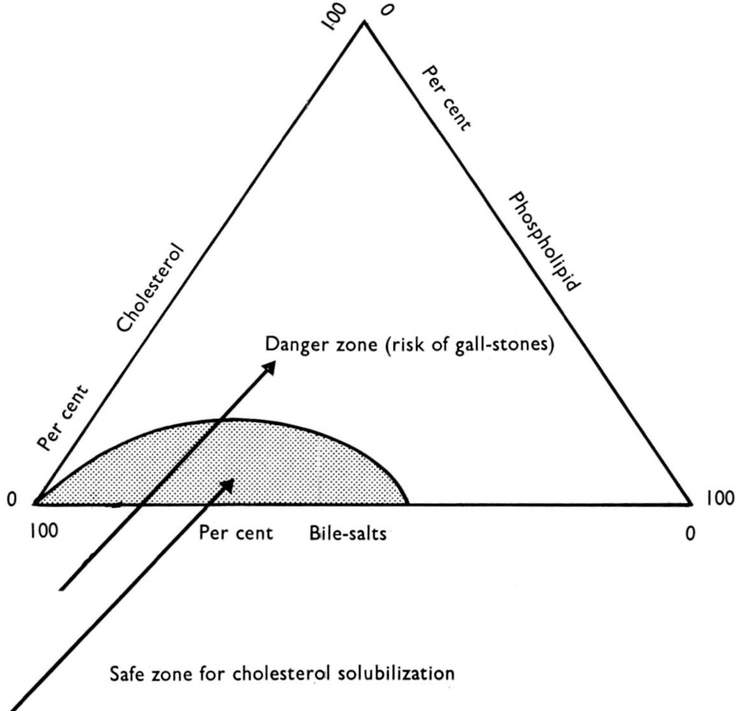

Fig. 56. The concept of triangular co-ordinates to explain the precipitation of cholesterol. (Small, D. M., *New Engl. Jl Med.* (1968), **279**, 588.)

Donald Small and his colleagues in Boston have introduced the concept of triangular co-ordinates to explain the precipitation of cholesterol when the concentration of bile-salts and phospholipid diminishes. Values of the three major biliary components within the shaded area (*Fig. 56*) permit solubilization of cholesterol whilst values outside are accompanied by precipitation.

OTHER FACTORS IN GALL-STONE PRODUCTION

There are remarkable racial differences. Increasing affluence and caloric intake are related to an increasing incidence of gall-stones. A family history of predisposition to gall-stone formation is common. Discovery often follows pregnancy, but the relationship is a difficult one to prove and may be more clearly related to the fact that it is the symptoms of gall-bladder disease rather than the stones that are aggravated by pregnancy. Hormonal factors may be responsible for delayed gall-bladder emptying in females. Bacterial infection is now considered a less important factor than it used to be though obviously it could play a part in stone formation by increasing cellular desquamation and mucus production. Actinomycetes have been demonstrated in the centre of gall-stones—their function in the formation of stones is unknown. It must not be forgotten that in a young person the presence of gall-stones should suggest a careful search for both ileal disease and haemolysis. Further, in patients with known haemolytic disease the symptoms of gall-stones may be wrongly confused with those of the abdominal symptoms of a haemolytic crisis.

PATHOLOGY

Appearance of Stones

1. PURE

   a. Bilirubin. Multiple, small, dark green or black, rarely radio-opaque.
   b. Cholesterol. Single or multiple, often large, yellow, and if pure, not radio-opaque.

2. MIXED

   Multiple, faceted, dark brown, often radio-opaque.

Appearances of Gall-bladder

A gall-bladder which is contracted by a thickened wall showing prominent cholesterol deposits on the mucosal surface is known as a 'strawberry gall-bladder'. The gall-bladder may sometimes be distended and filled with mucus if the cystic duct is obstructed by a stone.

Appearance in the Rest of the Biliary Tract

If they are obstructed the bile-ducts may dilate and show signs of infection, and this may also involve the hepatic parenchyma.

CLINICAL PICTURE

Gall-stones may cause no symptoms. Symptoms are usually dependent on the migration of a gall-stone into the cystic duct and the onset of inflammatory changes in the gall-bladder.

The patient with gall-stones is often female, middle-aged and parous, and suffers from bouts of upper abdominal discomfort and distension related to the taking of food and particularly fats. She attempts to relieve her discomfort by belching and by taking alkaline mixtures. These symptoms are not diagnostic and many a patient with such a history has lost her gall-bladder to the surgeons but kept her symptoms.

Symptoms of impaction and of acute cholecystitis are much more characteristic. The patient complains of severe pain in the epigastrium, the right upper abdomen, or under the costal margin. It is boring and steady, though on occasions colicky. The pain may radiate to the epigastrium, the lower abdomen, and, most characteristically, into the back by the angles of the scapulae and to the right shoulder. Left-sided pain occurs in about 5 per cent of cases. The patient is restless, nauseated, and vomits. A previous history of vague dyspepsia, flatulence, and distension, so common in many other conditions, is of little diagnostic value.

Examination may reveal a restless patient, tachycardia, and right upper abdominal tenderness and guarding. Murphy's sign—tenderness, and 'catching' of the breath on inspiration—may be present, and hyperaesthesia may be demonstrated over the sensory dermatome to which pain is referred. Difficulty arises when pain is referred to the right iliac fossa or to the left side of the abdomen.

DIAGNOSIS

The differential diagnosis of acute cholecystitis includes pleurisy and pneumonia, appendicitis, renal infection, pancreatitis, and perforation of a peptic ulcer. Myocardial infarction and the pain of hepatic engorgement secondary to congestive cardiac failure may cause difficulty.

Apart from the history and a complete clinical examination, help may be obtained from the following tests:

1. A plain radiograph of the abdomen may reveal the presence of gall-stones. These have to be differentiated from calcified costal cartilages and lymph-glands as well as from calcification in the liver, pancreas, adrenals, and kidneys. Only a small percentage of gall-stones are radio-opaque (about 15 per cent).

2. The blood will show a raised white count with a polymorph leucocytosis.

3. Where the clinical picture is confusing it is important to exclude other possible causes of pain by examination of the urine, electrocardiography, and chest radiography.

4. Cholecystography is not indicated in the acute stage of the illness, but will be helpful following recovery. The presence of stones appearing as filling defects in the gall-bladder, or failure of gall-bladder opacification, both support the diagnosis. An alternative approach is intravenous cholangiography which is much more specific for gall-bladder disease than oral cholecystography. Further, it demonstrates the calibre and the presence of obstruction in the duct system. It can be used in the acute stage of the disease via an infusion technique if there is diagnostic difficulty.

TREATMENT

The treatment of acute cholecystitis is rest in bed with adequate sedation and analgesia. Local warmth to the abdomen is helpful. Morphine is best avoided because it has a constricting effect on plain muscle in the sphincter of Oddi. The most satisfactory analgesics—because they produce no

change in common-duct pressure—are phenazocine (Narphen) and pentazocine (Fortal) which are given in a dose of 2–3 mg. and 30–45 mg., by i.m.
injection respectively. Food is withheld and fluids only are permitted by
mouth.

In the usual case without evidence of complications, antibiotics are not
indicated. Following recovery from an attack of cholecystitis, radiographic
studies of the gall-bladder should be made. In general, repeated attacks of
pain coupled with radiographic evidence of gall-stones or poor gall-bladder
function should be an indication for cholecystectomy in an otherwise fit
patient. The occurrence of jaundice is an indication for surgery after the
attack has subsided. Recently it has been shown that gall-stones can be
dissolved by giving oral bile-salts (chenodeoxycholate). The treatment is
expensive and at the moment experimental.

COMPLICATIONS OF ACUTE CHOLECYSTITIS ACCOMPANYING GALL-STONES
(*Fig. 57*)

1. Acute Gangrenous Cholecystitis and Empyema of the Gall-bladder
The rise of pressure caused by inflammatory exudate in the gall-bladder
obstructed by a stone may lead to devitalization of the wall, which becomes
gangrenous and perforates. If this does not happen, the gall-bladder,
which is filled with purulent bile and stones, becomes acutely inflamed
and there is an overlying peritoneal reaction. Thus, patients developing
an empyema usually have persistent pain and evidence of local peritoneal

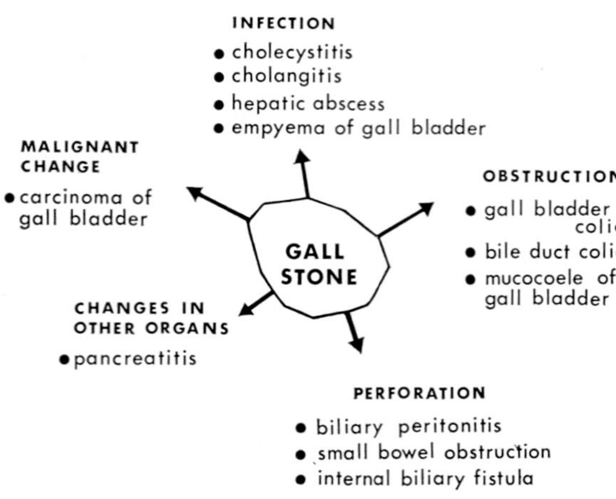

Fig. 57. Possible complications of gall-stones.

irritation. They develop a swinging temperature and become toxic and ill.
A mass can sometimes be felt in the right upper quadrant, but muscle
guarding makes palpation difficult. Perforation is accompanied by signs
of peritonitis and shock. In elderly patients the signs and symptoms of
gall-bladder necrosis and empyema may be few.

TREATMENT

Careful clinical observation is necessary. Persistence of pain and vomiting, shock, and increasing toxicity are important signs of continuing inflammation. Antibiotics are indicated (e.g., tetracycline, chloramphenicol, or penicillin with streptomycin) in prolonged cases and the serum amylase must be measured to exclude pancreatitis. Surgical intervention, though difficult and often dangerous, should not be delayed where there is evidence of progressive disease. In these circumstances cholecystostomy—drainage of the gall-bladder—and removal of stones may be preferable to cholecystectomy.

2. Cholangitis (*Fig. 58*)

If a gall-stone enters the common bile-duct it may pass into the duodenum or may obstruct the bile-duct and produce an infection of the biliary tree. This may cause a characteristic clinical syndrome. It used to be thought

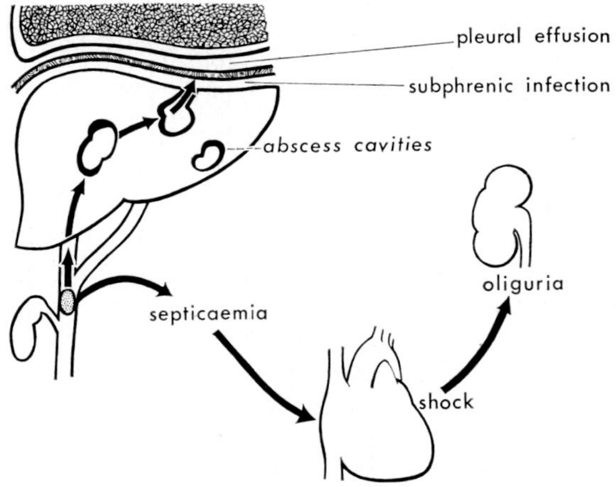

Fig. 58. Complications of cholangitis.

that the cholangitis was due to ascending infection from the gut, i.e., 'ascending cholangitis'. This has been questioned particularly because neoplastic biliary obstruction is so rarely complicated by cholangitis. It seems more likely that infection results from activation of a nidus of inflammation in a previously damaged gall-bladder.

The patient complains of attacks of severe right upper abdominal colic which radiates to the back and shoulders, and is accompanied by rigors. Vomiting and jaundice occur, the latter mild at first but deepening rapidly if biliary obstruction is complete.

Examination reveals a pyrexial, ill, and restless patient, who has faint jaundice and hepatomegaly. The gall-bladder is not palpable but the liver is tender. The urine contains bile and the faeces are paler than usual. The liver function tests show evidence of obstruction, such as a raised alkaline phosphatase and bilirubin. Rapid deterioration due to shock and oliguria occurs in some, and there is a fairly high incidence of *Escherichia coli* septicaemia. This organism may also be obtained from the infected bile, from liver biopsy material, and from duodenal aspirate. In some cases frank suppuration results in multiple intrahepatic abscess cavities and infection of the subphrenic and pleural cavities.

Treatment with full doses of tetracycline or chloramphenicol, or penicillin with streptomycin, in most cases effectively lessens pain, pyrexia, and jaundice. Rifampicin—an antibiotic of high molecular weight—is concentrated in bile. Though it must be given by i.m. injection, this compound is in our experience of great value in severe biliary tract infection. Measures to promote biliary flow, such as oral or duodenal instillation of magnesium sulphate, are of doubtful value. In those cases not responding satisfactorily, surgical exploration of the common bile-duct, with removal of stones and biliary drainage, is necessary at the acute stage.

After disappearance of the jaundice, radiological visualization of the bile-ducts and gall-bladder must be achieved in order to decide whether elective surgical treatment is necessary. Even if little pain has been experienced the common duct may contain numerous stones, and these must be removed. Sometimes the common duct is drained, and operative cholangiography is necessary to make sure that no stone remains.

3. Gall-stone Ileus

A fistulous communication between the inflamed gall-bladder and the small bowel may result in extrusion of gall-stones into the alimentary tract, and then obstruction of the duodenum causes symptoms which resemble those of pyloric stenosis, except that the vomit contains bile. Sometimes the stone, having traversed the wider jejunum, obstructs the distal small gut, in which case abdominal colic, distension, and vomiting are the main symptoms, and fluid levels are seen on the plain radiograph. The diagnosis is suggested by right upper abdominal pain typical of acute cholecystitis followed by small-bowel obstruction. The obstructing gall-stone may be radio-opaque or may be demonstrated by outlining it with barium. Gas in the biliary tree indicates a fistulous connexion between gall-bladder and gut. After decompression of the small bowel by aspiration, and replacement of fluid loss intravenously, the treatment is surgical.

4. Pancreatitis

Acute pancreatitis. (*See Chapter 16.*)

COMPLICATIONS OF CHRONIC CHOLECYSTITIS

Carcinoma is an occasional complication if gall-stones are present.

There is some evidence to suggest that in patients with coronary artery disease attacks of angina may be potentiated by gall-bladder disease. Cholecystectomy then may lessen the severity and frequency of angina.

Special Types of Chronic Cholecystitis

The association between haemolytic disease and recurrent gall-stone (pigment) formation must not be forgotten, and tests of red-cell survival and red-cell fragility may be necessary if gall-stones are found in young patients. Chronic cholecystitis occurs commonly in patients with brucellosis, and chronic typhoid infection of the gall-bladder is a well-known sequel of typhoid fever. Treatment with ampicillin or trimethoprim-sulphamethoxazole (Septrin) may be effective in treating carriers as high doses of chloramphenicol are potentially dangerous. Biliary surgery may also be required.

Carcinoma of the Gall-bladder

AETIOLOGY

Since this lesion is nearly always found with gall-stones, most authorities believe that the irritative action of the stones causes a malignant change. However, although gall-stones are common, carcinoma of the gall-bladder is rare. Perhaps the infection which may accompany gall-stones is an important aetiological factor.

PATHOLOGY

The common tumour is an adenocarcinoma derived from glandular elements, but a small percentage is of squamous-cell origin. The gall-bladder may be thickened and contracted from previous cholecystitis, but it is enlarged if the tumour obstructs the cystic duct. Though usually infiltrative, papillomatous and colloid tumours are sometimes found. Neighbouring tissues, particularly the liver and bile-ducts, are involved early, no doubt due to their rich lymphatic and vascular connexions.

CLINICAL PICTURE

The patient is usually an elderly female who gives a history of bouts of pain or dyspepsia attributable to cholecystitis. The two important symptoms are attacks of right upper abdominal pain and obstructive jaundice. Loss of weight and failure of health, which come on quickly, may not be noticeable in obese elderly subjects. There may be hepatic enlargement as well as the local mass of the tumour itself. It is a challenge to the clinician that the diagnosis is rarely made before laparotomy.

Accompaniments and Complications

Cholangitis and hepatic abscess may complicate obstruction of the bile-ducts. Fistulae to the small bowel, and rupture causing peritonitis or widespread peritoneal dissemination of tumour, may occur.

DIAGNOSIS

If there is no jaundice, carcinoma of the colon or kidney may be suspected, but when icterus develops, a carcinoma of the pancreas or carcinomatosis of the liver is thought to be most likely.

11

There are no tests which specifically indicate a neoplasm of the gall-bladder, although very rarely a small tumour may be demonstrable by cholecystography in patients without jaundice. Tests of liver function in icteric cases merely show the features of biliary obstruction.

ASSESSMENT AND TREATMENT

Laparotomy is indicated after the administration of vitamin K, but the majority of cases are inoperable. It may be possible to remove the tumour and the right lobe of the liver, but such surgery is difficult and rarely possible.

Stricture of the Bile-ducts

AETIOLOGY

Usually due to operative trauma at the time of cholecystectomy and to the collection of bile around the ducts, or to probing and intubation of the common bile-duct, benign strictures only occasionally develop spontaneously. Gall-stones in the common duct may cause ulceration which leads to the formation of a stricture. Once this has formed, the hazard of repeated surgical operations to relieve obstruction is that of further stenosis and stricture.

PATHOLOGY

Operative trauma usually causes a stricture at the juncture of the cystic and common hepatic ducts. This is of variable length and the duct below is collapsed. In sharp contrast, the duct system, both extrahepatic and intrahepatic, above the stricture is dilated and inflamed. The liver is enlarged and may show the presence of a fine biliary cirrhosis secondary to the obstruction and infection. Portal hypertension with splenomegaly and abnormal collateral channels or ascites may be found in advanced cases.

CLINICAL PICTURE

The disorder is commonest in females. If after cholecystectomy and choledochotomy, prolonged and profuse drainage through an external biliary T tube is followed by cholangitis and jaundice when the tube is removed, a stricture must have developed, or a stone been left in situ.

A biliary stricture may not show itself, however, until some time after operation. Attacks of right upper abdominal pain and discomfort are accompanied by pyrexia, headache, or even frank rigors, during which the patient feels hot or cold and shivery and sweats profusely. As jaundice appears the patient notices darkening of the urine during attacks. Pale stools, attacks of diarrhoea, and pruritus may be noted.

Helpful investigations include:

1. Liver function tests which show the features of obstructive jaundice and sometimes also those of liver cell dysfunction.

2. Increased faecal fat excretion.

3. Intravenous cholangiography (providing the patient is not jaundiced) may allow identification of the stricture or stones, and may show dilatation

of the bile-ducts. Transhepatic or endoscopic cholangiography may also be helpful, as in this way delineation of the site and extent of the stricture or strictures is made. Aspiration of bile which is subsequently cultured may also give valuable evidence concerning the presence and antibiotic sensitivity of biliary infection.

4. A liver biopsy may show evidence of cholangitis with bile retention and polymorphonuclear infiltration in portal tracts. It may also show evidence of cirrhosis.

5. A test for mitochondrial antibodies performed with the patient's serum is always negative in spite of secondary biliary cirrhosis. This is useful in the distinction from primary biliary cirrhosis where a positive result is seen in over 90 per cent of patients.

Accompaniments and Complications

Attacks occur at varying intervals and some patients develop permanent liver damage. Secondary biliary cirrhosis may be responsible for episodes of bleeding from oesophageal varices, hepatic coma, oedema, and ascites.

ASSESSMENT AND MANAGEMENT

The repair of a stricture is not easy, and multiple operation scars bear witness to this. If biliary drainage cannot be re-established, attacks of cholangitis will continue and liver damage will result. If at choledochotomy a stone is found which is known to have been present for some time, the possibility of stricture formation may be anticipated by performing a choledocho-duodenostomy.

When a stricture has formed, the operation of choice is excision followed by anastomosis of the two ends of the bile-duct. In order to exclude stones, operative cholangiography may be helpful once the bile-duct has been defined. Hepatico-jejunostomy (anastomosis of the jejunum to the common hepatic duct) with entero-enterostomy or Roux-en-Y anastomosis of the jejunal loop is an alternative operation where the bile-duct is unsuitable for end-to-end anastomosis. Dilatation of the stricture may be effective, particularly if the stricture is a high one or of minimal degree. An anastomosis is often fashioned over a prosthesis—a T tube or Y-shaped tube. If only the hepatic ducts are healthy, they may be anastomosed to the jejunum with the aid of an appropriate prosthesis.

If the patient is ill with deep jaundice, preliminary external drainage of the biliary tree above the stricture may allow liver function to improve and inflammation to subside, so that the stricture can be tackled more easily and with less risk at a second-stage operation.

Results are good in about 60 per cent of cases; the rest develop further evidence of biliary obstruction, infection, and liver damage. Operative mortality in good hands is about 5 per cent. Where there is incomplete relief of biliary obstruction attacks of cholangitis should be treated with antibiotics, which should be taken at the first warning of an attack so that its severity is reduced. The serum alkaline phosphatase level is a good guide to the completeness of surgical relief.

So serious are the effects of bile-duct stricture that great care must be taken when operating upon or probing the biliary tract, and sepsis must at all times be prevented. Should damage to the bile-duct occur it should be repaired promptly before a stricture can form.

Tumours of the Bile-ducts

With the exception of those arising from the ampullary region, neoplasms of the bile-ducts are rare. Benign tumours (adenoma, papilloma) do not cause symptoms other than those of biliary obstruction.

Carcinoma of the bile-ducts is somewhat more common in men than in women and the patients are usually elderly. There is no known factor of aetiological importance and the association with gall-stones is not nearly as close as it is with cancer of the gall-bladder. Some cases are reported complicating liver fluke infestation and ulcerative colitis.

PATHOLOGY

The tumour is most commonly found at the bifurcation of the common hepatic duct, but the lesion can arise from any part of the duct system. Macroscopically, the lesion may appear as a stricture, a papilloma, or a diffusely infiltrating lesion. It may be so small that its presence may be missed. If there is complete biliary obstruction the bile-ducts proximal to the lesion are dilated and the liver enlarged. Microscopically, the lesions are either adenocarcinomata or squamous-cell growths. The smallness of biopsy fragments may make an accurate diagnosis difficult.

CLINICAL PICTURE

Obstructive jaundice is of early onset and it is progressive. There may be pain of an intermittent or colicky nature in the upper abdomen and weight-loss, anorexia, diarrhoea, and pyrexia. The rigors of cholangitis may occur.

Examination usually reveals an elderly patient with obstructive jaundice, and the preoperative diagnosis is usually that of cancer of the head of the pancreas.

Tests are not helpful in making the diagnosis for they merely indicate obstructive jaundice. Slight anaemia, leucocytosis, and a raised sedimentation rate are slightly more specific. The only completely diagnostic tests are transhepatic or endoscopic cholangiography and examination of the duodenal contents for cancer cells. If transhepatic cholangiography is performed it is done as a preliminary to some operative attempt as a by-pass operation to relieve biliary obstruction. The major diagnostic difficulties are the differentiation of this condition from primary biliary cirrhosis and chronic obstructive jaundice due to drugs. The absence of mitochondrial antibodies from serum in bile-duct carcinoma and in drug-induced cholestasis and their invariable presence in patients with primary biliary cirrhosis may be useful diagnostically.

TREATMENT

The outlook is poor because of the inaccessibility of the lesion. However, since they grow slowly, palliative surgery with external drainage of the biliary tract above the neoplasm, or intubation through the growth, may be compatible with a reasonably comfortable life for several months.

OTHER LESIONS OF THE BILE-DUCTS

Primary Sclerosing Cholangitis

This is a rare disease of unknown aetiology in which there is a diffuse patchy sclerosis of the extra- and intrahepatic bile-ducts and gall-bladder by a chronic fibrotic process. Though some cases may occur in association with ulcerative colitis or with diseases such as fibrosing mediastinitis, diffuse retroperitoneal fibrosis, and Riedel's thyroiditis where excessive fibrosis occurs, others have no such accompaniments.

The disease is commonest in middle-aged subjects.

The clinical picture may be extremely variable, particularly when it is associated with retroperitoneal fibrosis (*see* p. 364). Biliary stenosis produces attacks of cholangitis, jaundice, and pyrexia. The liver is enlarged and tender and the liver function tests show obstruction. Needle biopsy of the liver does not usually show any helpful diagnostic features and laparotomy and cholangiography are required. The former shows chronic fibrosis and narrowing of the bile-ducts whilst the latter shows multiple areas of narrowing in the intra- and extrahepatic ducts with intervening 'beading' where the ducts are comparatively normal. Biopsy of the bile-duct if this is possible or biopsy from the gall-bladder may show evidence of dense fibrosis and lymphocytic infiltration. The diagnosis can only be made with certainty in the absence of gall-stones or previous biliary surgery. Involvement of the bile-ducts should be diffuse and bile-duct carcinoma must be carefully excluded. Occasionally the association with ulcerative colitis may be of diagnostic help.

Treatment consists of antibiotics for active infection of the biliary tree and in some cases relief of biliary obstruction by surgery or T-tube drainage. Corticosteroids may be helpful. The prognosis is uncertain but many patients live for 6 or more years before succumbing to the effects of liver failure and secondary biliary cirrhosis.

Choledochal Cyst

This is a dilatation of the common bile-duct, probably of congenital origin. Attacks of abdominal pain, tumour, and obstructive jaundice, particularly when they occur in young female subjects, should make one suspect this lesion. The dilated bile-duct produces a tumour in the right upper abdomen which may be visible on a plain radiograph of the abdomen and may displace the barium-filled stomach. An intravenous cholangiogram may also be helpful. Treatment is excision of the cystic swelling followed by anastomosis of the bile-duct to the jejunum or duodenum.

Biliary Dyskinesia

Some clinicians believe that abnormal motor activity of the biliary tract causes symptoms such as pain, flatulence, and abdominal discomfort. Manometry of the gall-bladder and bile-ducts has been used to show states of hyperkinesia and hypokinesia. Sphincterotomy to correct biliary hyperkinesia is not recommended by clinicians in this country, who hold that dyskinesia is not an important source of symptoms.

FURTHER READING

Gall-stones
RAINS, A. J. HARDING (1962), 'Researches concerning the Formation of Gall Stones', *Br. med. J.*, **2**, 685.
SMALL, D. M. (1968), 'Gallstones', *New Engl. J. Med.*, **279**, 588.

Cancer of Bile-ducts and Gall-bladder
FORTNER, J. G., and PACK, G. T. (1958), 'Clinical Aspects of Primary Carcinoma of the Gall Bladder', *Arch. Surg., Chicago*, **77**, 742.
KUWAYTI, K., BAGGENSTOSS, A., STAUFFER, M. H., and PRIESTLEY, J. T. (1957), 'Carcinoma of the Major Intrahepatic and Extrahepatic Bile Ducts exclusive of the Ampulla of Vater', *Surgery Gynec. Obstet.*, **104**, 357.
WHELTON, M. J., PETREILI, M., GEORGE, P., YOUNG, W. B., and SHERLOCK, S. (1969), 'Carcinoma at the Junction of the Main Hepatic Ducts', *Q. Jl Med.*, **38**, 211.

Primary Sclerosing Cholangitis
THORPE, M. E. C., SCHEUER, P. J., and SHERLOCK, S. (1967), 'Primary Sclerosing Cholangitis, the Biliary Tree, and Ulcerative Colitis', *Gut*, **8**, 435.

Biliary Stricture
MAINGOT, R. (1960), 'Surgical Aspects of Non-malignant Strictures of Bile Ducts', *Proc. R. Soc. Med.*, **53**, 545.

Choledochal Cyst
HORNE, L. M. (1957), 'Congenital Choledochal Cysts', *J. Pediat.*, **50**, 30.

Chapter 16

Diseases of the Pancreas

PANCREATIC PHYSIOLOGY

THE PANCREAS produces 1–4 litres of fluid per 24 hours (usually $1\frac{1}{2}$–2 litres). The principal enzymes in this juice are *amylase* (which hydrolyses glycogen and starch), and *lipase* which hydrolyses neutral fat to fatty acids and glycerides, providing there is an optimal concentration of bile-salts present. *Trypsin*, *chymotrypsin*, and *procarboxypeptidase* are protein-splitting enzymes and are secreted in an inactive (zymogen) form. Their activation depends on a small-bowel factor—enterokinase.

Pancreatic juice also contains sodium, potassium, chloride, and bicarbonate. The latter is present in the highest concentration (approx. 100 mEq. per litre) and responsible for its high *p*H (6–8) compared with gastric acid. The secretion of pancreatic juice is under the control of two hormones, secretin and pancreozymin/cholecystokinin. Secretin is released by hydrogen ions from the duodenal wall and it causes secretion of a pancreatic juice low in enzymes and high in bicarbonate, whilst pancreozymin which is produced by the gastric antrum and duodenal mucosa produces a small volume of enzyme-rich juice. Pancreozymin is identical with the gall-bladder-contracting enzyme cholecystokinin. Nervous control is via the vagus nerve, stimulation of which produces pancreatic secretion.

Pancreatitis

AETIOLOGY

At the Symposium on *Aetiology and Pathology of Pancreatitis* held in Marseilles in 1963 a classification of pancreatitis as below was proposed:

I. Acute pancreatitis.
II. Recurrent acute pancreatitis (in which the pancreas returns to normal between attacks: removal of a precipitant, e.g., biliary disease or alcoholism may be curative).
III. Recurrent chronic pancreatitis.
IV. Chronic pancreatitis.

In types III and IV the disease is progressive, the difference between them depending on the presence of recurrent or persistent pain.

It is becoming increasingly clear that a non-bacterial inflammation of the pancreas can occur in association with a number of vascular, endocrine, nutritional, and hereditary disorders. As there is little apparent connexion between these groups it is best to review them separately.

1. *Hereditary Pancreatitis*

A rare familial type of pancreatitis has been described occurring in young persons which has a relapsing course and is associated sometimes with amino-aciduria. It is thought to be inherited as a Mendelian dominant.

2. *'Mechanical' Pancreatitis*

In patients where there is a common opening of the biliary and pancreatic ducts it is postulated that bile or duodenal juice can gain an entrance to pancreatic ducts and initiate an acute inflammatory process. This probably accounts for a small percentage of cases of pancreatitis.

3. *Disease of the Biliary Tract*

This, particularly gall-stones and cholecystitis, is a most important factor in perhaps a third of all cases of pancreatitis. The exact way in which it provokes the disease is unknown, but, experimentally, regurgitation of bile is a potent cause of pancreatitis. Biliary infection seems a more likely precipitant.

4. *Alcoholism*

This may produce increased pancreatic secretion whilst duct obstruction by proteinaceous material and sphincter spasm aid gland autodigestion. American observers particularly stress the importance of alcoholism. It seems to be less common in this country.

5. *'Metabolic' Pancreatitis*

This is being increasingly recognized in association with essential hyper-lipaemia and with hyperparathyroidism. The cause is unknown, but it has been suggested that in hyperparathyroidism an elevated tissue-calcium concentration activates trypsin and leads to pancreatic autodigestion.

Other Factors of Importance

Protein-splitting enzymes, e.g., trypsin, are probably not the sole cause of the pancreatic digestion associated with pancreatitis. It is, however, possible that trypsin can act as an activator of enzymes such as phos-pholipase-A and elastase. Phospholipase-A is known to act on lecithin (found in bile) to produce highly toxic compounds—lysolecithin and lipocephalin—which can injure cell membranes. Bile may be important in producing a lipid substrate for this enzyme. It is likely that *vascular factors*, such as thrombosis and atheroma, may play a part, and that sometimes ischaemia may be the major cause of pancreatitis. This would certainly explain the segmental distribution of the disease as sometimes seen at operation and post-mortem. Infection is rarely of importance, though the pancreatitis complicating *mumps* is an exception to the rule. *Hypothermia* is sometimes associated with pancreatic destruction, and *auto-immunity* has been implicated. Diet itself may be of importance. Certainly malnutrition can cause degenerative lesions in the pancreas, and both destruction and calcification of the gland are found in those countries where malnutrition is common. Pancreatitis may occur *postoperatively*, particularly after operations on the stomach and biliary tract, in which case ischaemia and trauma to ducts are both presumably of importance. There is also some evidence to suggest that *corticosteroid* drugs may cause pancreatitis.

In this country the aetiology of acute pancreatitis (types I and II) is uncertain in one-quarter of the cases. Nearly a half are associated with gall-stones, either in the gall-bladder or common duct. Less than one-twentieth are due to postoperative or other trauma and less than 1 in a 100 is associated with alcoholism.

On the other hand, chronic pancreatitis (types III and IV) appears to be more closely related to alcoholism, and gall-stones are less commonly associated with this type of disease.

Acute Pancreatitis

PATHOLOGY

Pancreatic enzymes activated by the spread of inflammation from the duct system to the parenchyma cause oedema, haemorrhage, and destruction of the gland (*see Fig. 60*). There is often a peritoneal exudate of blood-stained fluid and necrosis of fat in the mesentery.

Microscopically, the gland is heavily infiltrated with inflammatory cells, and the area of necrosis and haemorrhage may be widespread or localized to certain areas.

CLINICAL PICTURE

In this country the disorder is commonest in those prone to gall-bladder disease, such as women in middle life. Attacks are of all grades of severity. In severe cases the onset, which may follow a heavy meal or a bout of alcoholism, can be catastrophic, with epigastric upper abdominal and back pain, collapse, and persistent vomiting. Pain may radiate to the shoulder-blades and slight jaundice may be noticed.

Very ill patients may have a cyanotic tinge and air-hunger. The pulse is rapid, the blood-pressure low, and on examination of the abdomen there is upper abdominal guarding. Discoloration and lividity of the loins and around the umbilicus may be seen (Grey-Turner's sign) but this is rare.

The patient who is not so severely shocked merely complains of steady upper abdominal pain radiating into the back. Rarely, subcutaneous fat necrosis may be seen in the skin.

The diagnosis may be difficult because certain abdominal and thoracic conditions can produce a similar clinical picture. Amongst these are per-foration of a peptic ulcer, acute cholecystitis, and a mesenteric vascular occlusion. Thoracic conditions to be excluded include pericarditis, acute myocardial infarction, and a dissecting aneurysm of the aorta.

The following tests are helpful in proving the diagnosis:

1. *Serum Enzyme Tests*

The serum amylase is invariably elevated and is usually greater than 500 and often more than 1000 Somogyi units per 100 ml. (normal less than

200 units). There are other disorders, such as perforation of a peptic ulcer or peritonitis, in which there may be a moderate elevation of the serum amylase and renal failure may also elevate it. Values of more than 1000 units are pathognomonic of pancreatitis. The serum lipase is also raised.

2. *Urinary Enzyme Tests*

Tests of urinary amylase may be helpful, providing that the answer is expressed with due regard to the 24-hour urinary volume. The urinary amylase elevation drops more slowly than the blood elevation and may be of diagnostic help in this respect.

3. *Amylase in Peritoneal Fluid*

The exudate in the abdomen of patients with pancreatitis is rich in amylase. A few millilitres of fluid obtained with a needle and syringe from the abdominal cavity are valuable for enzyme tests, particularly when blood-levels are returning to normal at the end of the acute phase.

4. *Other Blood Tests*

Serum calcium may be low if there is extensive fat necrosis. The serum potassium may be low if there is vomiting or elevated if there is extensive tissue necrosis and renal damage. The serum glucose may rise in one-quarter to two-thirds of patients but glycosuria is less common. However, the combination of a high serum amylase and a raised blood-sugar is particularly suggestive of acute pancreatitis. Hypoglycaemia can also occur. There is a polymorph leucocytosis, and there may be biochemical evidence of liver cell damage. In young patients amino-aciduria should be looked for. The serum fibrinogen may be prognostically helpful (*Fig. 60*).

5. *Radiographs*

A plain film of the abdomen is as valuable in this disorder as in all acute abdominal emergencies. It may show:
    a. Evidence of gall-stones.
    b. Fluid levels, particularly in loops of small gut adjacent to the pancreas in the left upper abdomen.
    c. It will exclude conditions such as intestinal and gastric perforation.
    Other radiographic studies are contra-indicated in the acute phase, but in some instances intravenous or infusion cholangiography is indicated provided that jaundice is minimal. A chest radiograph may show a pleural effusion.

6. *Other Tests*

An E.C.G. often shows T wave inversion, ST deflexion, and other changes caused by alteration in serum electrolyte levels or hypotension. These must be distinguished from those of myocardial ischaemia.

A rare associate of acute pancreatitis is hyperlipidaemia (type I hyper-lipoproteinaemia) and the serum lipids may then be elevated and the serum milky on naked eye inspection.

Accompaniments and Complications (Figs. 59, 60)

Shock, renal impairment, and disturbances of electrolyte balance are common. Disease of the biliary tract is likewise part of the clinical picture. Alcoholic patients may have cirrhosis. An abscess may form, or fluid

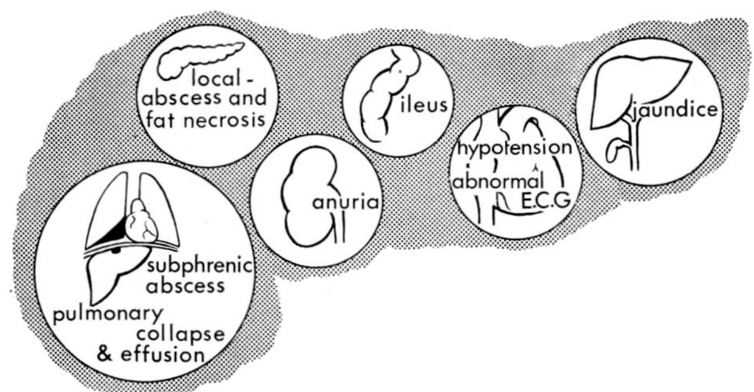

Fig. 59. Complications of acute pancreatitis.

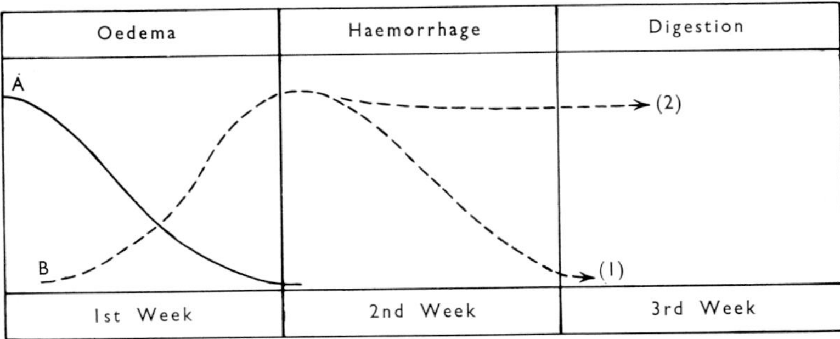

Fig. 60. Natural history of pancreatitis. **A,** Serum enzyme and **W.B.C.** counts/level—raised at outset. **B,** Evidence of tissue destruction serum fibrinogen level —highest 7–10 days. (1) Usually returns to normal. (2) Continued high level— bad prognosis.

collecting in the lesser sac may develop into a pancreatic pseudocyst. Tetany may occur if there is a considerable reduction in serum calcium or magnesium. The possibility of hypoglycaemia being present and needing treatment must be borne in mind.

MANAGEMENT AND ASSESSMENT

The treatment of acute pancreatitis is governed by the following rules:
1. The reduction of pancreatic secretory function.
2. The avoidance of surgical intervention.
3. A close watch on electrolyte and fluid balance.
4. The treatment of pain and shock.

1. *Reduction of Secretory Function*

Oral medication and food are not given, and the contents of the stomach are aspirated continuously. Pancreatic activity mediated by the vagus can be diminished by the use of anticholinergic drugs such as atropine, probanthine, or poldine. Treatment by 'anti-enzymes', on the supposition that much of the pancreatic damage is mediated by active protein-digesting enzymes trypsin and chymotrypsin, has been tried with an extract of bovine parotid gland, Trasylol. This preparation in an initial i.v. dose of 200,000 units has recently been shown to be effective in reduction of mortality.

2. *Surgery*

Unless for the drainage of abscesses or the treatment of biliary obstruction this is best avoided. If the diagnosis is made at laparotomy the abdomen should be closed, unless obvious gall-bladder disease calls for drainage of the biliary tree.

3. *Maintenance of Electrolyte and Fluid Balance*

Frequent determinations of serum electrolytes and measurement of vomit and urine are essential, and deficiencies are made good intravenously.

4. *Treatment of Pain and Shock*

Corticosteroid drugs are used with two objects in view: first, to combat shock, and secondly, with the aim of limiting the inflammatory process. Most clinicians feel that they should be used if shock is severe, and the fact that many feel that corticosteroids can cause pancreatitis should not deter one from using them in a bad case. Pain is treated by analgesics. Morphine is said to be contra-indicated because of its constricting action on the sphincter of Oddi, and pethidine, though not free from this side-effect, is usually preferred. It should be given in regular hypodermic doses of 100 mg. 6-hourly. Probably the safest drug to use is pentazocine hydrobromide (Fortral) which is both an effective analgesic and without a constrictor effect on plain muscle. It is given by i.m. injection 30–45 mg. 6-hourly. Splanchnic block has been tried for cases where pain persists despite full doses of analgesics. Antibiotics such as the tetracyclines have been shown to prevent secondary infection.

PROGNOSIS

In most series the mortality is of the order of 10 per cent. Cases due to alcoholism and those which follow surgery are at greater risk.

Apart from the hazards of the illness itself the possibility of recurrent attacks makes a careful search for an aetiological factor an important part of the follow-up. After the acute phase passes, biliary disorders should be treated and alcoholic habits curbed.

Chronic Pancreatitis

PATHOLOGY

The disease is patchy or generalized. The gland is usually so hard and fibrotic that malignant disease is simulated. Pseudocysts may be present.

Histologically, there is fibrosis and destruction of glandular tissue. Small ducts may show dilatation and squamous metaplasia with inspissation of retained secretions and the formation of duct stones. Calcification may be found in the fibrotic stroma of the gland.

CLINICAL PICTURE

Males are more commonly affected than females, which may reflect the importance of alcoholism as an aetiological agent. The illness is characterized by attacks of severe abdominal pain which often spreads to the back and shoulders and from which the patient seeks relief by sitting up to lean forward. Attacks may last up to twenty-four hours or more. Between attacks the patient is well or may suffer from a variable dyspepsia. With each attack endocrine and exocrine failure of the pancreas proceeds.

Diabetes, which is usually mild, may be first noted during a bout of pancreatic destruction, and in the absence of glycosuria the glucose tolerance curve may be abnormal. Steatorrhoea, caused by failure of pancreatic lipase production, is suggested by attacks of diarrhoea with loose, pale, bulky, and offensive stools. As destruction of the gland proceeds, attacks of pain may diminish, and steatorrhoea, wasting, cachexia, and diabetes become the prominent features. In some patients the disorder may be painless from the start and will then manifest itself only by exocrine and endocrine failure. Occasionally ascites may result from this disorder.

The *diagnosis* may be difficult unless the patient is seen during an attack. The following tests are helpful:

1. *During a Bout of Pain*

The serum amylase and lipase are elevated and the biochemical abnormalities of acute pancreatitis may be found.

2. *Between Attacks of Pain*

a. Provocation Enzyme Tests. Serum amylase or lipase may be measured after stimulating the pancreas by secretin, and giving morphine to prevent the exit of secretion into the duodenum. In normal subjects they rise, but if the gland is destroyed they do not. The duodenal contents can also be analysed after an injection of secretin and/or pancreozymin has been given, but it is a procedure which needs much practice before results become reliable. The volume of pancreatic juice recovered from the duodenum, the bicarbonate content, and the enzyme content are measured (*see Chapter 24*). In the presence of chronic pancreatitis, enzyme and bicarbonate levels are low. The Lundh Test meal may be helpful.

b. Tests showing overt or latent diabetes, including serum insulin levels after a glucose tolerance test.

c. A fat balance (*see* p. 422) may show steatorrhoea, and microscopy of the stools may reveal undigested meat fibres and fat globules. The presence of steatorrhoea without other significant evidence of malabsorption is particularly suggestive of a pancreatic cause.

d. Radiographic Studies. A plain film may show calcification of the gland or duct stones. The former may consist of a few deposits, most often in the head and body, or may outline the whole pancreas. Gall-stones may be seen.

Barium studies, though usually normal, may be of value in the identification of pseudocysts which displace the barium-filled stomach forwards. Cholangiography may show biliary tract disease or, rarely, reflux of dye into the pancreatic duct. (Rarely bone X-rays may show evidence of areas of sclerosis due to fat atrophy in the bone-marrow.)

e. The blood-count is usually normal. Megaloblastic anaemia hardly ever complicates the steatorrhoea of chronic pancreatitis. In recent years it has been recognized that some patients with chronic pancreatic deficiency may develop an excessive accumulation of iron in the tissues. This is associated with increased alimentary absorption of iron—a lesion corrected by pancreatic extract.

f. Pancreatic scintiscanning using the amino-acid ^{75}Se-selenomethionine which is actively taken up by the pancreas may show in this disorder either a reduced uptake or, more rarely a localized abnormality associated with infarction, cyst formation, or abscess.

It must be remembered that tests which support the diagnosis of chronic pancreatitis do not identify its cause. Biliary disease, alcoholism, hyperparathyroidism, hyperlipaemia must, if present, be defined. Haemochromatosis may cause diabetes but does not cause steatorrhoea, and there is no pancreatic calcification (*see Chapter 13*).

ASSESSMENT AND TREATMENT

Treatment is medical in the first place. Alcoholism should be controlled and other causative conditions should be treated. Acute exacerbations are managed in the same way as acute pancreatitis. Between bouts the following measures should be taken.

Diet should be bland and meals small and regular. Avoidance of overeating and abstinence from alcohol are important. Patients with steatorrhoea who have troublesome diarrhoea can usually be relieved by a low-fat diet. Opinion seems divided about the value of pancreatic extracts which are quickly inactivated by gastric juice, and which have no certain effect on faecal losses of fat and protein. As pancreatic digestion takes several hours frequent (even hourly) and fairly large doses (up to 20 g.) of pancreatin should be taken throughout the day. Most patients improve clinically and some will benefit from pancreatin (5–10 g.) given with meals. The most suitable form of pancreatic replacement therapy seems to be with Cotazym, the contents of 2–3 capsules of which are sprinkled over each main meal. The preparation contains lipase, trypsin, and amylase. The lipase content of each capsule is sufficient to digest 17 g. of dietary fat. Nutrizym, a further preparation, also contains protein-splitting bromelains in the wall of the capsule.

Diabetes, though usually mild, may need treatment.

Regular analgesics should be avoided as there is a strong possibility of drug addiction. If the patient fails to benefit from a régime such as outlined, and particularly if attacks are severe and frequent, surgical therapy should be considered. It must, however, be appreciated that surgery does not guarantee freedom from symptoms and each case must be considered on its merits. The following procedures are in current use:

1. *Operations on the Biliary Tract*

Disease of the biliary tract should be corrected wherever possible. On the assumption that spasm of the sphincter of Oddi is liable to increase biliary reflux into the pancreatic duct system, sphincterotomy is popular. Results, however, are very variable.

2. *Operations on the Pancreas*

The present tendency is to search for duct stenosis by probing or by operative or endoscopic pancreatography. The dilatation of stenosed ducts or the anastomosis of the duct system to the jejunum may be effective. Since the whole of the system may be involved at many points this type of operation may not be feasible. Another possibility is resection of the tail of the pancreas and re-anastomosis of the body to the gut (caudal pancreatectomy). In cases where the disease is crippling and where the gland is uniformly involved total pancreatectomy may be considered. In those patients where pseudocyst formation has occurred this lesion should be treated by surgical drainage into the gut.

3. *Operations on the Stomach*

Partial gastrectomy will reduce the output of secretin and thus, theoretically, may prevent attacks.

The prognosis in chronic pancreatitis is uncertain and the importance of eliminating alcoholism cannot be overstressed.

Mucoviscidosis: Fibrocystic Disease of the Pancreas (*Fig. 61*)

AETIOLOGY

The disease is inherited as an autosomal recessive with an incidence of about 1–2000 in a Caucasian population. It has been shown that serum from patients and from heterozygote carriers can inhibit ciliary action in the gills of a fresh-water mussel, *Dreissena polymorpha*, but the precise significance of this is unknown. Sweat from an affected patient can also inhibit Na-resorption from rat parotid gland. It seems possible that some abnormality of ground-substance mucopolysaccharide interferes with glandular electrolyte secretion. This could perhaps explain two of the three basic underlying defects of the disorder:

1. Abnormal electrolyte secretion from mucus glands.
2. Abnormal mucus.
3. A suspected abnormality of the autonomic nervous system.

Such a change in ground substance might inhibit the transfer of water and electrolytes into the glandular lumina with the resultant production of an isotonic secretion but with a higher organic (mucus) content such as occurs in the pancreas. A reverse abnormality might explain the increased sodium and water concentration in sweat as there would be interference by a similar mechanism with entry of sodium and water into proximal sweat-duct cells with a resultant increase in sweat volume and sodium excretion.

PATHOLOGY

There is a widespread disorder of mucus-secreting glands in the alimentary tract, pancreas, respiratory mucosa, and biliary tract. An abnormally viscid mucus causes swelling of glandular acini and thus secondary mechanical and infective complications follow. In the *pancreas* there is destruction and fibrosis of glandular tissue and the formation of retention cysts. In the *biliary tract*, obstruction may cause biliary cirrhosis. In the *lung*, infection secondary to bronchial obstruction causes bronchitis, bronchopneumonia, and bronchiectasis, and staphylococci are the most important organisms. Death occurs from the effects of lung sepsis and pancreatic malabsorption.

CLINICAL PICTURE

This is extremely variable.

1. In the newborn, if intestinal obstruction from meconium ileus has to be relieved surgically, the prognosis is very poor.

Perforation of the gut may then be associated with diffuse peritoneal calcification.

2. In babies and young children the disease is noticed first because of a failure to thrive, repeated respiratory infections, or steatorrhoea. After repeated chest infections, emphysema and bronchiectasis become established and there is clubbing of the fingers. The steatorrhoea causes abdominal distension, wasting, and rectal prolapse.

The high salt content of the sweat may lead to salt depletion in hot weather. The appetite is usually preserved.

3. Observations have shown that adult relatives of those with the classic disease may frequently have 'chronic bronchitis' and asthma, a high incidence of peptic ulceration, incidents of vasomotor collapse and dehydration, and even myocarditis and choroiditis.

DIAGNOSIS

The combination of diarrhoea and respiratory infection should suggest the possible diagnosis. Helpful tests include the following:

1. *Analysis of Sweat*

Patients have a high sodium and chloride concentration in their sweat.
Samples may be collected in a plastic glove after the body has been warmed,
or, more simply, a finger-print on an agar plate impregnated with silver

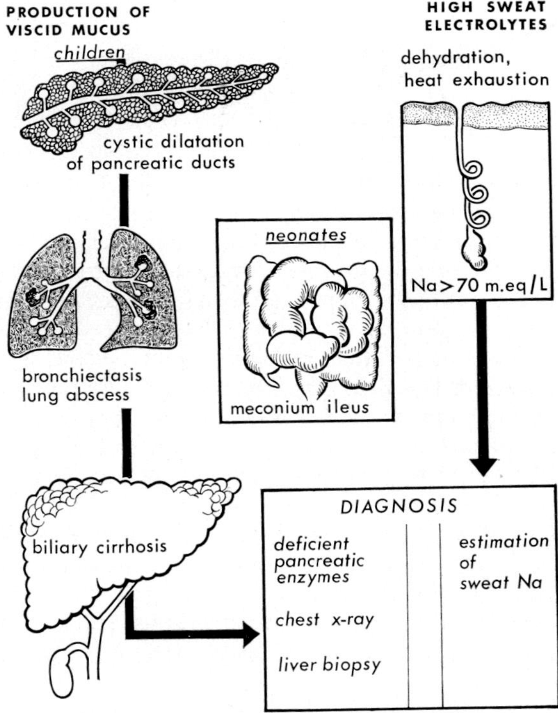

Fig. 61. Fibrocystic disease of the pancreas.

nitrate may be used as a screening test. The sweat contains 70 mEq.Na/l.
or more (normal = 60). Since heat may upset young patients iontophoresis
may be used, employing pilocarpine. Other body fluids, e.g., saliva, may
be more readily obtained in many young children.

2. *Tests of Pancreatic Exocrine Function*

These are difficult to perform in young children, and for this reason
evidence of trypsin and amylase deficiency is usually sought by examination of faeces and duodenal aspirate. Diabetes is rare, but the reason for
this is not known.

3. *Radiography of the Chest and Sinuses*

This may show signs of infection, lung collapse, emphysema, bronchiectasis, or pneumonic consolidation.

4. *Bacterial Examination of the Sputum*
Staphylococci, *Haemophilus influenzae*, or streptococci are usually revealed.

5. *Steatorrhoea*
This can be confirmed.

6. *Mucosal Biopsy*
Intestinal or rectal *mucosal biopsy* may show changes in mucus glands.

ASSESSMENT AND TREATMENT

Those patients with the fully developed clinical disorder need treatment (1) for the persistent chest infection, and (2) of the steatorrhoea.

1. Before the advent of antibiotics these patients did not survive, but because of the introduction of antibiotics effective against staphylococci, survival to adult life is now not rare. A recent report puts this as high as 70 per cent. The overall importance of the staphylococcus in the initiation and progression of pulmonary damage has been confirmed and the importance of continuous therapy with agents effective against this organism emphasized. Terminal lung infection with *Pseudomona aeruginosa* may occur, but the basis of therapy is the use of agents such as penicillin, cephaloridine, cloxacillin, and Fucidin, supplemented by aerosols and mist tents, together with sputum-liquefying agents, expectorants, and physiotherapy.

2. The failure of pancreatic exocrine function requires a high-protein, low-fat diet with the addition of Cotazyme or Nutrizym. Fat-soluble vitamin supplements must also be given, and a high salt intake encouraged.

3. Portal hypertension associated with a complicating cirrhosis may require surgical treatment and is obviously a serious complication.

TUMOURS OF THE PANCREAS

Neoplasms of the pancreas may cause a variety of clinical syndromes:
1. Non-insulin-secreting adenomas→ (1) Zollinger-Ellison syndrome
                                                              (2) Pancreatic pseudocholera
2. Insulin-secreting adenoma   → Hypoglycaemia
3. Carcinoma of pancreas and   → Obstructive jaundice, intestinal
    carcinoma of ampulla   bleeding, etc.

1. Zollinger-Ellison Syndrome

This is a rare disorder but one of great interest. It is due to hyperplasia or adenomata of non-insulin-secreting islet cells of the pancreas. Tumours are usually seen in the body and tail of the pancreas but, rarely, may occur outside the gland. Many of the tumours are locally malignant and some metastasize particularly to the liver.

Clinically, the disorder is characterized by intractable peptic ulceration or, less commonly, by profuse diarrhoea and potassium depletion. Peptic ulceration recurs after surgery and often involves the jejunum. Many patients have multiple operations, and complications such as perforation or haemorrhage are common. Peptic ulceration is caused by intense gastric hypersecretion and the gastric mucosa is hypertrophied. A 12-hour collection of gastric juice may produce more than 2 litres and about 200 mEq. of HCl and the basal 1-hour collection (BAO) usually yields 20–40 mEq. of acid (*see* p. 72). The maximal acid output (MAO) after pentagastrin yields a further but small increase and the ratio BAO/MAO = >0·6 (normal <0·6). It is hardly surprising that ulceration of the stomach and proximal jejunum occurs with such quantities of acid, and that diarrhoea results from the effect of this secretion on the rest of the small bowel where bile-salts and enzymes are inactivated.

The disorder has been shown to be due to the secretion of large amounts of gastrin (the hormone normally produced by the gastric antrum—gastric G-cells) by the tumour cells (δ-cells of the pancreas). A certain percentage of the cases where there is no tumour may be associated with hyperplasia of gastric G-cells.

DIAGNOSIS

Unless there is a high index of suspicion, cases will be missed. Recurrent haematemesis, anastomotic ulcers, or primary jejunal ulcers should arouse suspicion. The cause of chronic watery diarrhoea and steatorrhoea may not be immediately apparent, and chronic potassium depletion leading to renal impairment may further confuse the clinician.

The fasting gastric contents are conveniently collected overnight, and the volume, pH, and acid output measured. The administration of pentagastrin makes little difference to the volume or acid output, presumably because the stomach is already working at full pressure. Radiographs may show multiple ulcers in the upper gastro-intestinal tract and mucosal hypertrophy of the stomach. Bioassay of gastrin activity in urine and blood also shows high levels in the fasting state and though high levels are found in pernicious anaemia there is unlikely to be clinical confusion.

Rarely, multiple adenomata in the pituitary, parathyroid, and adrenal cortex occur with the pancreatic tumour, and thus a variety of endocrine functions may be disturbed in the same patient.

TREATMENT

The identification of a tumour should be followed by enucleation and total gastrectomy. This is because a significant percentage of tumours are malignant or multiple and the patient is likely to succumb from the complications of ulceration unless the target organ is removed. If no tumour is found, the body and tail of the pancreas are removed. If operation is not possible or if symptoms recur, treatment with anticholinergic drugs may be helpful.

Pancreatic Pseudo-cholera

A further pancreatic disorder has been described in which the patient has profound watery diarrhoea and hypokalaemia with normal or reduced gastric acid production. This syndrome is due to production by the tumour of an unknown hormone (possible secretin or enterogastrone) which interferes with water and electrolyte absorption in the small bowel. The treatment is surgical resection where this is possible.

2. Insulin-secreting Adenoma

The clinical picture produced by an insulin-secreting (beta-cell) adenoma of the pancreas depends on the production of hypoglycaemia.

Classically, attacks of hunger, faintness, weakness, profuse sweating, blurred vision, dysarthria, and confusion occur after exercise or between meals. Attacks are prevented and relieved by the taking of glucose or a meal.

The tumour, which is usually single, causes no local symptoms but may be invasive in 15 per cent of cases. Tumours may occasionally be ectopic, but most are found in the body or tail. The patient is usually in middle life, and the physical and mental symptoms of hypoglycaemia are such that it is not unknown for them to be thought psychoneurotic. Whipple described a characteristic triad of clinical features: (*a*) attacks of weakness and confusion and sweating, (*b*) their precipitation by fasting, and (*c*) their relief by glucose or other sources of carbohydrate.

Profuse sweating and tachycardia are the important physical signs, but convulsions and coma with positive Babinski responses may occur. In others the diagnosis may be extremely difficult and a close relationship of symptoms to fasting may be missing. Mental disturbances may be a prominent part of the clinical picture as may epileptiform convulsions.

The diagnosis of hypoglycaemia can be made from the blood during an attack, the glucose level being invariably below 50 mg. per 100 ml. Relief of symptoms by the injection of intravenous glucose is also important. The differential diagnosis includes other causes of hypoglycaemia and the psychoneuroses. Hypoglycaemia from hepatic and adrenal causes and that complicating galactosaemia may be recognized easily, but the main diagnostic difficulty occurs with the so-called 'functional hypoglycaemia' in which there is an excessive insulin response which is perhaps due to vagal over-activity. Distinction from the hypoglycaemia associated with tumours of the liver and retroperitoneal tissues must also be made. The symptoms are not so dramatic as with an insulinoma, and both coma and other neurological complications are rare. Helpful tests in the diagnosis of insulin-secreting adenoma are:

a. A blood-glucose level below 50 mg. per cent with high serum insulin levels.

b. The provocation of attacks and hypoglycaemia by starvation for 36 hours. Only water and unsweetened drinks are allowed during the test, which must be carried out in hospital. E.E.G. recordings are useful in detecting neurological deterioration before this is manifest clinically.

c. Hypoglycaemia can be precipitated by intravenous tolbutamide. Persistent hypoglycaemia lasting 1–3 hours after injection is very suggestive of insulinoma (*see Chapter 24*). Glucagon and L-leucine have been used in a similar fashion. Raised insulin and growth hormone levels are seen with these tests. The insulin response to i.v. tolbutamide is seen within 5 minutes of the injection and is particularly helpful. I.V. glucose must be available during this test which is potentially dangerous.

d. The glucose-tolerance test gives widely varying results, but may show fasting hypoglycaemia, a poor rise after glucose, and subnormal levels for from 2 to 3 hours. It has been replaced by the more specific tests.

e. Coeliac axis angiography is particularly helpful as these tumours though small (maximal size about 3 cm.) are vascular and are readily demonstrated. Multiple tumours may also be shown.

f. Pancreatic scintiscanning may also be helpful.

TREATMENT

Surgery is indicated if there is good evidence of insulinoma. Usually a careful search will reveal the tumour in the pancreas, but ectopic foci must not be forgotten, and in the event of multiple adenomata of the pancreas being found, the body and tail of the gland must be removed. It is most important to exclude a multiple adenoma syndrome so that studies of gastric secretion, calcium metabolism, and X-rays of the pituitary fossa may be required preoperatively. Resistant hypoglycaemia may respond to diazoxide.

3. Carcinoma of the Pancreas and Ampullary Region

Because of their different prognosis and clinical features it is of some importance to differentiate between carcinoma of the head and body of the pancreas and neoplasms arising from the peri-ampullary region.

PATHOLOGY

Carcinoma of the pancreatic glandular tissue occurs more commonly in the head of the gland (75 per cent) than in the body and tail (25 per cent). The growth is derived from duct epithelium and is thus an adenocarcinoma; more rarely, acini derived from glandular tissue are present. The stromal reaction varies and a hard scirrhous growth is the result of fibrosis. Peri-ampullary adenocarcinomata are derived either from the duodenal mucosa, the epithelium overlying the ampulla, or the terminal parts of the main pancreatic or common bile-ducts. Histological features do not usually allow one to differentiate between the sites of origin, and local invasion makes this more difficult still. The growth may vary greatly in size, and small lesions are easily missed unless the duodenum is opened so that the ampullary region can be inspected.

CLINICAL FEATURES

a. Carcinoma of the Head of the Pancreas

Males past middle life are most commonly affected. The initial symptoms include abdominal pain, fatigue, weakness, and loss of weight. Because of the position of the growth, obstruction of the common bile-duct occurs early, causing obstructive jaundice, pale stools, dark urine, and pruritus. Completely painless jaundice occurs in perhaps 25 per cent of patients. Pain may be felt in the epigastrium and may radiate to the back, or may be aggravated by food.

The liver is often enlarged, and sometimes the distended gall-bladder can be felt. Though unusual, it may be possible in thin patients to feel the pancreatic tumour itself.

In those cases where physical signs are absent and jaundice has not developed, diagnosis can be very difficult, and it must be remembered that a negative barium examination does not exclude carcinoma of the pancreas.

Helpful tests are those aimed at confirming the presence of obstructive jaundice, those related to pancreatic function, and those showing the tumour itself.

i. Rarely, there may be intermittent glycosuria and the glucose tolerance curve is of diabetic pattern.

ii. The stools may contain occult blood if the growth ulcerates the duodenum.

iii. A barium meal may show distortion of the duodenal loop or duodenal stenosis. A lateral film may reveal forward displacement of the stomach. Even when no obvious abnormality is shown in the films, altered motility of the duodenum, when observed by the radiologist, can be an important sign. Retroperitoneal insufflation of carbon dioxide and tomography have been used to aid the radiological diagnosis, but hypotonic duodenography seems to be more helpful. Duodenoscopy has a place in the diagnosis of lesions invading the duodenal loop, when cannulation of the ampulla may help to define the level of biliary obstruction.

iv. The duodenal aspirate can be examined cytologically for malignant cells after the injection of secretin. If the pancreatic duct is obstructed the volume is reduced, but the bicarbonate and enzyme concentration is unchanged. The presence of blood in the aspirate may also be suggestive.

v. Pancreatic scanning with ^{75}Se-selenomethionine may also be helpful.

vi. The serum amylase is raised occasionally when the pancreatic duct is obstructed.

vii. The E.S.R. is moderately raised.

viii. Prior to operation the duct system of the liver may be outlined by the technique of transhepatic cholangiography. This localizes the site of common bile-duct obstruction and helps to differentiate the lesion from a growth of the hepatic ducts or from biliary obstruction due to stones. It is being replaced by endoscopic cholangiography.

TREATMENT

The radical operation of pancreaticoduodenectomy is a major procedure which is not often possible, and even after an apparently successful excision patients rarely survive for more than a year. The average survival of all cases is about seven months. Operations such as cholecystojejunostomy, which allow bile to flow into the gut, are very useful for they relieve jaundice and pruritus and so make the patient's remaining life more comfortable.

Before surgery, prothrombin deficiency must always be corrected by parenteral vitamin K.

b. Carcinoma of the Ampulla of Vater

The following are the clinical and pathological features which may help to differentiate an ampullary carcinoma from a neoplasm of the head of the pancreas. Tumours in this site may originate from the bile-duct, the small-bowel mucosa, or the pancreatic duct.

i. The clinical course is more rapid with less prominent symptoms of anorexia, abdominal pain, and weight-loss.

ii. Jaundice is of early onset and, because of necrosis of the obstructing growth, may fluctuate.

iii. Haemorrhage into the small bowel is more common and may be dramatic. The combination of obstructive jaundice and intestinal haemorrhage should suggest an ampullary neoplasm.

iv. Radiological changes in the duodenal loop occur early in the course of the disease, and studies of exfoliative cytology may reveal malignant cells. In view of the fact that pancreatic duct obstruction occurs less frequently with ampullary than with pancreatic growths, tests of exocrine pancreatic function may be normal.

v. Duodenoscopy is helpful in visualization of these tumours and biopsy can then be taken for confirmation of diagnosis.

TREATMENT

The main difference between pancreatic and ampullary growths is that in the latter surgery is more likely to be curative. Radical pancreaticoduodenectomy, which has a mortality of about 7 per cent, gives in this disease a 30 per cent survival over five years.

c. Carcinoma of the Body and Tail of the Pancreas

In marked contrast to growths of the head and ampullary region, growths of the body and tail do not involve the bile-duct until late, so jaundice is not an early feature. The chief symptom is pain referred to the back, boring in character, relieved by sitting up, and aggravated by lying down. Loss of weight, anorexia, and loss of energy may also occur. Patients may be referred for 'back strain', or, worse still, after a series of negative investigations, referred to a psychiatrist, so great may be the difficulty of diagnosis. It is usual for the patient to have had symptoms for six months before the diagnosis is made.

Jaundice usually indicates that the lesion is inoperable. A feature of some interest is the occasional occurrence of multiple thromboses in superficial or deep veins and arteries, which, if they occur, may suggest the diagnosis, though they are also found with other neoplasms. Occasionally the tumour may be palpable. Slowly growing tumours may invade and occlude the splenic vein and haemorrhage from resultant varices may thus be the initial presentation. Rarely a bruit audible on abdominal auscultation results from this occlusive process.

There are no tests which show a consistent abnormality, though pancreatic scintiscanning may with further experience be an exception to this rule, and the same may be said for coeliac axis angiography, pancreatic tomography, and endoscopic pancreatography.

Serum amylase and routine radiology do not help, although serum lactic dehydrogenase and tests of islet function such as the glucose and tolbutamide tolerance tests may be helpful.

The E.S.R., which should be done in all patients with obscure abdominal pain, is raised.

PANCREATIC CYSTS

True cysts may occur in the substance of the pancreas, but more important are the 'pseudo' cysts which form from the outpouring of fluid into the lesser sac of the peritoneum. They develop after an attack of pancreatitis. The condition presents as a swelling in the upper abdomen which transmits pulsation from the aorta, and which may be obviously cystic. The cyst may be drained into the upper small bowel or stomach.

ANNULAR AND ABERRANT PANCREAS

These two conditions result from developmental abnormalities of the pancreas. The former gives rise to duodenal obstruction and it may produce symptoms similar to pyloric stenosis. This may occur within the first few days of life or may be deferred, rarely, to adult life. In the former case the clinical picture may be indistinguishable from that due to duodenal atresia. Later it may mimic congenital pyloric stenosis, though the vomitus in pyloric stenosis does not contain bile. In adults the features are indistinguishable from those of peptic ulcer causing pyloric narrowing, and peptic ulceration may complicate this lesion. Barium studies confirm the slow gastric emptying and gastric dilatation, and also reveal dilatation of the first part of the duodenum. Treatment is surgical—either dividing the constricting pancreatic tissue or performing a by-pass operation.

Ectopic areas of pancreatic tissue are found in the stomach and duodenum and usually cause symptoms in adult life. Symptoms include those of peptic ulceration, pyloric stenosis, and alimentary bleeding. Barium studies may demonstrate such lesions, the most characteristic finding being a polypoid tumour. Surgical removal of these foci is recommended because of the possibility of complications such as haemorrhage.

FURTHER READING

Acute Pancreatitis
RICHMAN, A. (1956), 'Acute Pancreatitis', *Am. J. Med.*, **21**, 246.
TRAPNELL, J. E. (1968), 'Pancreatitis—Acute and Chronic', *Br. J. Hosp. Med.*, **1**, 181.
Chronic Pancreatitis
GROSS, J. B., and COMFORT, M. W. (1956), 'Chronic Pancreatitis', *Am. J. Med.*, **21**, 596.
HOWAT, H. T. (1965), *Second Symposium on Advanced Medicine*, p. 301. London: Royal College of Physicians.
Surgery of the Pancreas
WARREN, K. W. (1961), 'Surgery of the Pancreas', *Proc. R. Soc. Med.*, **54**, 1119.

Fibrocystic Disease
ANDERSEN, D. H. (1938), 'Cystic Fibrosis of the Pancreas and its Relation to Coeliac Disease', *Am. J. Dis. Child.*, **56**, 344.
D'SANT AGNESE, P. (1961), 'Cystic Fibrosis of the Pancreas', *Ann. intern. Med.*, **54**, 482.
GRACEY, M., and ANDERSON, C. M. (1970), 'Childhood Malabsoptive Disorders of Increasing Importance in Adult Life', *Jl R. Coll. Phys.*, **4**, 305.

Hereditary Pancreatitis
GROSS, J. B., GAMBILL, E. E., and ULRICH, J. A. (1962), 'Hereditary Pancreatitis', *Am. J. Med.*, **33**, 358.

Carcinoma
KIBLER, C. E., and BERNATZ, P. E. (1958), 'Operative Experience with Carcinoma of the Body and Tail of the Pancreas', *Proc. Mayo Clin.*, **33**, 247.
NIGHTINGALE, E. J., BOYD, L. J., and MERSHEIMER, W. L. (1958), 'Observations on Pancreatic Carcinoma, a Study of 100 Cases', *Am. J. Gastroent.*, **29**, 612.

Zollinger-Ellison Syndrome
HOWE, G. T. (1968), 'Zollinger-Ellison Syndrome', *Br. J. Hosp. Med.*, **1**, 190.
SIRCUS, W. (1964), *First Symposium on Advanced Medicine*, p. 397. London: Royal College of Physicians.
ZOLLINGER, R. M., and CRAIG, T. V. (1960), 'Endocrine Tumours and Peptic Ulcer', *Am. J. Med.*, **29**, 761.

Annular Pancreas
MOORE, T. C. (1953), 'Annular Pancreas', *Surgery*, **33**, 138.

Heterotopic Pancreas
MARTINEZ, N. S., MORLOCK, C. G., DOCKERTY, M. B., WAUGH, J. M., and WEBER, H. M. (1958), 'Heterotopic Pancreatic Tissue involving the Stomach', *Ann. Surg.*, **147**, 1.

Chapter 17

The Small Intestine—Malabsorption

STRUCTURE

THE EPITHELIUM of the small bowel is well adapted to its function of absorption. Apart from the length (approximately 6 m.) the villous structure of the mucosa ensures a large absorbing surface, facilitating close contact between substances in the lumen of the gut and the blood and lymphatic vessels of the villi. A schematic representation of the villous lining is shown in *Fig. 62*.

The villi and the intervening crypts are covered by a single layer of cells through which absorption takes place. This layer consists of tall columnar cells and a smaller number of mucus-producing goblet cells. In the crypts themselves two further types are observed, Kulchitsky or argentaffin cells (named because of their ability to take up silver stains) which secrete serotonin, and Paneth cells containing granules of uncertain nature. The columnar cells, continually replaced by division of cells in the crypts, migrate along the villus and eventually are shed into the intestinal lumen. The columnar cell layer is therefore in a continual state of replacement. The integrity of the columnar cell layer is aided by lateral interdigitations and adhesions between cells.

The central 'core' of the villus or lamina propria contains a central leash of blood-vessels, lymphatics, and nerves as well as a few plain muscle-fibres. These are enmeshed in loose connective tissue continuous with that of the mucosa. Outer muscular and peritoneal layers complete the structure of the small intestine, the muscle layers in particular being well supplied with nerve filaments.

The process of absorption is largely one of transfer across the columnar cell layer, the outer border of which is thrown up into numerous cyto-plasmic projections or *microvilli*. The microvilli (or brush border) are in turn in close contact with an amorphous layer—the glycocalyx—which is the site of important digestive enzymes particularly concerned with disaccharide absorption.

The known absorptive processes are based on two different principles:

1. Simple water-soluble substances of low molecular weight are absorbed by *diffusion*. This is dependent on the fact that there is a higher concen-tration of the substance to be absorbed in the intestinal lumen than in the blood-stream. The process continues as long as this difference exists, and the mechanism cannot be saturated by increasing the load. There is no specific site for diffusion, which therefore begins in the upper gut at the

first point of contact between mucosa and absorbable material. The mechanism is important for the absorption of low-molecular-weight substances such as certain drugs and water-soluble vitamins. The process is non-energy-requiring and takes place through small pores in the cell wall.

2. More complex substances are absorbed by *active transport mechanisms*. This, unlike diffusion, is dependent on the provision of energy by the

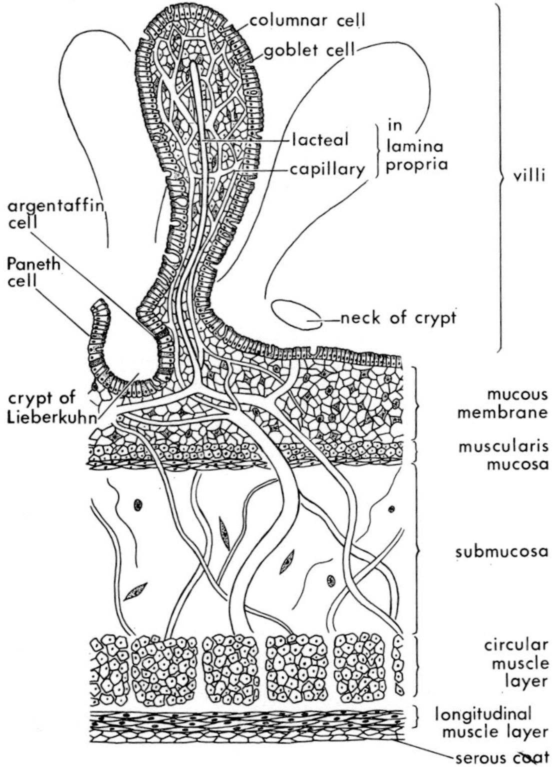

Fig. 62. The wall of the small bowel.

cellular membrane across which absorption is taking place. The mechanisms are specific for the substance absorbed and can work against a concentration gradient. Just as there are in the renal tubule specific areas for reabsorption of particular chemicals from glomerular filtrate, there are probably in the gut receptor areas for the active transport and absorption of complex substances. In the case of vitamin B_{12} and bile-salts, for example, a specific site for absorption has been demonstrated in the distal small bowel.

It is possible that in certain circumstances both mechanisms operate for a single substance. In the case of vitamin B_{12} it can be shown that very large and unphysiological doses can be absorbed by diffusion in the upper gut, whereas normal physiological amounts are absorbed after conjugation with intrinsic factor by a highly specialized mechanism of active transport in the ileum.

Other mechanisms involved include *pinocytosis*, a process by which particles of lipid are engulfed by the brush border, and *facilitated diffusion*. This latter term is given to a process which, though basically one of diffusion, seems to be performed more rapidly than simple diffusion, though there is no absorption against a concentration gradient as in active transport. In fact by far the major part of the absorption of dietary nutriments, water, and electrolytes depends on active transport mechanisms.

THE ABSORPTION OF INDIVIDUAL FOOD SUBSTANCES

1. FAT ABSORPTION

For fat absorption to take place there is an initial splitting of dietary long-chain triglycerides to long-chain fatty acids, monoglycerides, and glycerol under the action of intestinal and pancreatic lipases. For these to act effectively fat must be emulsified by bile-salts. Bile-salts together with glycerides, fatty acids, and lecithin form micelles, that is molecular aggregates, which solubilize lipid material. The micelle with its entrapped lipid is then known as a mixed micelle. The luminal pH and concentration of bile-salts are critical for effective micelle formation and it is conjugated bile-salts which are important in this respect.

Entry of lipid into the intestinal cell is the next phase. An engulfing process on the part of the cell membrane may be important here. It is not known in what form fat enters the cell. However it enters the cell, the next process is one of re-esterification, i.e., a rebuild-up of triglycerides from absorbed fatty acids, utilizing glycerol formed from the acetylation of 1,3-glycerophosphate. Coated with lipoprotein, long-chain triglycerides are then transported as chylomicrons into intestinal lymphatics. Short- and medium-chain triglycerides are absorbed more readily and are absorbed directly into the portal blood-stream. They do not require bile-salt intervention in this process. Malabsorption of fat may thus be due to decreased emulsification and micelle formation (bile-salt lack and abnormal pH), decreased lipolysis (lipase deficiency), decreased entry into intestinal cells (mucosal disease), and decreased chylomicron formation or impaired lymphatic absorption (lymphatic obstruction).

2. CARBOHYDRATE ABSORPTION

Hydrolysis of starch by salivary and pancreatic amylase leads to the production of mono- and disaccharides. The latter are split by enzymes in the brush border of the small bowel to constituent monosaccharides—the enzymes responsible being lactase, maltase, and sucrase. It is as monosaccharides that carbohydrate enters the portal circulation—the process being one of active transport, though certain sugars such as fructose are exceptions. Structural characteristics of monosaccharides may determine the speed of this process and an adequate concentration of Na ions is also essential. It is currently believed that movement across the cell is by means of an intermediate carrier which is part of the cell wall possessing particular attachment sites for particular monosaccharides. It is in the supply of energy for the transport process of the carrier and its sugar across the cell to the serosal side that Na and ATP (adenosine triphosphate) are required.

3. PROTEIN ABSORPTION

Following digestion by peptidases and trypsin the resulting amino-acids are absorbed by active transport. The L-isomers of naturally occurring amino-acids are more rapidly absorbed than the D-isomers. Competition also exists between amino-acids for absorption; this is presumed to represent affinity within structurally similar groups of amino-acids (neutral, acidic, basic) for a common protein carrier. In certain instances it has been shown that a defect of amino-acid absorption exists both in the kidney and in the small gut—a classic example of this situation being cystinuria, where the increased urinary excretion of cystine, methionine, lysine, and ornithine is matched by a similar pattern of malabsorption of the same amino-acids in the small bowel. Another clinical example of this dual type of transport defect is Hartnup disease.

It seems likely that peptides may also be absorbed as such, the initial hydrolysis to dipeptides occurring at the brush border, with subsequent intracellular hydrolysis of the dipeptides formed. Protein itself may also be absorbed unchanged and this is certainly so in the neonate. It must be remembered that the majority of protein undergoing absorption is of endogenous origin from the breakdown of epithelial cells, digestive secretions, etc.

4. ELECTROLYTE AND WATER ABSORPTION

These substances are also absorbed by active transport mechanisms. The active movement of Na results in subsequent transport and absorption of chloride and bicarbonate. Water absorption seems closely associated with the phenomenon and may occur between the intercellular spaces between the intestinal epithelial cells. The energy required for these processes is provided by the metabolism of glucose so that there is interdependence of glucose and Na absorption on each other. The process of water and electrolyte absorption is maximal in the lower small bowel.

5. VITAMIN B_{12}

Brief mention must be made of vitamin B_{12} absorption. This vitamin is absorbed in physiological amounts via a carrier substance intrinsic factor (I.F.)—M.W. 50,000—secreted by gastric parietal cells. The complex of vitamin B_{12} (extrinsic factor: E.F.) and I.F. (E.F.I.F.) is transported to the ileum where the combination is split and the two components are separately absorbed. Vitamin B_{12} is then bound to globulin and carried to organs such as the liver.

Larger doses of vitamin B_{12} can be absorbed by simple diffusion.

6. FOLIC ACID

Dietary folate consisting largely of conjugated pterylglutamates is split by intestinal conjugases to simpler folate derivatives, i.e., folic monoglutamate, etc., before absorption occurs. Absorption then seems to occur more readily than can be explained by simple diffusion and perhaps an active process is operative.

7. IRON ABSORPTION

Iron absorption occurs chiefly in the proximal small intestine. Iron exists in the intestinal cell after absorption in two forms—a bivalent non-ferritin 'transport' iron and a trivalent ferritin storage iron. Iron deficiency or iron overloading directs iron into the appropriate form depending on whether the emphasis is on absorption (transport) or storage. Storage iron can be lost by the shedding of intestinal cells while transport iron is rapidly absorbed. The co-ordinating mechanism for this mucosal control is unknown—it is *not* due to the controlling mechanism of an iron-binding protein (apoferritin). Ferrous iron (Fe^{++}) is more readily absorbed than ferric (Fe^{+++}). There is also considerable variation in the rate of absorption of organic and inorganic iron. Organic (food) iron may be malabsorbed particularly where there is diminished contact with intestinal ferments or with intestinal hurry. Organic iron of animal origin is generally more readily absorbed than iron from vegetable sources.

8. BILE-SALT ABSORPTION

The bile-salts in human bile, which are derived from cholesterol, are the glycine and taurine conjugates of one trihydroxy bile acid (cholic acid) and two dihydroxy bile acids (chenodeoxycholic and deoxycholic acid). The latter is formed by bacterial dehydroxylation of the trihydroxy cholic acid, whilst chenodeoxycholic acid is a primary dihydroxy bile acid. The ileum is the site of bile-salt absorption, so that the intraluminal concentration of bile-salts is highest in these areas where fat absorption occurs. The total bile-salt pool is small ($c.$ 4 g.) and an effective recycling system from ileum to liver is essential for effective fat absorption. The total bile-salt pool exchanges several times during each meal. Ileal disease or resection depletes the bile-salt pool producing steatorrhoea, whilst the resulting entry of bile-salts into the colon interferes with the colonic absorption of salt and water and results in a watery diarrhoea (cholerhoeic enteropathy). The picture is thus often mixed. In liver disease bile-salt depletion may cause malabsorption. In the blind-loop syndrome bacterial overgrowth leads to bile-acid deconjugation. Whether the steatorrhoea is due to the high levels of free, i.e., unconjugated, bile acids, which may have a 'toxic' effect on the small intestinal mucosa, or to the intraluminal deficiency of conjugated bile acids is not decided.

9. CALCIUM

Calcium absorption is via an active process and this occurs mainly from the upper small bowel. Parathormone and vitamin D facilitate this process whilst interference with fat absorption has the opposite effect. Vitamin D is malabsorbed in the presence of steatorrhoea for it needs micelle formation and an intact lymphatic system in the gut. Unabsorbed fatty acids may also precipitate calcium salts as insoluble soaps in the lower small bowel with resultant increased faecal calcium loss. The localization of calcium absorption in the duodenum and upper jejunum perhaps explains the frequency of bone disease in disorders such as coeliac disease and its comparative rarity in ileal disease, e.g., in Crohn's disease.

Tests of Small Bowel Function

Until recently the only tests of small bowel function available for general use were those directed at detecting defects of fat absorption—steatorrhoea. With improving facilities for investigation, it has now been possible to test the function of various parts of the small gut.

Reviewing these tests briefly, they would appear to be divisible into those reflecting function of the upper, mid, and lower small bowel.

Tests of absorption of water-soluble substances such as xylose, glucose, and folic acid reflect function of the upper small bowel because these substances are rapidly absorbed from the first part of the small gut they enter. Low blood-levels or low urinary excretion of these substances usually means a defect in the upper small bowel, as most classically seen in the 'sprue syndrome' (*see* p. 258). Fat absorption is a function of a variable area of the mid small gut, but heavy loads of dietary fat are absorbed more distally. A fat balance is therefore a test of mid small gut function which can be altered by structural changes or enzymes deficiencies and alteration of bacterial flora.

The lower small bowel has been shown to be the specific site of vitamin B_{12} absorption. The use of ^{58}Co vitamin B_{12} has therefore been a valuable diagnostic tool in the detection of distal bowel function and abnormal bile-salt metabolism may be found in ileal disease or resection.

Disorders of the villus brush border either may be detected by tests of disaccharide absorption, e.g., failure of the blood-glucose level to rise after an oral load of lactose suggests lactase deficiency, or can be confirmed by enzyme estimation in mucosal specimens.

Intubation techniques allow the measurement of the intestinal absorption of any substance by any part of the small bowel which can be intubated and perfused. Absorption is related to changes in the concentration of a non-absorbable marker, e.g., polyethylene glycol.

Malabsorption Syndrome

It is theoretically justifiable to apply the term 'malabsorption syndrome' to any condition in which there is impaired alimentary absorption of single or multiple substances. Thus it would be perfectly reasonable to call pernicious anaemia, in which there is malabsorption of vitamin B_{12}, a malabsorption syndrome, but in practice we tend to reserve the term for conditions of multiple malabsorption. As the most dramatic effect of such a state is steatorrhoea we think loosely of malabsorption and steatorrhoea as synonymous, but the latter is invariably accompanied by a failure to absorb and by resulting deficiency of other substances such as calcium, folic acid, and protein. It is therefore only a clinical label for the identification of the whole syndrome.

Steatorrhoea

Steatorrhoea is the passage of excessive fat in the stools, and in moderate and severe cases they are abnormal to the naked eye. They are loose and watery, or bulky and paler than normal. Some patients will volunteer that the stools look greasy, most admit that they are more offensive than usual, and many note that the stools are difficult to flush from the toilet. Undigested food may also be seen. In mild cases the stools may appear normal, and looseness is only noted after a fatty meal. Steatorrhoea can often be suspected by inspection of the stools or a faecal smear from a finger-stall. In normal subjects excretion of fat in the faeces is of the order of 2 g. per day, but since there may be fluctuations from intestinal hurry, diarrhoea, and intercurrent illness the daily upper limit of normal fat excretion is placed at 6 g. Greater amounts than this, whether there are symptoms or not, indicate steatorrhoea. In very severe cases the faecal fat content may be greater than that in the daily diet, indicating that the faecal fat is partly endogenous—arising from cells of the intestinal mucosa.

THE ACCOMPANIMENTS OF STEATORRHOEA

Where malabsorption of fat is sufficient to cause steatorrhoea, other deficiencies are usually found. The following are the possible accompaniments (*Table 19*). They may not all be found together and they tend to be more severe where there is a diffuse upset of intestinal function as in sprue and adult coeliac disease.

This list indicates the way in which the malabsorption of a particular substance may dominate the clinical picture and first bring the patient to seek medical advice.

Patients with malabsorption may make their first attendance in almost any hospital department.

Deficiencies as yet unrecognized may be discovered by new biochemical methods.

AETIOLOGY

1. Deficiency of biliary and pancreatic secretions, e.g., chronic obstructive and liver cell jaundice, chronic pancreatitis (*see Chapters 9 and 16*).

2. After gastrectomy (*see Chapter 8*).

3. Abnormal bacterial activity in the small gut, e.g., jejunal diverticulosis, stricture and blind loop in the small bowel, jejunocolic fistula (*Fig. 63*), Whipple's disease.

Table 19. ACCOMPANIMENTS OF STEATORRHOEA

SUBSTANCES MALABSORBED	POSSIBLE EFFECT
1. Fat	Steatorrhoea
2. Protein	Loss of weight
	Oedema
	Osteoporosis
	In children, failure to grow
3. Water	Nocturia
4. Calcium and vitamin D	Osteomalacia
	Tetany
	Secondary or tertiary hyperparathyroidism
5. Vitamin K	Bleeding tendency
6. Potassium	Lassitude
	Muscle weakness
	Tetany
7. Iron	Anaemia
Folic acid	Glossitis and anaemia
Vitamin B_{12}	Neuropathy, anaemia, and glossitis
8. Other vitamins	Pellagra, beriberi, dry skin, etc.
	Glossitis

4. Disease of the small bowel wall and mesenteric lymphatics, e.g., Hodgkin's disease, Crohn's disease, lymphosarcoma, amyloidosis.

5. Defect of gut mucosa, coeliac disease, adult coeliac disease, tropical sprue ('sprue syndrome').

6. Small bowel resection.

7. Drugs, phenindione, and antibiotics such as neomycin.

8. In some endocrine diseases, e.g., Addison's disease, thyrotoxicosis.

9. In certain patients with extensive skin disease or in relation to specific skin diseases such as dermatitis herpetiformis and possibly rosacea.

10. Deficiency of intestinal enzymes, mainly the disaccharides, e.g., alactasia.

11. Intestinal worms and parasites.

12. Rare and unclassified.

Steatorrhoea due to Abnormal Bacterial Activity

Normally the small bowel has a low content of luminal bacteria. Where there is gastric hypochlorhydria organisms of little clinical importance may inhabit the small gut but produce no symptoms.

In certain circumstances the small bowel becomes contaminated by a heavy growth of apparently harmful bacteria. The main situations in which this can occur are illustrated in *Fig. 63*. They depend on the existence of communication between small gut and a source of infection, or the presence in the intestinal circuit of an area of relative stagnation encouraging bacterial growth. All these defects, with the exception of gastrocolic fistula, are classified as 'blind loop syndromes', though not all are loops and some are not blind! Patients with anastomotic ulcer or carcinoma of the stomach may develop a gastrocolic fistula and intestinal stenosis may occur as a result of Crohn's disease or, more rarely, tuberculosis.

12

Recent work has suggested that organisms in the blind loop (often *Escherichia coli*, bifidobacteria, and bacteroides) can split conjugated bile-salts. The bile-salt depletion leads to a fall in their concentration below the critical micellar level with resultant steatorrhoea. The idea that deconjugated bile-salts are toxic to the mucosa is not supported by recent experimental observations. The splitting of conjugated bile-salts seems in particular to be a function of anaerobic enteric organisms, e.g., bacteroides.

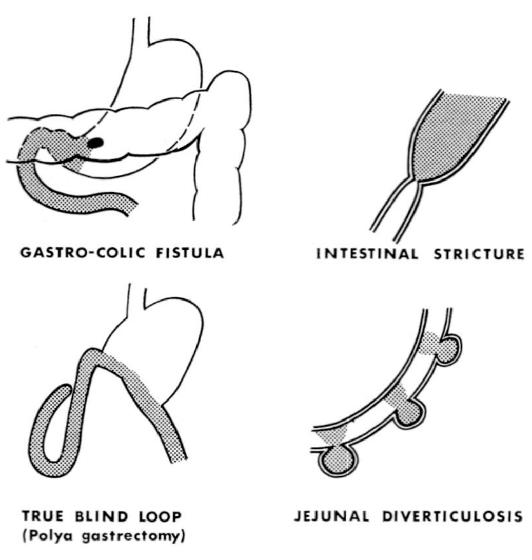

Fig. 63. Steatorrhoea due to abnormal bacterial activity.

CLINICAL PICTURE

This is dependent on the cause. Briefly, the possibility of this condition should be suspected in patients with malabsorption who have had an abdominal operation, particularly where this has involved gut resection and anastomosis, or partial gastrectomy of the Polya type. Simple laparotomy alone may cause the formation of adhesions and stenosis of small gut, but this is rare. Patients with jejunal diverticulosis are usually elderly females who have not as a rule had previous operations. Common symptoms are:

1. Diarrhoea, steatorrhoea, wasting, and signs of deficiencies.

2. Attacks of abdominal pain and rumbling, often with troublesome distension. These are particularly common in cases of jejunal diverticulosis or where there are strictures of the gut. Patients may occasionally complain of vigorous intestinal noises.

3. Anaemia is due to two factors:

a. There is often blood-loss in the stools from ulceration in a distended loop of gut. Iron deficiency is therefore not uncommon.

b. Megaloblastic anaemia due to vitamin B_{12} deficiency may occur. Bacterial growth in the gut leads to binding of vitamin B_{12} which is not available for absorption. (Body stores of vitamin B_{12} are therefore low.) In some patients with a blind-loop syndrome high levels of folate in the blood are found, and these are due to manufacture of this substance by organisms in the blind loop.

DIAGNOSIS

The diagnosis of malabsorption due to an abnormal bacterial population in the gut is often difficult. A past history of laparotomy is important and suspicion should be raised when cases of 'pernicious anaemia' present with diarrhoea, intestinal colic, and distension.

The diagnosis can be facilitated by the following tests:

1. Intestinal function tests (*see Chapter 25*) indicate normal upper gut function (providing the blind loop does not occupy this region) but reveal abnormal carbohydrate absorption, steatorrhoea, and malabsorption of vitamin B_{12}. The Schilling test is abnormal and is improved by antibiotic therapy. Unlike true pernicious anaemia, malabsorption of vitamin B_{12} is not corrected by the administration of instrinsic factor.

Note. In some cases there may be coexistent ileal disease or ileal resection so that vitamin B_{12} absorption cannot then be improved after antibiotics.

2. The blood may show iron-deficiency anaemia or macrocytosis with megaloblastic change in the marrow, and the vitamin B_{12} level in the serum may be low.

3. Occult blood may be found in the faeces.

4. A blind loop is demonstrated by careful radiological examination of the small bowel. In the case of a gastrocolic fistula, barium-enema examination is usually required. Examples of jejunal diverticulosis may easily be missed if too much contrast is given. Large blind loops may retain contrast hours after it has left the rest of the small gut.

5. Intestinal intubation reveals bacterial contamination of the small bowel—aerobic and anaerobic cultures must be performed and quantitation and antibiotic sensitivity are helpful. Significant concentrations of bacteria are of the order of 10^6 organisms per ml.

6. The urine may contain increased indoxyl sulphate-indican. This is a simple and useful test for possible intestinal bacterial contamination. On occasions it may be negative even when there is a significant contamination.

TREATMENT

The aim of treatment is that the patient's condition should be improved prior to surgical correction of the lesion, but patients may be old, frail, and wasted. A high-protein–low-fat diet and correction of anaemia are important. Antibiotics are not only of value in proving the diagnosis, but by correcting steatorrhoea are valuable in improving conditions prior to surgery. Lincomycin which is particularly effective against anaerobes may be helpful, together with ampicillin and tetracycline.

12*

In cases where it is impossible or unnecessary to correct the lesion surgically, e.g., extensive jejunal diverticulosis, antibiotics alone can be useful and administration does not necessarily have to be continuous. A long remission may follow a single course of antibiotics so that systemic vitamin B_{12} therapy may not be required, but vitamin B_{12} estimation is imperative. It has been well demonstrated that some patients with blind-loop syndrome—particularly that complicating partial gastrectomy—may develop a syndrome of extreme protein depletion. The physical signs include wasting, oedema, hypothermia, and apathy, whilst hair loss and depigmentation may also be seen. The salient investigational abnormalities include hypoproteinaemia, an increase in the ratio of non-essential to essential amino-acids in the serum, increased urinary urocanic acid in the urine after an oral load of L-histidine, and liver and pancreatic dys-function. It seems likely that severe protein depletion can be partly explained by the breakdown of dietary protein by anaerobic bacteria. The depletion responds to i.v. albumin infusions and to antibiotic therapy followed by surgical excision of the blind loop.

Steatorrhoea due to Disease of the Gut Wall and Mesenteric Lymphatics
Steatorrhoea may result from lymphatic obstruction secondary to disease of the gut or mesenteric lymphatics. Amongst the diseases causing this type of lesion are scleroderma, lymphosarcoma, Hodgkin's disease, and other malignant disorders, as well as inflammatory diseases such as tuber-culosis and Crohn's disease and the interesting condition of intestinal lymphangiectasia. Presumably lymphatic obstruction is the most important cause of this type of steatorrhoea, but multiple factors such as increased bacterial activity and mucosal changes may operate in some of them.

Diagnosis is usually made after radiological examination of the small bowel has revealed indistensible and thickened loops of gut. Biopsy of the affected area at laparotomy may be required, but a diagnosis is possible if there is evidence of the causative disease in other parts of the body. In the case of systemic sclerosis (scleroderma) changes in the facial appearance and tethering of the skin to the underlying tissues in the fingers is usually obvious, but occasionally the abnormality is confined to the intestinal tract, in which case skilled radiological studies may lead to the diagnosis which can be confirmed by biopsy. In some cases of scleroderma of the small bowel malabsorption is due to infection of stagnant loops of small bowel, i.e., a blind-loop syndrome is additionally present.

Intestinal lymphangiectasia may be suggested by oedema of the legs, a yellow thickening of the nails, and suggestive changes may be found in the small bowel X-rays with a fine 'cog wheel' pattern due to distended gut lymphatics. Distended lymphatics may be seen in small intestinal biopsy specimens. Steatorrhoea may accompany evidence of vitamin D deficiency and protein depletion as excessive protein loss occurs into the alimentary tract (protein-losing enteropathy). Treatment is difficult, but dramatic improvement may follow correction of deficiencies and institution of a low fat diet together with medium-chain triglyceride supplements. An attempt may be made to create an efficient drainage of intestinal lymph into venous channels by surgical techniques.

Whipple's Disease (*Fig. 64*)
The disease, first described by Whipple, is a rare disorder in which the main characteristics are diarrhoea with steatorrhoea, cachexia, and skin pigmentation, together with chronic polyarthritis and generalized lymph-gland enlargement. It is most often seen in middle-aged and elderly men.

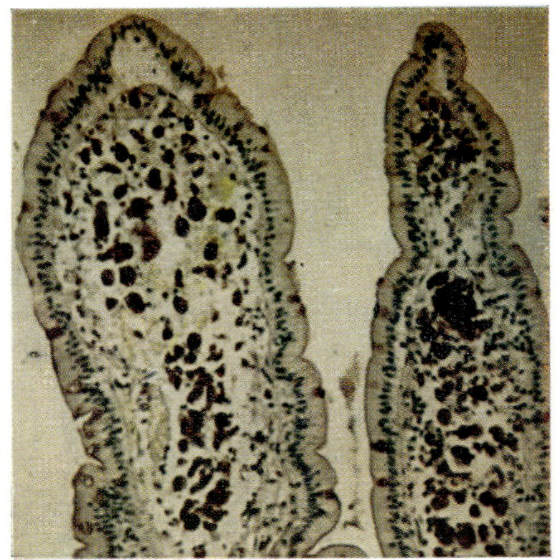

Fig. 64. PAS-positive material in villi of Whipple's disease.

Microscopical examination of the small bowel mucosa shows distension and ballooning of the villi. This may be recognizable under the dissecting microscope. The lamina propria is densely infiltrated by mononuclear cells with a 'foamy' cytoplasm which on staining with PAS reveals positive magenta inclusions. Dilated lymph-channels are also seen in the villi. The nature of this material (PAS positive), which is quite characteristic, is unknown, but it consists of a protein carbohydrate complex. Similar cells with PAS-positive material may be found in peripheral and mesenteric lymph-nodes and less commonly in liver, heart, lungs, etc.

Examination of material under the electron microscope has shown intracellular 'cigar-shaped' bacteria in the jejunal mucosa. Culture techniques have yielded variable results but the most consistent organism grown has been a *Diphtheroides* and *Streptococcus faecalis*. These could, however, be contaminants. Antibiotics have been shown to produce a remission in this once fatal disorder. If culture techniques are employed, tests of bacterial sensitivity to antibiotics may be useful. An initial course of systemic penicillin and streptomycin followed by 2 or 3 months' treatment with tetracycline produces a dramatic remission in most patients even though the precise bacteriological cause is uncertain. Occasionally in non-responsive cases corticosteroids may be needed. The old concept of the disease as one due to lymphatic obstruction by an abnormal fatty material ('lipodystrophy') is untenable.

Steatorrhoea caused by an Abnormal Small Bowel Mucosa

By far the commonest and most important groups of disease causing steatorrhoea in this country are those with an associated mucosal abnormality. These include:

a. In infants and children, coeliac disease.

b. In adults, a condition variously described as adult coeliac disease, non-tropical sprue, or idiopathic steatorrhoea. The third name is misleading because something of the pathological cause of the disease is now known. It tends to be used to describe those cases of sprue syndrome where there is no definite history of previous coeliac disease.

c. Tropical sprue, a similar disorder seen in the tropics in selected areas.

d. A certain number of chronic diseases such as skin disease, diabetes, ulcerative colitis, parasite infestation, etc., may for reasons unknown be associated with a flat intestinal musoca.

For the convenience of pathological description all four of these diseases can be grouped together as the *sprue syndrome* (*Table 20*).

Table 20. THE SPRUE SYNDROME—TERMINOLOGY

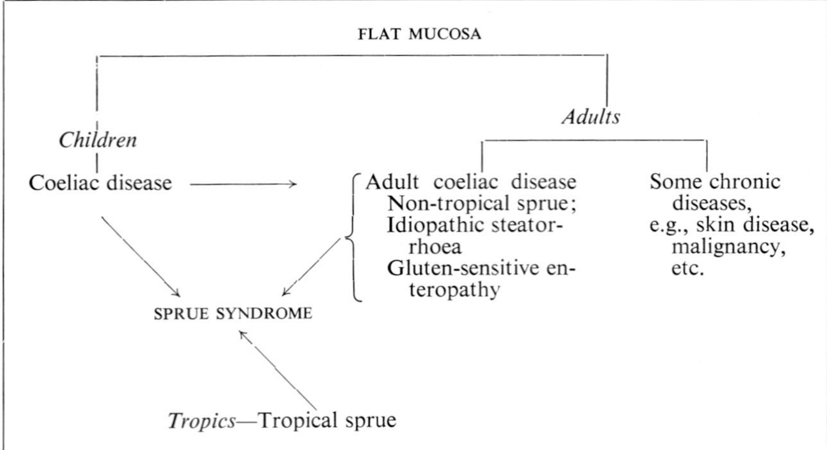

THE PATHOLOGICAL FEATURES OF THE SPRUE SYNDROME

The recognition of the mucosal changes of the sprue syndrome was made possible by the use of peroral mucosal biopsy of the small intestine. Previously Paulley had noticed histological changes in specimens obtained at laparotomy.

Changes can usually be detected even with the naked eye in a mucosal specimen obtained by biopsy (*Fig. 65*). The 'lush' appearance of the mucosal surface is missing and under the dissecting microscope the cause for this is seen to be a loss of villi. The mucosa appears flat or the surface is thrown up into a convoluted or ridged form. Microscopically, dramatic changes are seen in gross cases where there is complete loss of the villous surface ('subtotal villous atrophy') and an increased thickness of the mucosal layer due to infiltration of the submucosa by inflammatory cells and to glandular (crypt) hyperplasia. The cells of the epithelium are often flattened and show vacuolation of the cytoplasm, variable nuclear size, and less prominent or abnormal microvilli. In other cases, though the mucosal layer is thickened and shows chronic inflammatory change, shortened and misshapen villi may be present. Normal villi are about 450 μ in height, but if they are 100–300 μ 'partial' villous atrophy is recorded. Either subtotal or partial villous atrophy may be found in the sprue syndrome. In coeliac disease the lesion is certainly a diffuse one which affects the upper gut most and the lower gut less. Biopsy material will not

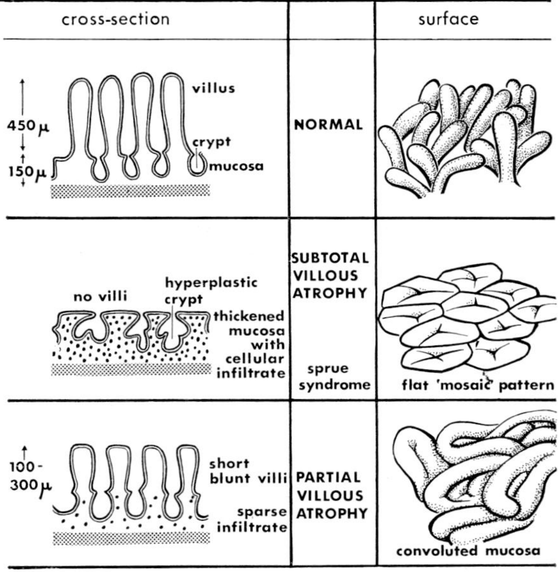

Fig. 65. The mucosal lesion of the sprue syndrome.

distinguish between tropical sprue and adult or juvenile coeliac disease, neither does the degree of histological change correlate well with the clinical picture, but as a rule patients with severe steatorrhoea are likely to show subtotal atrophy, whilst those with isolated absorption defects, such as for folic acid, show less severe changes. A better correlation is probably between the extent of the intestinal abnormality along the small bowel and the severity of malabsorption.

Nature of the Defect responsible for Malabsorption
The cause of malabsorption in coeliac disease is unknown. The part played by gluten in bringing about mucosal damage is of great importance

and one effect of this damage must be a reduction in absorptive surface. Another factor is probably a deficiency of enzymes required for absorption, and it has been shown that the surface of the 'coeliac' mucosa is deficient in certain enzyme systems. Certainly lack of protein-splitting enzymes (peptidases) could be responsible for failure of gluten digestion, although evidence suggests that deficiency of this type of enzyme is the result rather than the cause of the disease. Attention has also been given to the possibility that mucosal damage is potentiated by release of lysosomal enzymes which are present in higher than normal amounts in coeliac mucosa. Changes are also found when the mucosa is studied by the electron microscope. Enlarged mitochondria suggest disorganization of the absorptive mechanism.

It has been shown that in coeliac disease the process of cell division and migration from the crypts is accelerated. This means that there is a great increase in the extrusion of 'villous' cells into the gut lumen, and this fact has been demonstrated by detection of increased loss of DNA into the bowel lumen. This loss of cells may be one of the reasons why villi do not form. Certainly the epithelial cells are grossly abnormal when compared with the regular columnar cell layer found in normal persons.

Other secondary factors may be important. It has been demonstrated that, in tropical sprue at least, intestinal *bacteria* are important, and in the other variants of the sprue syndrome abnormal intestinal contents may encourage bacterial growth.

Disordered motility may quicken or slow the rate at which intestinal contents are propelled through absorptive areas of the gut. *Folic acid deficiency* may accentuate mucosal damage and aggravate malabsorption.

Whatever the factor or factors responsible, the initial disorder must be related to the effects of gluten. Because there is a higher than normal incidence of coeliac disease in close relatives of propositi an inherited disorder may sometimes determine gluten sensitivity. The present concept seems to favour an abnormal sensitivity to gluten and as a result immuno-logical damage to small bowel mucosa at the site of contact with dietary gluten.

a. Coeliac Disease in Children

This is the chronic disease of children.

AETIOLOGY

The classic studies of Dicke showed that patients with this disease are abnormally sensitive to gluten, which is a protein found in the germ of wheat, rye, and barley grain. Withdrawal of gluten from the diet not only leads to clinical but to histological improvement. Experimental work suggests that the toxic fraction of gluten is gliadin. Gliadin contains glutamine, also possibly harmful to the mucosa.

There is no information concerning the state of the small bowel mucosa before the symptoms of the disease are apparent. It seems likely that the small intestinal damage results from an immunological reaction to gluten or some subfraction of it. A family history of the disease is sometimes obtained though the pattern of inheritence is uncertain.

PATHOLOGY

Apart from the mucosal changes and a variable dilatation of the small intestine there are no important changes in the gut, but as a result of the disease there may be severe wasting and fatty infiltration of the liver.

CLINICAL PICTURE

The disease begins gradually, between the ages of 6 months and 2 years. With the tendency for early introduction of carbohydrate into the infant's diet symptoms may commence as early as 3 months. Anorexia, irritability, and diarrhoea with pale bulky stools are soon followed by loss of weight. In contrast to the wasted limbs and pinched facies, the abdomen is protuberant, soft, and tympanitic. Muscle tone is poor and anaemia may be obvious. If not treated the failure to grow is soon obvious.

Accompaniments and Complications

Hypoproteinaemia may cause oedema and hypocalcaemia cause tetany. Rickets may develop. In contrast with the adult disease, megaloblastic anaemia of any severity is uncommon.

DIAGNOSIS

Though the diagnosis is rarely difficult, the disease has to be distinguished from the other important cause of steatorrhoea at this age, which is fibro-cystic disease of the pancreas, but in that case the history dates from birth and there is a story of respiratory infections and the appetite is preserved.

The tests used to confirm the presence of malabsorption due to coeliac disease are identical with those indicated for use in adult cases (*see* Adult Coeliac Disease, *infra*). Some of these may be difficult to carry out at this age. Radiological evidence of delayed growth is obtained from radiographs of the feet and carpus to show centres of ossification. The ossification of epiphyses is often fragmentary.

PROGNOSIS AND TREATMENT

Before the introduction of the gluten-free régime there was an appreciable mortality, and in those who survived, permanent sequelae, such as rickets and stunting of growth, were common. The response to a gluten-free diet is so rapid that within a few days there is a noticeable change in the child's outlook and well-being, as well as an improvement in appetite. The diarrhoea and abdominal distension decrease.

There is no certainty as to how long a gluten-free diet should be continued, but probably this should be maintained for life. Certainly it is essential for this treatment to be continued until body growth is complete. Until the effects of dietary gluten restriction on the incidence of complicating neoplasms is fully known, lifetime gluten restriction seems the sensible approach. The return of diarrhoea and abdominal distension means that gluten sensitivity persists. Some children are sensitive to such small amounts of gluten that the addition of an ordinary biscuit may produce obvious deterioration. It is wise to give extra iron, folic acid, calcium, and vitamin D to ensure that deficiencies do not develop.

b. Adult Coeliac Disease

AETIOLOGY

About one-third of the patients have a history suggestive of coeliac disease in childhood. Two-thirds give no such history and it is not known whether the mucosal lesion antedates the onset of symptoms.

PATHOLOGY

The mucosal lesion is identical with that seen in other varieties of the sprue syndrome. On naked-eye examination the intestine is thin and dilated but microscopically some hypertrophy of muscle-fibres in the bowel wall and increased lipofuscin pigmentation may be seen. The intestinal lesion decreases in severity as it is traced distally to the ileum, but in severe cases the latter may be abnormal. The large bowel shows no changes.

CLINICAL PICTURE

The disease may appear at any age, males and females being equally affected. Increasing numbers of patients aged 60 years and over are being diagnosed, but most patients are young adults or middle-aged. In those with a history of coeliac disease symptoms either continue from childhood or, more commonly, abate in adolescence only to relapse in adult life.

The presenting symptom is usually diarrhoea with steatorrhoea, but most patients complain of lassitude, depression, and loss of weight. Abdominal pain is not usually a problem, but attacks of abdominal distension and colic with vomiting may simulate small-bowel obstruction. Loss of energy is usually accompanied by glossitis or skin rashes of a 'pellagroid' type. Nocturia may occur as well as symptoms of anaemia.

On examination the patient is wasted and the face, particularly in males, is so changed by the absence of buccal fat that it looks like an inverted triangle. The facial skin is fine and pigmented. Various erythematous or pellagroid rashes may affect the arms and legs, where the skin is sometimes rough and lichenified. Fairly intense pigmentation of the whole body is not uncommon, and finger clubbing quite usual. The tongue is often red, smooth, and fissured, and there may be signs of iron deficiency such as angular stomatitis, koilonychia, and pallor. In contrast to the wasting of the face and limbs, the abdomen is distended, doughy in consistency, and often hyperresonant.

Accompaniments and Complications (*Fig. 66*)

A certain degree of anaemia, which is either sideropenic and microcytic or megaloblastic, due to folic acid or, rarely, vitamin B_{12} deficiency, occurs in most patients.

Dependent *oedema* is associated with malabsorption of protein as well as increased intestinal loss (protein-losing enteropathy). *Bone disease* is caused by deficiency of calcium, vitamin D, and protein, and, histologically, osteomalacia, osteoporosis, secondary and tertiary hyperparathyroidism can occur. Adults usually complain of vague rheumatic pains, but severe localized pain may be due to 'pseudo fractures'. Hypocalcaemia causes overt or latent *tetany*. Paraesthesiae in the limbs suggests a *peripheral neuritis*, but perhaps due to the rarity of severe vitamin B$_{12}$ deficiency *subacute combined degeneration of the cord* is not usual.

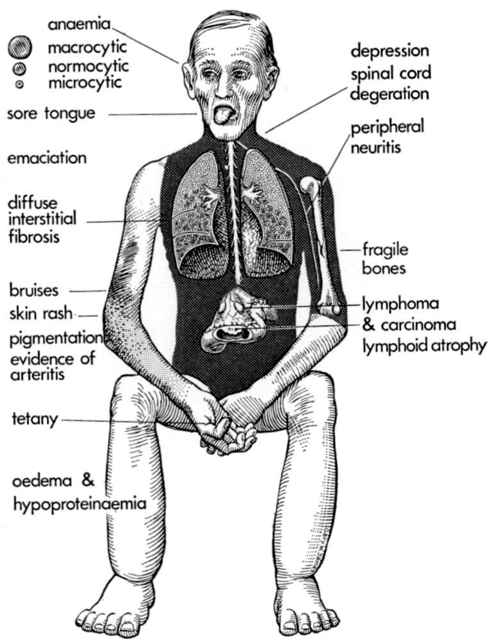

Fig. 66. Complications of coeliac disease.

A neuropathy of unknown cause is associated with posterior column and peripheral nerve involvement in the legs and causes progressive difficulty with walking. Proximal myopathy also occurs. A variety of changes are noted histologically in the brain and there is also an increased incidence of psychotic illness. The cause for the neuropathy is unknown and there is not necessarily an improvement with strict gluten restriction. Muscle weakness and lethargy may be due to hypokalaemia. Deficiency of vitamin K is sometimes of such severity as to cause spontaneous bleeding. Infertility is a further possibility. This responds to gluten restriction. There is no doubt that a reticulosis or carcinoma is an occasional complication of coeliac disease. The reticulosis is usually Hodgkin's disease and the site intestinal or abdominal with extension in some cases to mediastinal and peripheral lymph-glands. The onset of reticulosis is with failure of health, abdominal pain, diarrhoea, and in some cases intestinal perforation. Treatment is usually unrewarding and death may occur within 6 months. There is some evidence to suggest that reticulosis may be more common in those who relax dietary gluten restriction. Allied to this condition may be the widespread lymphoid atrophy (particularly of the spleen) with Howell-Jolly bodies in peripheral red blood-cells seen in some patients, and the abnormalities of lymphoid function and immuno-globulin concentration (particularly low serum IgM and high or low serum IgA) which are also found. A widespread disorder of lymphoid tissue could be associated with an increased tendency to neoplasia.

Of the carcinomata there is certainly an increase in oesophageal and small-bowel growths and again strict gluten restriction may have a protective effect.

Simple ulcers of the small bowel may also be seen. The cause is unknown but perforation may occur and diagnosis from reticulosis may be difficult. An arteritis with skin ulceration and as association with cryoglobulinaemia is also recognized and others postulate an increased incidence of inter-stitial pulmonary fibrosis.

DIAGNOSIS

This is straightforward in the classic case with severe steatorrhoea, but in those suffering chiefly from bone-thinning or anaemia the link with the causative intestinal disorder may be overlooked. The following diagnostic tests are helpful.

a. Tests of the absorptive function of the upper small intestine are abnormal. The glucose tolerance curve is 'flat' and the xylose absorption test shows a low excretion (less than 35 per cent in 5 hours) in the urine after an oral dose of 5 g. Folic acid absorption is impaired. It should be noted that the glucose tolerance test is sometimes flat for reasons other than poor absorption from the jejunum.

b. A fat balance may show steatorrhoea. This is best performed on a 100-g. fat diet so that intestinal 'reserve' is stressed. Tests of radioactive fat excretion may be helpful, but in general have not replaced chemical fat estimation. Anorexia may reduce fat intake and excretion in the stools so that steatorhoea is missed.

c. Lower small-bowel function is sometimes abnormal so that vitamin B_{12} uptake may be reduced and serum B_{12} levels low. There are, however, other factors which may interfere with vitamin B_{12} absorption.

The Blood

The peripheral blood-film may show an anaemia which is often both hypochromic and macrocytic. The bone-marrow will show megaloblastic haemopoiesis in about 30 per cent of cases. The serum iron level is often low, and the B_{12} level sometimes reduced. FIGLU (formiminoglutamic acid) excretion after a histidine load may be measured in the urine and the folate (folic acid) level in serum or red blood-cells can be measured by microbiological methods (*Lactobacillus casei*). The megaloblastic anaemia of adult coeliac disease is usually caused by folic acid deficiency secondary to its malabsorption. This can be shown by a folic acid absorption test (*see* p. 425). A further possible though disputed cause for folic acid deficiency in coeliac disease is lack of intestinal conjugases with subsequent failure of splitting of dietary folate complexes.

The Blood Chemistry

The serum potassium is often low owing to increased loss in fluid faeces and there may be an associated alkalosis. This deficiency may aggravate anorexia, abdominal distension, and lethargy. An E.C.G. may show flattened T waves and prolongation of QT complexes if there is hypokalaemia. The serum calcium may be low or normal if the parathyroids are functioning normally, and the serum phosphate is often reduced for the same reason, while alkaline phosphatase is elevated if there is osteomalacia. Magnesium deficiency may occur. The serum iron is often low, even if anaemia is not apparent.

Radiographic Studies

Radiographs of the skeletal system may show abnormalities. Bonethinning is best seen in films of the hand bones or the vertebrae. New techniques of measuring bone density may facilitate the earlier recognition of bone-thinning. Pseudo-fractures—slit-like areas in the cortex of long bones, scapulae, and pelvis—can be seen in some patients with osteomalacia, and the subperiosteal erosions of secondary or tertiary hyperparathyroidism are best seen in the phalanges and metacarpals; films of the teeth may demonstrate reabsorption of the lamina dura.

Studies of the bowel with a flocculable medium merely show clumping of contrast. This is suggestive but not absolute evidence of steatorrhoea. Details of mucosal pattern are best obtained with a relatively nonflocculable medium such as Raybar. In typical adult coeliac disease the small gut is dilated, the mucosal folds thickened, and the normal 'feathery' pattern lost.

Biopsy Studies

A biopsy from the iliac crest is sometimes valuable in confirming the presence of bone disease. Biopsy of the jejunal or duodenal mucosa is an essential step in confirming the diagnosis of adult coeliac disease.

Studies of Protein Metabolism

Tests designed to estimate loss of endogenous protein from the bowel utilizing albumin or compounds of similar molecular size, such as polyvinyl pyrollidone labelled with ^{131}I, may show increased losses of protein into the gut. The serum albumin and globulin may be reduced and albumin turnover studies reflect the increased breakdown or impaired synthesis of protein.

13

Out-patient Tests for Adult Coeliac Disease

In patients with symptoms suggestive of steatorrhoea certain screening tests may indicate whether hospital investigation is required so that fat balance and other studies can be made. Xylose absorption and FIGLU tests are helpful as is a red cell or serum folate test. The FIGLU test is invariably positive in patients with adult coeliac disease and the folate low. A radiological examination of the small bowel is also useful in excluding other causes of steatorrhoea, and in some cases giving positive evidence of the sprue syndrome.

ASSESSMENT AND TREATMENT

As with childhood coeliac disease there is a beneficial effect from a gluten-free diet. Unlike the childhood condition, however, the response to the withdrawal of gluten is often delayed and the full therapeutic benefit may not be seen for several months. However, in severe cases the response is accompanied by a lessening of diarrhoea, increased appetite and weight, and a great improvement in mental outlook. Tests of intestinal absorption improve and there may be histological improvement as well. Seventy per cent of patients can be controlled by a gluten-free régime providing they persist with it.

There is also a place for a high-protein–low-fat diet in the treatment of mild cases of steatorrhoea in elderly patients. On this régime most patients pass fewer stools and the improvement may be sufficient to control diarrhoea without the disadvantage of tedious diet.

Occasionally, antibiotics can improve bowel function and lessen diarrhoea.

A hard core of patients with adult coeliac disease does not respond to gluten withdrawal, and if symptoms are severe, corticosteroids can be tried. The improvement in small-bowel function and control of diarrhoea is rapid, but as soon as the drugs are withdrawn, relapse occurs. Aggravation of bone disease is obviously a hazard in patients treated in this way. The mechanism by which corticosteroids work is unknown, but they have been shown to improve the efficiency of intestinal absorption and to improve mucosal histology. The nature of the lesion in patients with coeliac disease refractory to treatment is unknown. Many are undoubtedly not examples of coeliac disease and most observers would say that failure to respond to strict gluten withdrawal means that the patient does not have the disease. Others feel that the occasional patient with coeliac disease enters a refractory phase. Interest has centred in this group on the possibility of pancreatic failure, lack of intestinal Paneth cells, or latent reticulosis as the cause of this syndrome.

Whatever the basic treatment the following supplements may be required to correct specific deficiencies.

a. Folic acid, 5–10 mg. t.d.s., and oral or systemic iron for anaemia. Vitamin B_{12} is not often required, but care must be taken to ensure that the serum B_{12} levels do not fall when folic acid is given, as in that case there would be a danger of cord damage.

b. Calcium as calcium lactate or effervescent calcium-Sandoz (4 tabs— 1600 mg.—80 mEq. of calcium) daily, and calciferol 50,000 units intramuscularly every month, for the control of tetany and osteomalacia. Osteoporosis may be improved by anabolic steroids.

c. Vitamin K, 10 mg. intramuscularly at monthly intervals, will correct prothrombin deficiency, and water-soluble vitamins (Tab. Vitaminorum Co.) can be given orally.

d. Simple symptomatic treatment of diarrhoea, e.g., with codeine phosphate 30 mg. t.d.s. or Mist. Kaolin 15 ml. t.d.s., may also be needed.

c. Tropical Sprue

This illness occurs in such tropical countries as India, China, and Puerto Rico. There are a few reports of its occurrence in Africa. In endemic areas the incidence is patchy; there may be a marked variation in the number of patients from town to town or even from house to house. In some areas such as southern India the disorder is very common. The basic aetiology is unknown, but an abnormal bacterial flora in the small bowel is the most likely provocative factor. It affects both white and coloured patients and the former may have symptoms some years after returning from the tropics. The parts played by diet and alimentary infection in producing abnormal bacterial activity in the gut cannot yet be assessed.

The disease begins with diarrhoea, steatorrhoea, loss of weight, ankle swelling, and a sore tongue. Studies of small-bowel absorptive power demonstrate the diffuse mucosal changes. There is impaired glucose, fat, vitamin B_{12}, and folic acid absorption and, as a result of the latter, megaloblastic anaemia often occurs.

Intestinal biopsy shows identical changes to those of adult coeliac disease, though on the whole histological changes are less severe and diagnosis must be based on the history of residence in a 'sprue' area. The good response to antibiotic therapy is also diagnostic. A chronic form with anaemia due to vitamin B_{12} deficiency may present long after removal from a sprue area.

There are three main lines of *treatment*:

a. Folic acid therapy may lead to an improvement in the diarrhoea and usually cures the glossitis and megaloblastic anaemia. It is important to remember that vitamin B_{12} deficiency is common in chronic tropical sprue and folic acid administration may then cause overt neurological damage. Careful clinical and serological monitoring of vitamin B_{12} status is essential.

b. Antibiotic therapy produces marked clinical improvement in about a half, and partial improvement in the remainder, of the patients. This treatment alone can produce a reticulocytosis and improves anaemia. Non-absorbable sulphonamides, chlortetracycline, chloramphenicol, or streptomycin have been shown to be effective. Presumably the clinical response is due to the removal of abnormal bacteria or their toxic products which have interfered with intestinal absorption. A remission is accompanied not only by improvement in intestinal function but by regrowth of normal villi.

c. Removal to a temperate climate. Although there is no knowledge as to why remissions tend to occur in temperate climates and no certainty that they will do so, it has been well known for many years in the Indian Army that transfer to a hill station will often cure sprue. Most patients with tropical sprue get better in time whatever is done. With folic acid, antibiotics, and a low-fat diet improvement is rapid. A gluten-free diet does not help.

d. Other Mucosal Disorders

Amyloid deposits in the mucosa may cause steatorrhoea, and the condition can be diagnosed by biopsy. Infiltration of the bowel wall and lymphatics by Hodgkin's disease or systemic sclerosis may also interfere with absorption.

Steatorrhoea due to Intestinal Resection

There is little doubt that the small bowel is sufficiently long for there to be a considerable intestinal 'reserve', so that even a large resection may not impair absorptive function. Massive intestinal resection leaving 2 feet of small intestine is compatible with a healthy life.

Ischaemic necrosis of the gut from occlusion of the branches of the superior mesenteric artery is the usual reason for massive resection, and the cause in elderly patients is usually embolism or atherosclerotic thrombosis, and in younger patients polyarteritis nodosa. The other reasons for resection are traumatic damage, strangulation, and Crohn's disease.

In massive resections the increased bulk of the intestinal contents causes the gut to dilate and to hypertrophy, and an increase in absorptive function has been demonstrated by perfusion studies in the remaining gut.

CLINICAL PICTURE

Owing to regional differences of absorptive function and motility (distal motility is less vigorous than that of the proximal bowel) the clinical picture varies.

Patients with *distal* bowel resection may develop megaloblastic anaemia from inability to absorb vitamin B_{12}, and they may be troubled by steatorrhoea from bile-salt loss. In some patients entry of bile-salts into the colon and by-passing of the ileal absorptive mechanism for these compounds may also produce an irritative watery diarrhoea (cholerhoeic enteropathy). Other patients with distal resections may be little troubled by diarrhoea. A section of 30 cm. of distal ileum is of the sort of order which may interfere with bile-salt metabolism. Those with large resections should always take a low-fat diet, otherwise diarrhoea with wasting, hypoproteinaemic oedema, and magnesium and calcium deficiency occurs. Children with this condition may fail to grow and because of increased oxalate absorption there is a danger of oxaluria and renal stones.

Useful Tests

1. Tests of proximal bowel function.
2. Estimate fat excretion during high- and low-fat diets.
3. Estimation of vitamin B_{12} uptake, and serum levels.
4. A blood-count and bone-marrow examination for megaloblastic change.
5. Estimation of serum proteins, potassium, calcium, magnesium, iron.
6. Barium studies will demonstrate the length and condition of the remaining gut and give some idea of intestinal transit time. Fluid levels which may be caused by liquid intestinal contents do not therefore mean obstruction.
7. Gastric hypersecretion with ulceration of the stomach is a complication of massive resection which may require investigation though evidence for its occurrence in man is fragmentary.

TREATMENT

A high-protein–low-fat diet is the basis of the treatment in those with diarrhoea after resection of the small bowel. Only too often one hears that patients with intestinal resection have been told to increase their fat intake to gain weight. This invariably results in increased diarrhoea with electrolyte and fat loss. Simple carbohydrate substances may appear to be an easily absorbable source of calories, but they often aggravate diarrhoea and a solid high-protein diet is better tolerated. Regular injections of vitamin B_{12} are required if the distal small bowel has been resected. Supplements of other vitamins and minerals will often be necessary. Hypoproteinaemic oedema can be lessened by diuretics and albumin infusions. Patients who fail to respond to this régime may be able to tolerate increased fat supplements in the form of medium-chain triglycerides. In those who prove to have diarrhoea without steatorrhoea a trial of the bile-salt chelating agent cholestyramine is worth while. Another therapeutic possibility with this type of diarrhoea is a dietary supplement of vegetable fibre such as lignin. A reversed loop of gut which acts as a brake to intestinal transit has been a surgical way of approaching severe diarrhoea following resection of the small bowel.

Steatorrhoea due to Drugs

Antibiotics, particularly neomycin, may cause steatorrhoea, which is accompanied by defects of carbohydrate and protein absorption. Doses higher than normal are more likely to precipitate this complication. An interesting feature is that the intestinal mucosa may come to resemble that of the coeliac syndrome, but the flattening disappears when treatment is stopped. Neomycin also produces steatorrhoea possibly by interfering with fat absorption (micelle formation) in the small-bowel lumen. Damage to the intestinal mucosa is presumably the basis of a similar malabsorption syndrome following irradiation to the bowel or the use of cytotoxic drugs. Phenindione has been reported as causing steatorrhoea, but this is rare and the mechanism is unknown. PAS is another possible cause.

Malabsorption due to Endocrine Disease

Addison's disease may be associated with malabsorption and cortisone is known to improve intestinal absorptive function in some malabsorption syndromes. Thyrotoxicosis is commonly associated with diarrhoea and sometimes there may be frank steatorrhoea. Recent studies in the thyrotoxic rat have failed to show any defect of fat absorption by isolated mucosal specimens but a great shortening of intestinal transit time. This could explain thyrotoxic malabsorption in man.

Malabsorption and Skin Disease

These seem to be linked in the following ways:

i. In severe generalized skin disease malabsorption and steatorrhoea may occur and abnormal disaccharidase activity may be demonstrated. The mucosal biopsy is abnormal and the malabsorption which is of uncertain cause will return to normal when the skin disease improves. The term 'dermatogenic enteropathy' has been applied to this group by Shuster.

ii. In malabsorption syndromes of various types skin disorders are not unusual. These include skin pigmentation, hyperkeratosis, and eczema. The skin abnormality may improve as the malabsorption improves. Care must be taken to distinguish skin involvement due to a reticulosis complicating coeliac disease.

iii. Some disorders of the skin also affect the bowel and cause malabsorption. Scleroderma is an obvious example of such an association and a recently identified one is dermatitis herpetiformis. This itchy vesicular eruption is associated with the small intestinal mucosal lesion of coeliac disease. Malabsorption of some degree and mucosal abnormality are found in 70 per cent of those affected. The fact that dermatitis herpetiformis can develop in patients with established coeliac disease suggests a close genetic relationship. Certainly in dermatitis herpetiformis some improvement of the skin condition and the malabsorption syndrome (including the jejunal histology) is achieved by dietary gluten restriction.

Disaccharidase Deficiency

A congenital deficiency of lactase in the brush border was described by Höltzel. It is associated in neonates with diarrhoea and failure to thrive after milk feeding. Glucose and galactose, the constituent monosaccharides, are, however, well tolerated and the disease is caused by failure to absorb the disaccharide lactose due to absence of hydrolysing enzyme. Sucrase deficiency is also a recognized congenital disorder and is due to absence of brush-border sucrase, whilst fructose intolerance is due to deficiency of hepatic ketose-1-phosphate.

Disaccharidase deficiency is also a feature of any disease which damages the intestinal brush border. It is therefore a complication of coeliac disease and tropical sprue. It occurs in skin diseases, hepatitis, intestinal infection, and ulcerative colitis, in fact wherever there is brush-border damage.

Diarrhoea, gurgling, and steatorrhoea are the clinical features and many patients will volunteer that milk aggravates these symptoms. The disease may be unassociated with symptoms until gastrectomy or other intestinal operations shorten intestinal transit times. Diagnosis is from the history and from the results of disaccharide-loading tests. After a lactose load of 50 g. the serum glucose fails to rise more than 20 mg. in the patient with primary or secondary alactasia, despite a normal rise when glucose and galactose are separately administered. Diagnosis can be verified by measuring enzyme concentrations in mucosal specimens and by noting in alactasia the acidic (low pH) reaction of the stools. Steatorrhoea may be found with either primary or secondary alactasia. In the former it is due to intestinal hurry caused by the osmotic effect of intraluminal lactose.

It should be noted that primary alactasia may not manifest itself until adult life and that there is marked ethnic variation. Though rare in Caucasians this is not so in Mediterranean and Negro populations. Dietary habits are obviously important in the clinical expression of the disease.

Alactasia can be treated by exclusion of milk and milk products from the diet. In primary alactasia this should control symptoms, but in secondary cases the primary disease may need treatment. In children coeliac disease may be more readily brought under control by dietary restriction of both gluten and lactose.

Worms and Parasites

Many infestations of the alimentary tract are associated with malabsorption. Giardiasis (*Giardia lamblia*) is an important cause of malabsorption, particularly in children with coeliac disease, kwashiorkor, and immune deficiency syndromes (*vide infra*). It may also be found in those returning from holidays in tropical and subtropical countries. Possibly a mechanical barrier produced by large numbers of parasites prevents access of nutriments to epithelial cells—or there may be villous damage. Giardiasis is diagnosed by examination of faeces and is treated with mepacrine or metronidazole (Flagyl). *Hookworm* is a common cause of anaemia but a rare cause of malabsorption in the tropics. This type of malabsorption is associated with partial villous atrophy. Diagnosis is by faecal microscopy for ova and treatment is with tetrachloroethylene (most successful for *Necator americanus*) or bephenium hydroxynaphthoate or a combination of both.

Strongyloides stercoralis is also sometimes associated with malabsorption due to invasion and thickening of the intestinal mucosa. Diagnosis is from examination of the faeces for larvae and treatment is with thiabendazole.

Other Rarer Causes of Malabsorption

In the Zollinger-Ellison syndrome malabsorption is probably due to inactivation of intestinal enzymes and bile-salts consequent upon the extremely low pH resulting from massive acid production by the stomach. In the *carcinoid syndrome* malabsorption may be a feature and this is generally ascribed to intestinal hurry consequent upon the action of serotonin. Damage to villi is the cause of malabsorption resulting from the use of antimetabolic drugs and from X-ray therapy to the abdomen, though it is possible that neoplasms themselves can affect cellular proliferation in the small intestinal mucosa and produce histological changes.

An interesting syndrome of malabsorption occurs with primary agammaglobulinaemia, but only in the acquired type and is of unknown cause. About half of such patients have malabsorption and in some patients there may be lymphoid hyperplasia in the small gut and elsewhere. There is a tendency, too, for lymphoma and thymoma to develop. It is possible that alimentary infection or infestation (giardiasis) could be a cause of this malabsorption which responds to immunoglobulin replacement and antibiotics.

Vascular disease of the small bowel either of the major vessels, e.g., atheromatous occlusion of the superior mesenteric artery, or of the small vessels such as occurs in polyarteritis nodosa may be a cause of steatorrhoea.

Diabetes, particularly when accompanied by evidence of peripheral neuropathy, can lead not only to diarrhoea but occasionally to steatorrhoea. The precise cause of this syndrome is unknown, but increased gut motility related to degeneration of intestinal ganglia and nerve plexuses in the wall of the gut is a likely mechanism, but small intestinal bacterial contamination may occur. A similar type of disorder occurring without diabetes is characterized by attacks of intestinal bloating due to gut distension and steatorrhoea. The latter may be a result of bacterial contamination of dilated intestinal loops and a partial improvement may follow antibiotic therapy. The disease has been called 'pseudo-obstruction of the small bowel' but the precise cause for the degeneration of intestinal nerve plexuses is unknown. The colon in this disorder is normal.

The syndrome of diarrhoea associated with medullary carcinoma of the thyroid has recently been described. Though principally associated with increased water and electrolyte loss mild steatorrhoea may be found. The condition presents as diarrhoea in a patient with thyroid enlargement and evidence of lymph-node involvement. Prostaglandins may be responsible for the increased bowel motility which is probably the basis of the diarrhoea and malabsorption. In A-beta-lipoproteinaemia there is a genetic defect in lipoprotein metabolism, a failure of chylomicron formation (and steatorrhoea), defective red cells, and brain damage.

Alpha-chain Disease

A number of cases of this interesting disease have been recorded in those of Mediterranean and Asian stock. Patients have malabsorption and a lymphoma of the upper small bowel. The cells of the lymphoma produce an abnormal IgA immunoglobulin lacking its light chains. The protein can be found in both serum and urine—there is no effective treatment.

FURTHER READING

Anatomy and Physiology
LASTER, L., and INGELFINGER, F. J. (1961), 'Intestinal Absorption. Aspects of Structure, Function and Disease of the Small Intestine Mucosa', *New Engl. J. Med.*, **264**, 1138, 1192, 1246.

Coeliac Disease
BOOTH, C. C. (1970), 'The Enterocyte in Coeliac Disease', *Br. med. J.*, 3, 725, and 4, 14.
COOKE, W. T. (1968), 'Adult Coeliac Disease', in *Progress in Gastroenterology* (ed.
GLASS, G. B. J.), vol. 1. New York and London: Grune & Stratton.
HOLMES, R., HOURIHANE, D. O'B., and BOOTH, C. C. (1961), 'The Mucosa of the Small
Intestine', *Post-grad. med. J.*, 37, 717.
PADYKULA, H. A., STRAUSS, E. W., LADMAN, A. J., and GARDINER, F. H. (1961), 'A Morpho-
logical and Histochemical Analysis of the Human Jejunal Epithelium in Non-tropical
Sprue', *Gastroenterology*, 40, 735.
RUBIN, C. E., BRANDBORG, L. L., PHELPS, P. C., and TAYLOR, H. C. (1960), 'Studies of
Coeliac Disease', *Ibid.*, 38, 28.
SHINER, M., and DONIACH, I. (1960), 'Histopathological Studies in Steatorrhoea', *Ibid.*,
38, 419.

Clinical
BADENOCH, J. (1960), 'Steatorrhoea in the Adult', *Br. med. J.*, 2, 879, 963.
COOKE, W. T., PEENEY, A. L. P., and HAWKINS, C. F. (1953), 'Symptoms, Signs and Diag-
nostic Features of Idiopathic Steatorrhoea', *Q. Jl Med.*, 46, 59.
FRENCH, J. M., GADDIE, R., and SMITH, N. M. (1956), 'Tropical Sprue. A Study of Seven
Cases and their Response to Combined Chemotherapy', *Ibid.*, 49, 333.
HAWKINS, C. (1961), 'Idiopathic Steatorrhoea', *Post-grad. med. J.*, 37, 761.

Blind Loop Syndrome
BADENOCH, J. (1960), 'The Blind Loop Syndrome', *Proc. R. Soc. Med.*, 53, 657.
TABAGCHALI, S., and BOOTH, C. C. (1970), 'Bacteria and the Small Intestine', in *Modern
Trends in Gastroenterology*, p.143. London: Butterworths.

Intestinal Resection
BOOTH, C. C. (1961), 'The Metabolic Effects of Intestinal Resection in Man', *Post-grad.
med. J.*, 37, 725

Whipple's Disease
FARNAN, P. (1959), 'Whipple's Disease—the Clinical Aspects', *Q. Jl Med.*, 52, 163.
RUFFIN, J. M., KURTZ, S. M., and ROUFAIL, W. M. (1966), 'Intestinal Lipodystrophy
(Whipple's Disease). The Immediate and Prolonged Effect of Antibiotic Therapy',
J. Am. med. Ass., 195, 476.
WHIPPLE, G. H. (1907), 'Hitherto Undescribed Disease characterised Anatomically by
Deposits of Fat and Fatty Acids in Intestinal and Mesenteric Lymphatic Tissue', *Bull.
Johns Hopk. Hosp.*, 18, 302.

Skin Disease and the Gut
MARKS, J., and SHUSTER, S. (1970), 'Small Intestinal Mucosal Attachments in Various
Skin Disease—Facts or Fancy', *Gut*, 11, 281.

Bile Acids
DAWSON, A. M. (1967), 'Bile Salts and Fat Absorption', *Gut*, 8, 1.
HEATON, K. W. (1969), 'The Importance of keeping Bile Salts in their Place', *Ibid.*, 10, 857.

Small Bowel Resection
DOWLING, R. H. (1970), 'Small Bowel Resection and By-pass—Recent Developments
and Effects', in *Modern Trends in Gastroenterology*, p. 73. London: Butterworths.

Skin Disease and Malabsorption
(*a*) Dermatitis Herpetiformis
SHUSTER, S., WATSON, A. J., and MARKS, J. (1968), 'Coeliac Syndrome in Dermatitis
Herpetiformis', *Lancet*, 1, 1101.
(*b*) Dermatogenic Enteropathy
SHUSTER, S., and MARKS, J. (1965), 'Dermatogenic Enteropathy. A New Case of Steatorrhoea', *Ibid.*, 1, 1637.

Chapter 18

Ileitis and Crohn's Disease

Acute Non-specific Regional Ileitis

AETIOLOGY

THIS DISEASE differs from classic Crohn's disease in that it is confined to the terminal ileum, it occurs chiefly in young patients or children, and it has a much better prognosis. Occasionally the disease may develop after the patient has been treated with drugs such as the tetracyclines, and it is possible that some cases may be due to *Yersina* (*Pasteurella X*) infection from animals. Many cases occur without any predisposing cause.

PATHOLOGY

The histological features are very similar to those of classic Crohn's disease, but eosinophil infiltration, oedema, lymphatic congestion, and lymph-node enlargement are prominent, whereas the fibrosis, linear ulceration, and shortening of the gut which are so characteristic of classic Crohn's disease are not seen. The disease never affects the anus, rectum, or colon.

CLINICAL PICTURE AND DIAGNOSIS

The symptoms are similar to those of appendicitis but the history of pain in the right iliac fossa may extend back for several days prior to the request for medical advice. Diarrhoea is often a feature, and the local pain and tenderness may be somewhat less than in acute appendicitis. A sausage-shaped mass may be felt if the abdominal wall is not too rigid. Leucocytosis may occur.

As a rule, the picture is too much like that of appendicitis for the surgeon to make a confident diagnosis, but he may suspect acute ileitis before embarking on laparotomy.

After opening the peritoneum the thickened red and tense terminal ileum is seen and sometimes peritoneal exudate and purpuric spots are conspicuous. If these also involve the caecum and other parts of the small intestine, the alternative diagnosis of Henoch's purpura should be considered. Acute mesenteric lymphadenitis causes a more widespread lymphadenopathy than is found in acute ileitis, and in the former only slight and patchy thickening of the ileum is noted.

TREATMENT

Since we know that more than half of the patients get better without specific treatment, most surgeons avoid any surgical procedure, but total resection of the diseased area followed by ileocolostomy can be successful. However, there are considerable risks in cutting and suturing diseased bowel, so most surgeons prefer to close the abdomen. Some may remove the appendix, but others, fearing the risk of abscess or wound fistula, will not do so.

After operation the patient is rested and given a semisolid or fluid diet. Penicillin and streptomycin can be given postoperatively, or long-acting sulphonamides, mainly with the aim of reducing the risks of secondary bacterial infection. Pain, tenderness, and fever usually subside within a week. Dietary protein is gradually increased and injections of B_{12} and other B vitamins may be given parenterally to guard against secondary deficiencies. After a month, if fever has subsided and the weight is increasing the patient will be ambulant and taking a full diet. By this time the E.S.R. is usually normal.

In cases where pain, tenderness, diarrhoea, or fever persist for longer than a week after operation, corticosteroids may be given. The oral route is adequate if diarrhoea is not profuse, but if malabsorption of steroid drugs appears likely, then corticotrophin or a depot steroid preparation should be given by injection. If steroid or corticotrophin therapy is started it should be continued in gradually decreasing dosage for 2 months at least, and to guard against osteoporosis oral calcium and vitamin D should be given with the steroid therapy.

A long convalescence is usually advised, and the patient is followed up for 2 years. Such precautions may be unnecessary—their value is unproven —but we know that some 20 per cent of the patients diagnosed as suffering from acute ileitis continue to have symptoms and later go on to develop classic Crohn's disease, and it seems worth while to take every possible precaution in the hope that this will not happen. A few cases have had further acute attacks of ileitis after appearing to recover from the first one.

Crohn's Disease

This disease, originally described as regional ileitis, is now known to involve, though rarely, the skin, oesophagus, stomach, duodenum, jejunum, colon, and anus. For this reason, the eponymous title is retained. Alternative descriptive names such as chronic granulomatous enterocolitis have not as yet found universal acceptance.

AETIOLOGY

The sex incidence is almost equal, the decade of maximal susceptibility being the third. There is a distinct genetic tendency to this disease, and multiple cases in a family have often been described. There is also a tendency for ulcerative colitis and ankylosing spondylitis, eczema, and polyarthritis to occur in the relatives of patients with Crohn's disease, just as it is known that ankylosing spondylitis and polyarthritis occur with significant frequency in the actual patients with Crohn's disease.

In the British population the prevalence seems to be about 1 per 8000, but the disease is known to be very uncommon in Japan and is probably rare in Africa and southern Asia. As with ulcerative colitis it appears to be commoner amongst Jews.

Lesions similar to Crohn's disease have been produced by lymphatic sclerosing agents and by feeding rats with sand, but it is very unlikely that similar processes are causative of the human disease. Some workers have derived a transmissible agent from Crohn's disease tissue.

A pointer to altered immunological responses comes from the fact that patients with Crohn's disease are commonly Mantoux negative and that many of them do not show a hypersensitivity response to skin patch testing with dinitrochlorbenzene. Recent studies have suggested that in Crohn's disease there is an imbalance between the activity of the lympho-cytes responsible for humoral immunity and those responsible for cellular immunity, and that macrophage function may be impaired.

PATHOLOGY

This is a necrotizing and ulcerative inflammatory process in which lym-phatic congestion and, later, fibrosis are marked features. When the disease affects the terminal ileum which is richly supplied with lymphoid follicles and mesenteric lymph-nodes, the gross lymphoedema and lymph-node enlargement are the most striking naked-eye features. Elsewhere in the gut, oedema and thickening of the wall, cobblestone or linear ulcera-tion of the mucosa, and the tendency to the formation of strictures is most noticeable. There is usually a fairly sharp line of demarcation between involved and healthy gut, and the disease rarely spreads beyond the ileocaecal valve. However, involvement of the rectum and segments of the colon is now increasingly recognized and differentiated from ulcerative colitis.

The whole small intestine may rarely be involved, and in other cases the whole colon and part of the small intestine are affected. Rare manifesta-tions are involvement of the duodenum and antrum, involvement of the skin of buttocks and groins, and a form of 'miliary' disease affecting the small intestine and mesentery. However, 90 per cent of cases have some involvement of the ileum, and only 10 per cent have disease confined to the large intestine. Disease confined to the terminal ileum accounts for about 30 per cent of cases. A frequent combination is disease in the ileum and disease of the anus. The latter has certain characteristic clinical features which will be described later, but the pathological features are fibrosis, fissuring, bluish skin tags, and fistulae. Multiple biopsies must be done to be sure of finding the typical 'sarcoid-like' lesions.

Microscopically, the appearances are those of a diffuse granuloma of the submucosa. Plasma cells, round cells, polymorphs—both neutrophil and eosinophil—are found, and sarcoid-like lesions containing giant cells are characteristic. The glandular structure is destroyed and the mucosa ulcerated. Draining lymph-nodes are also converted into granulomata with giant-cell systems. Peritoneal reaction may be serous or purulent, but if an abscess forms, it is more likely to burrow and penetrate other organs than to form a large collection. For this reason, fistulae may develop between small gut and large gut, bladder or abdominal wall.

CLINICAL PICTURE

Symptoms and signs vary a great deal according to whether the disease is early or late, and what parts of the gastro-intestinal tract are involved.

There are, however, certain cardinal features which occur in most cases of Crohn's disease:

Diarrhoea;
Loss of weight;
Low-grade fever;
Slight anaemia;
Raised E.S.R.

The mode of presentation is so variable that some cases will first be referred to a physician and others to a surgeon.

Such symptoms as may first be seen by a physician are:

1. Obscure loss of weight, appetite, and energy. Secondary amenorrhoea. Vague and fleeting abdominal pains with nausea, worse after meals. Bouts of diarrhoea. Pyrexia of unknown origin.

2. Troublesome and continuous diarrhoea with enhanced gastrocolic reflex and urgency of bowel action. Stools rarely contain visible blood, and may even appear yellow, frothy, and 'fatty'. Steatorrhoea may, in fact, be present. Weight-loss, low-grade fever, abdominal pain, and tenderness in the right iliac fossa may be found.

Such symptoms as may first be seen by a surgeon are:

1. Acute or subacute intestinal obstruction with central abdominal distension, violent pain and vomiting, radiographs showing dilated loops of small intestine.

2. Pain and tenderness in right iliac fossa, the acute form resembling acute appendicitis, the less acute resembling an appendix abscess, actinomycosis, or carcinoma of the caecum.

3. Perirectal sepsis and fistula formation.

COMPLICATIONS AND ACCOMPANIMENTS

These may be general or local. The general accompaniments can be grouped as follows:

1. Due to associated diseases and lesions, e.g., ankylosing spondylitis, polyarthritis, eczema, erythema nodosum, occasional ulcerative skin lesions, iritis, and episcleritis.

2. Due to the effects of the intestinal disease such as internal haemorrhage causing anaemia, hypoproteinaemic oedema, B_{12} and other B-vitamin deficiencies, infantilism in growing children and amenorrhoea in girls. Amyloid disease is a rare occurrence, but finger clubbing and pigmentation of the skin are not uncommon in severe cases.

Local Complications

These are subacute intestinal obstruction, ileo-ileal, ileocolic, ileovesical, and rectovaginal fistulae, abscesses, and skin fistulae around the anus, peritoneal or psoas abscesses.

The mechanisms of malabsorption in Crohn's disease may be due to either:

1. Diffuse involvement of small gut, thus lessening its absorptive surface.

2. Stagnation in a distended gut above a stricture giving rise to bacterial contamination and a blind-loop syndrome.

3. Contamination of ileal lumen by colonic organisms after an ileocolic fistula has developed.

4. Loss of absorptive surface after surgical resection.

INVESTIGATIONS

Simple screening tests, such as the observation of day and night temperatures while the patient rests in bed, the measurement of haemoglobin, and E.S.R. are invaluable. There is, in most active cases of Crohn's disease, a low-grade but measurable pyrexia, a fall of haemoglobin levels to below 12 g. per 100 ml., and a rise of E.S.R. to over 15 mm. per hour. The E.S.R. will tend to reflect the degree of activity of the disease.

Faecal occult blood-tests are often positive, but intermittently so. The stools may contain excessive fat and undigested meat fibres if a large area of the gut is involved, or if the jejunum proximal to the diseased area is much distended. These two factors, or the occurrence of an ileocolic fistula, are responsible for malabsorption.

The serum albumin is often reduced, and particularly so if there is malabsorption or marked loss of protein from deep-fissured ulcers in the small and large bowels. The α_2-globulin is usually raised.

Tests of intestinal absorptive capacity may indicate the areas most affected by the disease, for example, impaired absorption of xylose and other sugars indicates jejunal involvement, whereas poor uptake of labelled vitamin B_{12} is to be expected with the more usual ileal disease.

Radiological techniques for the detection and measurement of the extent of Crohn's disease are difficult. Most clinicians prefer to have both a barium enema and a study of the small intestine by ingested barium.

The enema is necessary to determine the presence and extent of colonic involvement, and if the ileocaecal valve is incompetent, as it is so frequently in Crohn's disease, the terminal ileum can be outlined by this method. The detailed barium study of the small gut should be made from 30 minutes to 5 hours after the ingestion of a small amount of a micro-suspension of barium. The rate of progress of the barium in the upper parts will indicate to the radiologist the time at which he is most likely to outline the lower ileal loops. The use of too much barium, its rapid passage, or undue dilution by succus entericus will all make interpretation difficult, and many radiologists prefer to pass a small tube into the jejunum and thus to fill the suspected segments with barium. This technique, the 'small-bowel enema', allows the distensibility, thickness, and fixity of the loops to be gauged more accurately (*Fig. 67*).

Intraluminal biopsy of the jejunum and ileum is of less value in Crohn's disease than in adult coeliac disease, but can be valuable in distinguishing between the two.

DIAGNOSIS

In its early stages the disease may be suspected, but is extremely difficult to diagnose. Many patients ultimately found to have Crohn's disease give a 5-year or even a 10-year history of malaise, loss of energy with abdominal

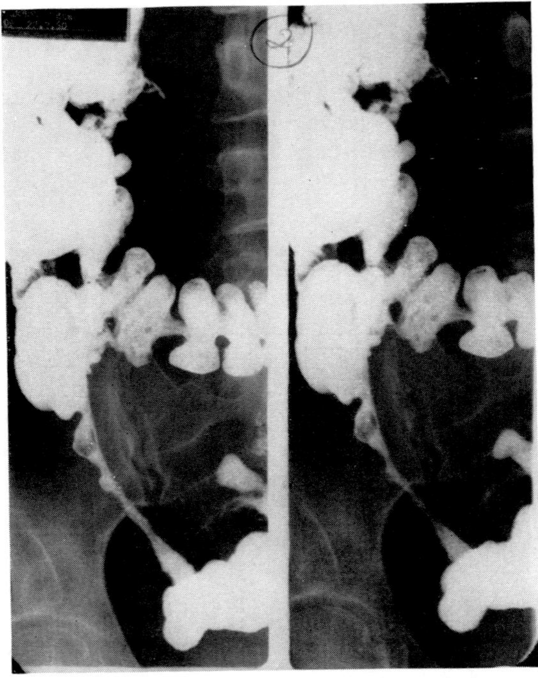

Fig. 67. Crohn's disease: barium series showing typical appearances ('string sign') in terminal ileum.

pains, and intermittent diarrhoea for which they may have consulted many doctors and even undergone radiological studies. The simple screening tests—haemoglobin, E.S.R., faecal occult blood, and measurement of evening temperature—are most valuable. If the clinical history and the screening tests suggest the possibility of Crohn's disease, the radiologist should be asked specifically to look for it, using the technique to which he is most accustomed. It is foolish to make ill-defined requests such as, 'Barium meal and follow-through, please'.

If a segment of narrowed, irregular, thick-walled, and fixed small intestine is found, then the diagnosis may, in some cases, be confirmed by laparotomy, but if surgical treatment is not contemplated therapy may be started in the reasonable certainty that no other disease is likely to produce such characteristic lesions of the small intestine.

If the disease involves the colon, the rectum, or anus, the differentiation from ulcerative colitis may be difficult. The radiological appearances of Crohn's disease of the colon are, however, in some cases characteristic. The visualization of longitudinal fissured ulcers is diagnostic, and the appearance of the descending colon is fairly typical of certain cases of Crohn's disease. If the disease affects the rectum, the sigmoidoscope shows a loss of vascular pattern, obvious submucosal oedema, and a lack of distensibility. Contact bleeding is uncommon and the mucosa is less red than in ulcerative colitis. When the anus is affected digital examination may reveal a fibrous stricture of the anal canal and a cobblestone surface of the oedematous rectal mucosa within. Bluish skin tags around a misshapen anus, and the scars of healed sinuses, or open fistulae, complete the characteristic clinical picture. Often a single biopsy of these areas is less reliable than the overall clinical appearances, but multiple biopsies should reveal the typical lesions. Colonoscopy may become a useful method of diagnosis.

TREATMENT

It is impossible to be dogmatic about the treatment of Crohn's disease and it is unrealistic to separate the medical and surgical phases of what may prove to be half a lifetime of care and management. There is, in fact, no treatment for the disease as such, but only treatment for the patient.

The main principles are as follows:

1. Provided that there is no evidence of intestinal obstruction or major abscess formation, always treat conservatively in the first place.

2. Try to avoid surgical operations, particularly resections, in patients with very active disease or in very poor general condition. First, try to improve the general condition and lessen disease activity.

3. In the presence of severe disease with peritoneal matting, it is wiser for the surgeon to isolate the diseased segments by anastomosing healthy bowel above to healthy bowel below, in such a way that the peristaltic wave does not drive the faecal stream past the anastomosis into the diseased area. Such an operation is known as a short-circuit with exclusion. It may be followed safely, months or years later, by excision of the damaged tissues.

4. No resection should be so extensive as to impair the absorptive power of the small gut—usually not more than half its length should be removed. The intestine often appears to be shorter than normal in Crohn's disease.

5. After resection, watch carefully in subsequent months or years for signs of recurrence above or below the original lesions, and treat such recurrence thoroughly, by the best medical means. Do not embark on further operations unless these are rendered absolutely necessary by virtue of obstructive complications.

Conservative Treatment

BEFORE SURGERY

With an acute or subacute onset, the régime outlined on p. 275 of this chapter should be followed. High-residue foods should be avoided because of the risk of bolus colic. Anaemia, protein deficiency, and avitaminoses should be defined and corrected. If after a few weeks the patient is failing to gain ground the surgeon and physician should consult to decide whether a prolonged course of corticosteroid therapy or an operation for exclusion or resection offers the best chance of control and the least risk. The decision will depend on the extent of the disease and its location, presence or absence of other diseases, and social and psychological factors.

If it is decided to employ corticosteroid therapy it is wise to employ fairly large doses for the first month. Prednisone 40 mg. a day should be given for 2 weeks and thereafter, if progress is satisfactory, reduced to 30 mg. a day for the next month.

If the patient has severe diarrhoea or malabsorption, oral steroids may not be well absorbed and it may be best to give a depot steroid such as 'Depo-Medrone' by injection on alternate days until the diarrhoea has lessened sufficiently to make it safe to change over to oral therapy. If the patient does well the dose of prednisone may then be cut by 5 mg. each month until the patient is taking a maintenance dose of 10–15 mg. daily. When giving corticosteroids to patients with diarrhoea, it is wise to give extra potassium. Potassium chloride 3 g. per day can be given, or effervescent potassium tablets dissolved in water may be better tolerated. The patient liable to malabsorption who is treated with steroids may develop osteomalacia or osteoporosis so that extra calcium in the diet or in tablet form should be given, and sometimes testosterone propionate intermittently to stimulate the assimilation of dietary protein into the body's stores.

If this treatment improves matters, it is always difficult to decide whether to continue steroids indefinitely or to stop them. Some guidance may be gained from symptoms, E.S.R., and haemoglobin level. As an alternative to steroids immunosuppressive drugs such as azathioprine have been tried, but they seem to offer no special advantages, and more recently steroids and azathioprine given together have given better results than steroids alone.

AFTER SURGERY

Any surgical operation on a patient with Crohn's disease should be followed by a long spell of convalescence. If the surgeon considers that he may have, of necessity, used in his anastomosis bowel which is in the early stages of the disease, then corticosteroid therapy may be started immediately after the operation. Otherwise it may be used later at the first sign of a recurrence. Undoubtedly corticosteroids help to control diarrhoea and other symptoms due to recurrence of disease in the colon or jejunum after a primary resection, but whether they make any fundamental difference to the disease process and to the prognosis is uncertain. The physician charged with the care of a patient who has had an operation for Crohn's disease should not only watch for signs of recurrence but also for signs of anaemia, malabsorption, and protein deficiency, and these deficiencies should, if possible, be corrected.

EVALUATION OF CORTICOSTEROID THERAPY IN CROHN'S DISEASE

It appears that corticosteroid therapy given in the first or subsequent attack does not lessen the chances of future surgery being necessary, but patients treated with corticosteroids before surgery do better subsequently than those who have surgery without prior treatment. The ideal patient for corticosteroid therapy is the patient with diffuse jejuno-ileitis in the exudative phase, the patient with miliary Crohn's disease, or the patient with ileocolitis. Corticosteroids will not prevent intestinal obstruction if fibrotic narrowing is already a feature before the start of treatment. In cases of Crohn's disease where diarrhoea is the main problem, steroid therapy nearly always improves the condition of the patient, and apparent cures are not unknown. Where Crohn's disease affects the anus and rectum only or a segment of colon, steroids are beneficial but surgery may eventually be necessary due to the development of fibrotic narrowing or fistulae. Local corticosteroids in Crohn's disease of the rectum are not so effective as in localized proctocolitis.

Azathioprine, a cytotoxic and immunosuppressive drug, is occasionally useful. Daily dosage régimes vary between 5 mg. per kg. for 2 weeks to 2 mg. per kg. for several months. The value of this and similar drugs is as yet unproven; therapeutic trials are in progress.

Surgical Treatment

Surgery is always necessary if the bowel becomes obstructed, if obstructive colic makes life a misery, if a large abscess has to be drained, or if a fistula has to be dealt with.

There is, however, a wide difference in the practice of different surgeons as to what may be called primary treatment. Some analyses suggest that patients who have a resection of the diseased area do better than those who have a by-pass with exclusion of the diseased area. It has to be remembered, however, that total resection is in many cases not feasible or safe, and that a simple analysis of cases so treated will include most of the naturally favourable cases. Basically, the surgeon's task is to treat the disease surgically when there are mechanical problems only susceptible of a mechanical solution, and the method used to overcome the mechanical problem should be both radical and safe. One surgical practice which nearly always leads to early recurrence of symptoms is the side-to-side anastomosis of ileum to transverse colon. This procedure does not prevent chyle and food being driven on to the diseased area by peristaltic action. End-to-side anastomoses are preferable and the distal loop of ileum may be brought out to the surface as a mucus fistula or sutured to the abdominal wound.

Patients will tolerate quite large resections of the jejunum, but if the whole ileum is removed then diarrhoea must be expected and vitamin-B_{12}

deficiency guarded against by regular parenteral treatment thereafter. Diarrhoea may occur after ileal resections because bile acids are mainly reabsorbed in the terminal ileum. Failure of ileal absorption leads to the loss of increasing amounts of bile acids into the colon. Bile acids have an irritant effect on the large colon and interfere with sodium and water absorption leading to diarrhoea—'cholerhoeic enteropathy'. Cholerhoeic enteropathy has been successfully treated by the use of bile-acid-binding resins such as cholestyramine.

Recurrences at 5 years after surgery occur in 60 per cent of cases but only 40 per cent require further surgery.

PROGNOSIS

Since the disease occurs mainly in young people, the expectation of life may be long, but the likelihood of continued morbidity is high. Probably only about 10 per cent of all patients with the chronic form of the disease are permanently cured. Seventy-five per cent battle on through a lifetime of major and minor recrudescences but die of some other disease. Less than 15 per cent die of Crohn's disease either as a result of surgical attempts to relieve their misery or from gradual wasting and starvation.

FURTHER READING

CROHN, B. B., and YARNIS, H. (1958), *Regional Ileitis*, 2nd ed. New York and London: Grune & Stratton.
EDWARDS, H. C. (1958), 'Crohn's Disease', in *Surgical Progress, British Surgical Practice* (ed. CARLING, SIR ERNEST, and ROSS, SIR JAMES PATERSON), p. 84. London: Butterworth.
LAW, D. H. (1969), 'Regional Enteritis', *Gastroenterology*, **56**, 1086.
LEADING ARTICLE (1970), 'Aetiology of Crohn's Disease', *Lancet*, **2**, 193.
LENNARD-JONES, J. E. (1970), 'Crohn's Disease', in *Modern Trends in Gastroenterology* (ed. CARD, W. I., and CREAMER, B.), p. 273. London: Butterworth.

Chapter 19

Other Diseases of the Small Bowel

a. Acute Gastro-enteritis (Infective Diarrhoea)

A NUMBER of bacteria are responsible for infective diarrhoea and in this country the most important are the Salmonellae, the Shigellae, certain Staphylococci, and Clostridia.

The disease is spread by faecal contamination of food and water either due to poor personal hygiene in food handlers or by means of insect vectors. Prepared foods left at room temperature are a particular source of danger because of rapid bacterial proliferation. Occasionally water-supplies may be contaminated by infected sewage. Viruses, particularly ECHO types 8, 11, 19, and 20, are implicated in some cases.

CLINICAL PICTURE

The illness is of acute onset, 6–24 hours after exposure, and with vomiting, fever, colicky abdominal pain, and diarrhoea. The stools are loose, offensive, and in severe cases may contain blood and mucus. In infancy and in debilitated patients dehydration and peripheral circulatory collapse may soon be precipitated, but the average case is usually of mild or moderate severity only.

DIAGNOSIS

This is suggested by the occurrence of several cases occurring together following known or probable exposure to contaminated food or drink. It is diagnosed by:

1. Stool culture or, more conveniently, culture of rectal swabs.

a. Salmonella food poisoning may be caused by a large number of different organisms; the most important is *S. typhimurium*. An animal source of infection is common—often from poultry or rodents.

b. Shigellae

Bacillary dysentery exists in two forms, Sonne dysentery (*Sh. sonnei*), which is mild, and Flexner and Shiga dysentery (*Sh. flexneri* and *Sh. shigae*), where the disease is usually more severe.

DIFFERENTIAL DIAGNOSIS

In this must be included ulcerative colitis where rectal bleeding is invariable and the characteristic sigmoidoscopic appearances are more extensive than those found in bacillary dysentery. In young children the possibility of intussusception must be remembered as a possible cause of symptoms.

TREATMENT

Most cases are mild and recover if oral feeding is stopped and copious fluids given. This may be supplemented by agents such as codeine phosphate or diphenoxylate to control diarrhoea. Antibiotics are not routinely required and indeed there is even evidence to suggest that complete eradication of the disease may be prolonged if they are used. However, in the very young, the elderly, and in those who are ill with pyrexia and severe symptoms, there is certainly a need for them, together with i.v. fluid replacement.

The most satisfactory drugs are sulphonamides, e.g., sulphadimidine 1 g. 6-hourly or neomycin and streptomycin. Traditionally, three negative rectal swabs or specimens of faeces are required before the patient can be declared free of the disease and therefore no longer a possible health risk to others.

b. Diffuse Ulcerative Jejuno-ileitis

This is a rare disease of unknown aetiology and apparently not related to Crohn's disease from which it differs histologically by the absence of granulomata.

CLINICAL PICTURE

Patients are usually middle-aged and the symptoms are in no way typical. Diarrhoea is a usual complaint often with the feature of small intestinal dysfunction, namely steatorrhoea. Accompanying this there are often attacks of colicky abdominal pain, fever, and considerable weight-loss. In view of the pain, fatty diarrhoea, and abdominal distension that accompanies it the presumptive diagnosis is usually Crohn's disease or abdominal lymphoma. Physical signs are usually absent, though distension, cachexia, and oedema are often prominent in a condition which may produce intermittent symptoms over some months or years.

Investigations

These point to the small bowel as the site of disease. There is steatorrhoea and hypoproteinemia due to protein loss from the gut. (1) Small bowel biopsy *fails* to reveal the classic subtotal villous atrophy of coeliac disease though partial villous atrophy is often present and may be patchy. (2) Radiology of the small bowel often shows increased clumping of barium and dilatation of small bowel loops, but no thickening or stricture formation such as is found in Crohn's disease. The mucosal pattern is often slightly coarser than usual. (3) At this stage laparotomy is often embarked upon and the jejunum is dilated and there is reddening and thickening of areas of small bowel with enlargement of mesenteric nodes. The nature of the condition is only revealed if a full-thickness biopsy of involved gut is taken where there are mucosal ulcers scattered throughout the small bowel averaging about 0·5–1 cm. in diameter with no specific pathological features and accompanied by areas of mucosal atrophy. The vascular supply to the gut shows no abnormality.

TREATMENT

As this disease is of uncertain origin treatment is empirical. The disease is a serious one, and in one series 9 of 13 patients died within 1–5 years of the onset of symptoms. Not infrequently the diagnosis is first made at autopsy, the patient having been too ill for laparotomy or having had a laparotomy examination of mesenteric nodes, etc., not establishing a diagnosis. Treatment with a gluten-free diet is unhelpful and the role of corticosteroid therapy uncertain, though remission of symptoms may follow their use. Treatment of hypoproteinaemia with a high-protein diet and albumin infusions may be required.

c. Ileocaecal Tuberculosis

This is now a rare disease in this country, but a certain number of cases occur in immigrants from India, Pakistan, and Hong Kong, and for this reason the disease remains of some importance. In most patients the disease is secondary to pulmonary disease, bacilli being swallowed and causing ulceration in the ileum and caecum. The reason for the predilection for this area of the intestinal canal is unknown, the usual reason given being the increased lymphoid tissue found in this area. The disease causes ulceration of the intestinal mucosa—classically circumferential ulcers which tend to produce stricturous lesions—and there is accompanying mesenteric adenitis, often with caseation. Gross thickening of the gut wall is often seen and the term 'pseudohypertrophic' is often used to describe this feature of chronic ileocaecal tuberculosis. Rarely, too, sinuses and fistulae may form. Another interesting point is the comparative rarity of the bovine tubercle bacillus as a causative agent, even in countries where cattle are infected.

CLINICAL PICTURE

This is entirely non-specific. The patient may be desperately ill with pyrexia and signs of gross cavitating disease in the lungs and complains of right-sided abdominal pain and occasional diarrhoea. In others the symptoms are entirely intestinal, with anorexia, weight-loss, and pain which may be colicky in nature and related to meals. A very helpful physical sign is the presence of a mass, often tender, in the right iliac fossa. The normal caecum is often palpable, so repeated abdominal examination may be required before this organic thickening is diagnosed. The patient's lungs must be carefully examined; features such as alcoholism or racial origin may make the diagnosis more probable.

INVESTIGATIONS

1. There is often an anaemia with a normal white count and raised ESR.
2. Chest X-ray is required in all cases and when tuberculous disease is found this may suggest the diagnosis of the abdominal symptoms.

3. Acid-fast bacilli must be looked for by direct examination and culture in sputum, gastric aspirate, and stools, though in the latter the yield (even with gross tuberculous disease) is of the order of 25 per cent. The Mantoux reaction is invariably positive though this is of little discriminative value.

4. Sigmoidoscopy may rarely reveal ulceration and lymphoid hypertrophy, and very rarely biopsy may show granuloma formation and acid-fast bacilli. Obviously the diagnosis from Crohn's disease can be difficult in the presence of granulomata without tubercule bacilli. Colonoscopy may also be helpful.

5. Radiology. Gross ileotuberculous disease may show radiological abnormalities. These include abnormalities of mucosal structure, stricture formation, and fistula formation as well as an irritable non-filling caecum. A pattern suggesting malabsorption—which may be verified and which is associated with partial villous atrophy—is sometimes seen. In contra-distinction to Crohn's disease the ileum in this disease is often dilated—due to stricture formation—rather than narrowed.

6. Occult blood tests in the stools are usually negative.

In many cases the diagnosis is still in doubt even when full investigations have been performed. Carcinoma of the caecum and Crohn's disease are the two other important diagnoses to consider in this country and there may be grave difficulty particularly with the former. For this reason the diagnosis is (rightly) made at laparotomy. Tubercles may be seen on the surface of the thickened gut, though the tuberculous origin may not be suggested until histology is available. Resection of the affected bowel is then not infrequently carried out. A postoperative pleurisy or chest signs may be further evidence to suggest a tuberculous origin.

TREATMENT

If the cause of symptoms is clear cut, 18 months' antituberculous therapy is required. This is best given as 18 months' PAS and INAH and 6 months' streptomycin therapy—the latter given three times weekly to prevent 8th nerve damage. If the affected bowel has been removed the same period of treatment is required. There is a danger that young patients may be wrongly diagnosed as having Crohn's disease and treated with cortico-steroids. This may lead to exacerbation of abdominal symptoms and activation of tuberculosis with miliary spread.

d. Eosinophilic Granuloma

This is a rare disease but one which may affect any part of the alimentary tract. In perhaps a third of patients there is a history of allergy. The allergy may be expressed as sensitivity to drugs and articles of food and on occa-sions symptoms may seem to follow ingestion of particular foods. It seems likely that a small percentage of cases are associated with parasitic infesta-tion of the gut and certainly cases due to infestation with the herring worm (*Eustoma rotundatum*) and *Strongyloides stercoralis* are recorded.

Pathologically there is thickening of the wall of the affected part of the alimentary canal which is most commonly the stomach. There is considerable tissue oedema, infiltration by sheets of eosinophils, and sometimes involvement of the serosal surface of the gut. In some cases obstruction (pyloric or intestinal) results. Ulceration and polypoid changes may also be seen as well as a necrotizing angiitis.

The symptoms are those of subacute gastric or intestinal obstruction, and thickening of the gut wall with serous exudation may produce a protein-losing enteropathy with oedema of the dependent parts or even anasarca. Rarely involvement of the serous coat of the gut may cause ascites.

Helpful diagnostic information may be obtained:

1. By careful attention to the patient's history and that of his family which may reveal evidence of allergy.

2. There is often a systemic eosinophilia.

3. Radiology may demonstrate mucosal thickening or irregularity and in those patients where infiltration and oedema has resulted in obstruction there may be added the features of pyloric or intestinal obstruction.

4. Gastric involvement can be diagnosed by endoscopy and biopsy.

TREATMENT

In patients with pyloric stenosis or in others who present acutely with intestinal involvement laparotomy may well be undertaken and the diagnosis only made on microscopy. The gross eosinophilic infiltration, oedema, and comparative rarity of ulceration and fibrosis distinguish it from Crohn's disease. Otherwise apart from avoiding offending foods and drugs corticosteroids usually produce a dramatic amelioration of symptoms. It should be noted that the intestinal features of angioneurotic oedema where abnormalities of complement activation are described and those of polyarteritis nodosa represent the extremities of a range of allergic disorders centred around this disease.

Disease of the Mesenteric Blood-vessels

The small intestine is supplied by the superior mesenteric artery. This vessel may be occluded in the middle aged and elderly by atheroma and in a younger age-group by emboli associated with mitral valve disease or myocardial infarction and by thrombosis complicating polycythemia, pregnancy, and the use of the contraceptive pill. Disease of small arteries such as polyarteritis nodosa may also be causative. The result of these conditions is ischaemia of the small gut and in severe cases necrosis due to gangrene. Ischaemia may also occur with patent vessels when perfusion is abnormal, as in heart failures and hypotension.

CLINICAL PICTURE

This may be acute, in which case the patient experiences all the features of an acute abdominal emergency with central abdominal pain, collapse, vomiting, and abdominal distension. In an elderly patient the diagnosis of mesenteric vascular occlusion should always be considered in this situation and in others a search for heart disease or coexisting arteritis should be sought.

In patients with more chronic symptoms the diagnosis may be more difficult. Pain is characteristically severe and peri-umbilical, often colicky in nature. It is worse after a meal (particularly a heavy one) and the patient is therefore afraid to eat, loses weight, and often becomes depressed. The diagnosis is often thought to be one of peptic ulcer or even cancer and a negative barium meal often relegates the patient to the diagnostic category of 'functional' dyspepsia. Other features of small-bowel ischaemia include attacks of diarrhoea, often with features of malabsorption. Physical signs are few, though there is often a history of vascular disease elsewhere (myocardial infarction, intermittent claudication) and murmurs which can be heard on abdominal auscultation may arise from a partially occluded superior mesenteric artery.

DIAGNOSIS

One must always suspect the presence of this disorder which is undoubtedly more common than previously thought. Proof of diagnosis may be obtained by superior mesenteric angiography. This may be a formidable procedure in an elderly person and is best reserved for those patients where there is diagnostic difficulty or where surgery is contemplated. Even the demonstration of superior mesenteric narrowing or occlusion does not mean that the patient's symptoms are definitely due to this cause and careful appraisal is necessary.

TREATMENT

Conservative management is indicated in the elderly. Reduction of the volume of meals and small frequent snacks may be very helpful. In those without severe generalized arterial disease operations to restore superior mesenteric flow may be required. Surgery (resection of ischaemic gut) is also required for acute superior mesenteric obstruction with complicating bowel necrosis.

Pseudomembranous Enterocolitis

This condition is of uncertain cause and indeed the precise aetiological factors responsible may be variable. The basic abnormality seems to be an ischaemic necrosis of a variable length of the mucosa of the intestinal canal and in extensive cases this necrosis may spread from oesophagus to rectum. Certain things are known about its causation. First, it often complicates some other debilitating disorder in an elderly person—examples of this include congestive cardiac failure—and a period of hypotension following myocardial infarction. Others have recently had an abdominal operation perhaps again complicated by hypotension or followed by the use of broad-spectrum antibiotics. A further group may result from mucosal ischaemia due to intravascular coagulation. The part played by bacteria in the initiation of this disease is uncertain. Some are claimed to be caused by the staphylococcus but in others it would seem that the bacterial damage is secondary and dependent on the basic defect of impaired mucosal blood-flow. Rarely the disorder is seen in gut proximal to an obstruction, again perhaps stressing the importance of mucosal ischaemia.

PATHOLOGY

There is a striking patchy or generalized mucosal necrosis seen maximally in the small bowel. The gut is hyperaemic, but on opening it is seen to be brownish yellow on its mucosal surface and in some areas there is a frank haemorrhagic necrosis. Under the microscope the superficial parts of the mucosal surface of the gut are necrotic, forming a pseudomembrane, whilst the rest of the bowel wall, though congested, is intact. The major blood-vessels are patent—the lesion seeming to be one of the mucosal microcirculation.

CLINICAL PICTURE

This is often dramatic. There is profuse watery blood-stained diarrhoea and abdominal distension and colicky pain. The patient becomes rapidly dehydrated, the body temperature, blood-pressure, and urinary output fall. The patient becomes apathetic, feeble, and often dies. The clinical picture simulates mesenteric vascular obstruction and in patients recently operated on paralytic ileus is a difficult differential diagnosis.

INVESTIGATIONS

1. Radiology—a plain X-ray of the abdomen shows dilated loops of small bowel with fluid levels.

2. Culture of the faeces is important in order to exclude those cases with a staphylococcal basis and in order to detect those patients who, having been treated with broad-spectrum antibiotics, have developed candidiasis.

TREATMENT

The outlook in this disease is poor—not only because the bowel is so widely involved but because, too, patients are often elderly and suffering from some underlying disease process or are recovering from an abdominal operation.

Broad-spectrum antibiotics should be withdrawn and the small percentage of patients with staphylococcal enteritis treated with an appropriate antibiotic, e.g., cloxacillin. Replacement of fluid volume is vital and plasma and normal saline may be used initially in order to do this, remembering of course the dangers of over-transfusion in this group. It is uncertain whether corticosteroids have a place in the treatment of the hypervolaemic patient with pseudomembranous enterocolitis, but they are usually given. Because of diagnostic difficulties some of these patients come to laparotomy—little is found except intestinal and peritoneal injection and the only purpose served is the proven patency of major intestinal vessels and the absence of gangrene. Many patients are fortunately too ill for laparotomy and survival depends on both the patient's intestinal 'reserve' and the effectiveness of replacement therapy which must correct deficiencies and compensate for the severe losses from diarrhoea and the enforced régime of intravenous feeding.

Though this syndrome may sound clear cut and precise there is often grave difficulty in making a firm diagnosis, which is often in fact first made at autopsy. Rarely changes in the rectal mucosa may help to confirm the diagnosis, though in any case non-specific changes are common in many chronic diarrhoeal states and too much reliance should not be placed on this.

Ulceration of the Small Bowel

Ulceration of the jejunum may be found in patients with the Zollinger-Ellison syndrome (p. 238) and may complicate the use of enteric-coated potassium chloride tablets. Jejunal ulceration is also reported in coeliac disease and its precise cause in this disorder is unknown. The ulcer may, however, perforate and obviously on occasions may be confused with malignant jejunal ulceration complicating coeliac disease. Diffuse small-bowel ulceration is seen in diffuse ulcerative jejuno-ileitis which has already been described.

Carcinoid Syndrome

Carcinoid tumours occur anywhere in the gut but are commonest in the appendix and terminal ileum. They are derived from argentaffin cells, have a characteristic yellow colour, and are usually 1–2 cm. in diameter. A certain percentage of these normally common tumours are malignant and metastasize to the liver and are then associated with a rare but characteristic set of symptoms and signs—'the carcinoid syndrome'. Some but not all of the clinical features of this disorder are due to the liberation of serotonin (5-hydroxytryptamine, 5-HT) into the blood-stream. Destruction of the serotonin by liver cells prevents the syndrome from developing unless tumour secretion is directly into hepatic veins—hence the importance of hepatic secondary deposits.

Tryptophan
  ↓
5-Hydroxytryptophan (5-HTP)
  ↓
5-Hydroxytryptamine (5-HT serotonin)
  ↓
5-Hydroxyindole acetic acid (5-HIAA) in urine.

CLINICAL PICTURE

There are variations in the clinical picture depending on the part of the gut from which the tumour arises, i.e., *foregut tumours* (bronchial, gastric, pancreatic) give rise to a classic carcinoid syndrome though unusual features include production by the tumour of 5-HTP (5-hydroxytryptophan), a particularly livid flush (*vide infra*), and a tendency for bone and skin metastases. *Midgut tumours* (small bowel, appendix, right colon) produce the classic carcinoid syndrome. *Hindgut tumours* (descending colon and rectum) rarely produce carcinoid syndrome even when they metastasize.

Symptoms include attacks of flushing and warmth particularly related to food and the taking of alcohol. The attacks are often distressing to the patient and they are accompanied by gurgling and abdominal borborygmi. Diarrhoea is a feature and the abdominal symptoms are the result of the stimulating effect of serotonin on intestinal smooth muscle. The skin flushing, on the other hand, is the result of activation of bradykinin by tumour kinins. Further features include attacks of bronchospasm, oedema, and skin rashes. The latter consists both of pigmentation of the skin as well as a dermatitis of exposed skin areas—pellagra. This latter is caused by diversion of the amino-acid L-tryptophan to serotonin production, consequently diminishing the production of nicotinic acid.

Signs of the disease may also include hepatomegaly—and possibly a separate tumour mass usually in the right iliac fossa as well as right-sided cardiac murmurs and even right heart failure. Murmurs are due to valvular fibrosis, probably as a result of serotonin which seems capable of exciting a fibrous tissue reaction both in the heart and in other areas, e.g., peritoneal cavity. It is important to note that patients are often in good health and despite the fact that they may have metastases in the liver the prognosis may be relatively good and survival for many years is not unknown.

DIAGNOSIS

The following tests are helpful:

1. The detection of increased 5-HIAA in the urine derived from 5-HT. Normal up to 10 mg. per 24 hours. Occasionally tests for 5-HTP and histamine may be required in atypical cases.

2. Biopsy of the liver may show typical nests of glandular cells with silver-staining granules.

3. Food, alcohol, or 1–10 μg. of i.v. adrenaline may be used to produce the typical flush.

TREATMENT

Symptoms may be controlled medically by avoiding dietary substances known to produce symptoms—the most obvious precipitant being alcohol. Antiserotonin drugs, such as methysergide, will control diarrhoea, and as catecholamines are potent triggers for flushing, antisympathetic drugs such as Dibenzyline and chlorpromazine may be helpful. Heart failure may require digitalis and diuretics and pellagra may require nicotinic acid therapy. Surgery may be effective in the removal of metastases if they are confined to one of the liver lobes (hepatic lobectomy) but caution must be exercised, as the operation is a major one and profound hypotension a possible complication. Further, prognosis may be favourable without surgical intervention.

DIVERTICULA

Duodenal Diverticula

These may be single or multiple. They often occur on the concave border of the duodenal loop where they may become quite large. Duodenal ulcers may also by their surrounding fibrosis cause traction diverticula.

Though generally symptomless it seems possible that duodenal diverticula can rarely:

1. Cause intestinal bleeding, though another source should always be sought.

2. Infection in a duodenal diverticulum may result in a blind-loop syndrome with diarrhoea and vitamin-B_{12} deficiency. This is, however, much more commonly a feature of multiple jejunal diverticula.

3. A duodenal diverticulum of the second part of the duodenum can rarely cause obstructive jaundice by compressing the common bile-duct.

Usually duodenal diverticula which are common can be ignored and no special treatment is required.

Jejunal Diverticula

These commonly develop along the mesenteric border of the small gut when they may be solitary or multiple. They can become quite large (*Figs. 68, 69*) and though sometimes symptomless and a chance finding at operation, autopsy, or abdominal radiology, they can be associated with two patterns of symptoms.

1. Perhaps due to a related disorder of peristalsis, attacks of abdominal pain, vomiting, borborygmi, and diarrhoea may result—and symptoms of

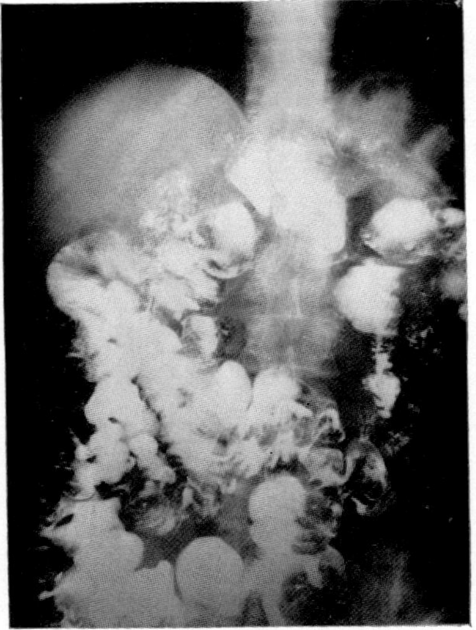

Fig. 68. Barium series of jejunal diverticulosis.

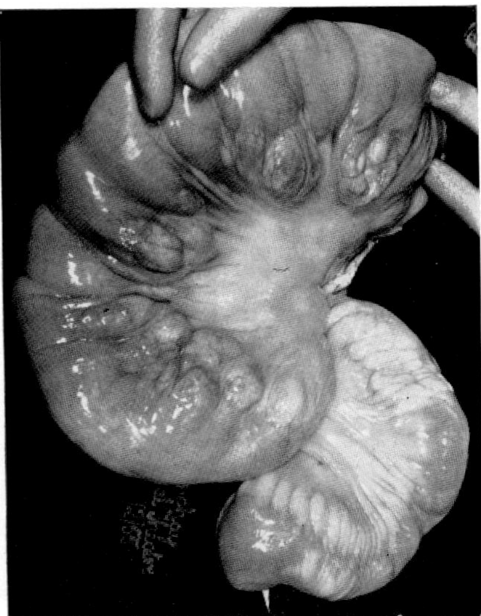

Fig. 69. Resection of 2 ft. of jejunum cured a severe state of malabsorption.

this sort in middle-aged or elderly patients should suggest this diagnosis as one of the possibilities and prompt a request for radiological examination of the small bowel. So often a barium enema is the only examination performed in patients with diarrhoea, in which case jejunal diverticula may be missed. Occasionally, bleeding from the diverticula or intestinal perforation may occur.

2. The most interesting aspect of this disorder is the occurrence of a malabsorption syndrome due to colonization of these pouches by bacteria (*see* p. 253).

Meckel's Diverticulum

This developmental abnormality occurs in about 2 per cent of normal subjects. It is situated on the antimesenteric border of the ileum about 45 cm. (18 in.) from the ileocaecal valve and is often occupied by gastric mucosa. This accounts for the majority of the symptoms which are due to formation of a peptic ulcer with resultant abdominal pain and bleeding (rectal haemorrhage and melaena and symptoms of chronic anaemia). The diagnosis should be considered in young patients with lower intestinal bleeding of unknown cause. Technetium scintiscanning can identify the diverticulum if gastric mucosa is present within it.

TUMOURS OF THE SMALL INTESTINE

1. Simple

Benign tumours of the small bowel are rare and include leiomyoma, lipoma, fibroma, and angiomata. The latter may bleed profusely. The gut may be involved in von Recklinghausen's disease (neurofibromatosis). The commonest simple small-bowel tumour is argentaffinoma of the appendix and ileum. Malignant degeneration and metastasis to the liver result in the carcinoid syndrome (*see* p. 291).

Special mention should be made of the Peutz-Jeghers syndrome which mainly affects the small bowel, though gastric and colonic involvement is well recorded. The condition is one of multiple small intestinal polypi, the lesions on histological examination being hamartomata, i.e., orderly collections of all the elements of the small intestinal wall. Associated with this there are changes in the skin, notably the appearance of small dark-brown or blue macules, resembling freckles, which are noted over the bridge of the nose, around and in the mouth, and on the lips and extremities.

CLINICAL PICTURE

There is usually a strong family history of this genetically determined disorder and although the patient may be referred to a dermatologist concerning the skin lesion, the multiple intestinal polyps cause either pain —due to small bowel obstruction—or intussusception or bleeding with the resultant symptoms of anaemia.

There is great argument concerning the malignant potentialities of the Peutz-Jeghers syndrome, and although one or two resultant carcinomata are described the risk seems small. This is important because surgery is only required if the patient has symptoms which cannot be controlled by conservative therapy—multiple resections of the small bowel lead to malabsorption, wasting, and serious metabolic deficiencies (*see* p. 291).

Other Conditions associated with Gastro-intestinal Polyposis
These, though not all affecting or even being confined to the small intestine, are conveniently summarized in *Table 21*.

Table 21. GASTRO-INTESTINAL POLYPOSIS

Name	Peutz-Jeghers syndrome	Gardner's syndrome	Familial polyposis coli	Canada—Cronkhite syndrome
Histology	Hamartoma	Adenomatous polypi	Adenomatous polypi	Mucosal cysts
Site	Small bowel, also colon and stomach	Mainly colon	Colon	Stomach and whole bowel
Associated disorders	Skin pigmentation	Skin tumours, i.e., sebaceous cysts, lipomata, peritoneal fibrous tumours. Bone tumours. Osteomata	None	Loss of hair and nails
Family history	Yes	Yes	Yes	No
Clinical manifestations	Skin changes. Alimentary bleeding. Alimentary obstruction	Skin and bone tumours. Rectal bleeding, etc.	Rectal bleeding. Diarrhoea	Malabsorption. Vomiting. Cachexia. Loss of hair and nails
Malignant change	No	Yes*	Yes	No
Treatment	Conservative or resection	Colectomy	Colectomy	May respond to i.v. feeding and ? surgical resection

* Association with carcinoma of ampulla of Vater.

2. Malignant Tumours

Carcinomata of the small bowel are unusual but when they do occur are usually found in the second or third part of the duodenum. Here they produce both intestinal obstruction and bleeding. Unfortunately they also have a very poor prognosis as metastasis to the regional lymph-nodes and peritoneum occurs early. Though surgery is required to relieve obstruction and bleeding, palliation only is possible, the 5-year survival being 10 per cent or less. This bad prognosis is not necessarily shared by ampullary carcinomata (*see* p. 243).

Reticuloses, on the other hand, are more commonly found in the jejunum and ileum. Lymphosarcoma is the commonest tumour, perhaps related to the increased lymphoid tissue in the lower small bowel. An important exception seems to relate to the malignant change accompanying some cases of coeliac disease. Here tumours of lymphoid tissue occur most frequently in the upper small bowel and Hodgkin's disease and reticulo-sarcoma are more frequent than lymphosarcoma.

The lymphoid tumours in general involve the small bowel secondary to generalized tumour spread and are very rarely primary gut tumours in the true sense of the word. The clinical picture produced is therefore one of generalized lymphoid neoplasia with symptoms due to this, e.g., pyrexia, anaemia, etc., and physical signs of generalized lymphadenopathy, hepatosplenomegaly, jaundice, etc. This is therefore not the place to consider the overall manifestations or the exciting possibilities of the aetiology and new methods of treatment that pertain particularly in relation to Hodgkin's disease.

The lymphomata produce ulceration and polypoid change in the gut lymphoid tissue. Extension through the gut wall leads to perforation and there may be lymphatic obstruction from involvement of the mesenteric lymph-nodes. Alimentary symptoms as opposed to general ones include abdominal pain, often colicky and mid-abdominal—anaemia due to intestinal bleeding—and dramatic symptoms—pain, peritonism, etc., due to perforation. Diarrhoea with steatorrhoea may also occur and ascites may result from peritoneal involvement or from lymphatic obstruction (chylous ascites).

Diagnosis is easy if the patient has obvious evidence of generalized reticulosis and should be considered in patients with coeliac disease who show clinical deterioration despite a strict gluten-free diet or in patients with a malabsorption syndrome proving refractory to treatment and presenting in middle age.

Helpful diagnostic tests include:

1. Radiology of the small bowel where polypoid filling defects—a non-specific malabsorption type of picture—or fistulous communications between loops of small bowel may all be demonstrated.

Lymphangiography may demonstrate both enlargement and abnormal structure of mesenteric and aortic lymph-nodes and this may on occasions be useful in assessing the effects of later therapy.

2. Biopsy is obviously the sheet anchor of diagnosis. Biopsy of the small intestinal mucosa usually shows only non-specific partial villous atrophy. A careful examination of the submucosal cellular infiltrate is, however, very worth while and occasionally suggestive of lymphoma. Biopsy must otherwise be taken from involved tissue. This may be from enlarged lymph-nodes, liver, or bone-marrow. At laparotomy, biopsy material should include other than mesenteric lymph-nodes which are in any case often enlarged because of non-specific changes. Abnormal tissue from the small bowel or a full-thickness surgical biopsy from one or more areas of even normal appearing small bowel are worth while.

Treatment of small intestinal lymphoma is difficult as the disease is usually generalized and the whole or a considerable length of gut is involved. Surgery is important for diagnosis and for resection of local areas which have perforated, obstructed, or developed fistulae. Massive resection is, however, rarely indicated as the after-effects are considerable and do not guarantee cure of the disease. Pulse therapy with multiple anti-mitotic agents may be helpful in some patients but here again long-term results due to the nature of the disease process are disappointing.

Pneumatosis cystoides intestinalis (Gas Cysts of the Intestine)

This is a rare but striking condition of uncertain cause in which gas-filled cysts occupy the submucosal and subserosal aspects of the stomach, small or large bowel. The major cause seems to be some break in the continuity of the intestinal mucosa, e.g., peptic ulcer or trauma following sigmoido-scopy, whilst others occur—particularly in the presence of respiratory disease such as asthma and emphysema—perhaps by gas tracking through the mediastinum into the mesentery and gut wall. Apart from the slight risk of pneumoperitoneum, other symptoms are rare but include diar-rhoea, steatorrhoea, and intestinal bleeding. Difficulty is sometimes en-countered in distinguishing gas cysts from rectal polyps when they occur in the lower large bowel—though they disappear on attempted biopsy! The radiological findings are usually characteristic with gas cysts tending to cluster in a segment of bowel and particularly in the ileocaecal region. Occasionally they may be large enough to simulate a pneumoperitoneum which, of course, can complicate their presence. Occasionally, too, evi-dence of the tracking of gas from thorax to abdominal cavity may be found. They require no treatment.

Leukaemia

The small bowel may also be involved by chronic leukaemia. Chronic lymphatic leukaemia may cause multiple polyps which may bleed or cause intussusception, whilst ulceration and anaemia due to intestinal bleeding may be features of chronic myeloid or chronic lymphatic leukaemia.

Protein-losing (Exudative) Enteropathy

Excessive loss of serum proteins into the alimentary canal is the cause—partial or total—of the hypoproteinaemia that complicates a wide variety of gastro-intestinal disorders. These include:

1. Diseases of the stomach, e.g., giant hypertrophic rugal folds; gastric carcinoma.

2. Diseases of the small bowel, e.g., coeliac disease; Crohn's disease; intestinal lymphangiectasia; intestinal reticulosis—in which ulceration and/or lymphatic obstruction are the operative features.

3. Disorders of the large bowel, e.g., ulcerative colitis.

4. Generalized diseases, e.g., cardiac failure; constrictive pericarditis.

The result of this protein loss is oedema which may be widespread, whilst the total and individual globulin fractions are also decreased with an attendant risk of infection. Wasting, skin cracking, follicular

14

hyperkeratosis, hair depigmentation, and lethargy—which are signs of generalized protein depletion—are often not present as it is the vascular protein compartment which is depleted in this syndrome.

Special mention should be made of the condition of intestinal lymphangiectasia as clues to its presence may be obtained from the family history (it is often present in several members of the same family) whilst lymphoedema, chylous ascites, and a yellowish discoloration of the nails may also be found. Leakage of lymph into the gut occurs from dilated and obstructed lymphatics and protein loss is due to the appreciable protein content of chyle. Dilated lymphatics may be found on intestinal biopsy—on the surface of the gut at laparotomy and by lymphangiography. Apart from protein loss these patients also have steatorrhoea and deficiency of fat-soluble (ADK) vitamins, in each case due to the failure of lymphatic absorption.

Diagnosis of protein-losing enteropathy may be difficult but should be suspected in patients with gastro-intestinal disease and generalized hypoproteinaemia, providing no other source of protein loss (e.g., skin, urine) is present. An ^{131}I albumin turnover would show a shortened half-life (hypercatabolic hypoproteinaemia) rather than the lengthened half-life found in patients with malnutrition due to gastric or intestinal resection (hypo-anabolic hypoproteinaemia). Tests are available for demonstration of increased protein loss into the gut, the tests depending on the use of an i.v. marker of molecular weight approximately that of albumin and its subsequent detection in the stools. The most commonly used substance is [131]polyvinylpyrrolidone (PVP), which is a synthetic substance with a molecular weight of about 40,000. Following i.v. injection normal subjects excrete less than 1 per cent of the radioactivity in the stools over 5 days. Difficulties may arise due to urinary contamination, particularly in female subjects.

Treatment of protein-losing enteropathy is obviously that of the cause and there may be a special place in intestinal lymphangiectasia for the use of medium-chain fatty acids which not only may decrease protein loss but they may also diminish steatorrhoea. This action reflects their easier and different route of absorption. A low-fat diet may also be helpful in reducing steatorrhoea. Corticosteroids and/or surgery may be needed to stop protein exudation in ulcerative and neoplastic diseases, whilst in intestinal lymphangiectasia reconstructive surgery on the major lymphatics and the establishment of effective lymphovenous anastamosis may be effective.

FURTHER READING

Small Bowel Ischaemia
BIRCHER, J., BARTHOLOMEW, L. G., CAIN, J. C., and ADSON, M. A. (1966), 'Syndrome of Intestinal Arterial Insufficiency (Abdominal Angina)', *Archs intern. Med.*, **117**, 632.

Diffuse Ulcerative Jejuno-ileitis
JEFFRIES, G. H., STEINBERG, H., and SLEISENGER, M. H. (1968), 'Chronic Ulcerative (Non-granulomatous) Jejunitis', *Am. J. Med.*, **44**, 47.

Carcinoid Syndrome
SJOERDSMA, A., and MELMON, K. L. (1964), 'The Carcinoid Syndrome', *Gastroenterology*, **47**, 104.

WILKINS, E. D., and SANDLER, M. (1963), 'The Classification of Carcinoid Tumours', *Lancet*, **1**, 238.

Intestinal Lymphoma
AUSTAD, W. I., CORNES, J. S., GOUGH, K. R., MCCARTHY, C. F., and READ, A. E. (1967), 'Steatorrhoea and Malignant Lymphoma. The Relationship of Malignant Tumours of Lymphoid Tissue and Coeliac Disease', *Am. J. dig. Dis.*, **12**, 475.
HARRIS, O. D., COOKE, W. T., THOMSON, H., and WATERHOUSE, J. A. H. (1967), 'Malignancy in Adult Coeliac Disease and Idiopathic Steatorrhoea', *Am. J. Med.*, **42**, 899.

Alpha Chain Disease
RAMBAUD, J. C., BOGNEL, C., PROST, A., BERNIER, J. J., LE QUINTREE, Y., LAMBLING, A., DANON, F., HUREZ, D., and SELIGMAN, M. (1968), 'Clinicopathological Study of a Patient with "Mediterranean" Abdominal Lymphoma and a New Type of IgA Abnormality (Alpha Chain Disease)', *Digestion*, **1**, 321.

Peutz-Jeghers Syndrome
DORMONDY, T. L. (1957), 'Gastro-intestinal Polyposis with Mucocutaneous Pigmentation (Peutz-Jeghers Syndrome)', *New Engl. J. Med.*, **246**, 1093.

Pseudomembranous enterocolitis
GOULSTON, V., and MCGOVERN, V. (1965), 'Pseudomembranous Enterocolitis', *Gut*, **6**, 207.

Intestinal Tuberculosis
ANAND, S. S. (1956), 'Hypertrophic Ileo-caecal Tuberculosis in India with a Record of 50 Hemicolectomies', *Ann. R. Coll. Surg.*, **19**, 208.

Pneumatosis Cystoides
HUGHES, D. I. D., GORDON, K. C. D., SWANN, J. C., and BOLT, G. L. (1966), 'Pneumatosis Cystoides Intestinalis', *Gut*, **7**, 553.

Eosinophilic Granuloma
SALMON, P. R., and PAULLEY, J. W. (1967), 'Eosinophilic Granuloma of the Gastro-intestinal Tract', *Ibid*, **8**, 8.

Protein-losing Enteropathy
GORDON, R. S. (1959), 'Exudative Enteropathy', *Lancet*, **1**, 325.

Chapter 20

Diseases of the Colon

DISEASES OF MOTILITY

Aganglionosis Coli (Hirschsprung's Disease)

THIS CONGENITAL disease of infancy and childhood is due to the absence of the normal ganglia and nerve plexuses in the wall of the colon which renders it non-propulsive. The condition is analogous to achalasia of the oesophagus, it has a strong familial tendency, and affects males more than females. Parents who have a child with aganglionosis should be warned that there is a 1 in 8 chance of a subsequent male child being similarly affected. Often the loss of ganglion cells is confined to the rectosigmoid segment. Faeces accumulate proximal to the aganglionic segment causing the colon to become enlarged (*Fig. 70*). The symptoms are obstinate

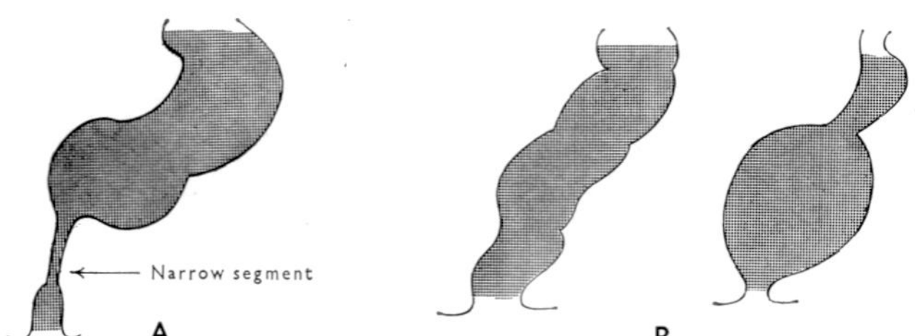

Fig. 70. Illustration of findings in barium enema in A, Hirschsprung's disease, and B, secondary megacolon.

constipation, distension, anorexia, intermittent vomiting, anaemia, and failure to thrive. Intestinal obstruction may occur in the newborn. Spurious diarrhoea and loss of blood from stercoral ulceration may occur. On examination the rectum is usually empty, but through the abdominal wall firm faeces can be felt in the distended colon. The child is wasted and anaemic. Good barium-enema films, though essential for diagnosis, are not easy to obtain because of the great difficulty in clearing the proximal colon beforehand. Bowel wash-outs may be required, but water intoxication from absorption of the fluid is a risk. The films should show the dilated colon above, the smooth immobile rectosigmoid segment, and a rectum of normal calibre. Under a general anaesthetic and through a sigmoidoscope a deep biopsy of the affected segment may be obtained and the lack of ganglia confirmed microscopically.

The treatment of aganglionosis is surgical. Where a large area of the colon is aganglionic the prognosis is poor and some form of ileorectal anastomosis or permanent ileostomy is required. In the commoner condition of aganglionosis confined to the upper rectum, various operations have been devised with the aim of preserving the sensitive rectal mucosa while cutting out and by-passing the aganglionic muscular coat. Preoperatively, anaemia should be corrected and nutrition improved by parenteral means if necessary, but it is useless to expect any great improvement of the child's general condition until after recovery from surgery, when a normal bowel action is usually restored, weight is gained, and growth proceeds.

Acquired Megacolon

The whole bowel may become atonic and dilated in some children who constantly ignore the impulse to evacuate a full rectum. Naturally such a condition takes years to develop and is common in the mentally defective or emotionally disturbed. The belly is distended as in Hirschsprung's disease, but in contrast to that condition the rectum is full of impacted faeces, which causes faecal leakage and soiling of the clothes and perineum. The anal region is fissured and excoriated.

The bowel should be cleared by repeated wash-outs, and its tone gradually restored by keeping it as empty as possible. This can only be done by the regular use of purgatives such as standardized senna (senokot) in doses adequate to secure a daily evacuation. If the co-operation of a child of normal intelligence can be retained, and if emotional conflicts and social difficulties can be resolved, it may, in the most favourable cases, be possible to restore the normal bowel habit, but more often in the mentally feeble patient the atony persists, and bowel wash-outs have to be repeated throughout life in order to prevent discomfort or intestinal obstruction.

Lazy Rectum

Some people, perhaps by force of civilized circumstance which inhibits the normal tendency for the full rectum to empty itself by the massive contraction of defaecation, develop an insensitive or lazy rectum which can retain faeces without provoking any desire to defaecate. Vague pelvic discomforts may be noticed or reflex symptoms such as headache and dizziness, but the bowel does not empty. Very often such patients resort to the irritant cathartics which cause intestinal cramps, nausea, and heartburn before they can empty the bowel.

The condition often develops in childhood as a result of faulty habits, rushed meals, social anxieties, and inadequate toilet facilities, but patients rarely complain of symptoms until adult life, by which time the reflex is completely lost. At the other end of life, elderly or enfeebled patients may lose the power to empty the rectum, which becomes distended by faeces and further weakened.

In early adult life, the condition is best treated by the patient co-operating in an attempt to re-establish normal emptying by utilizing the gastrocolic reflex. The rectum is more likely to contract after a meal, and at such times the patient must retire to the lavatory and insert a cathartic suppository, or if necessary, distend the rectum by a small enema from a disposable plastic bag, and wait for a contraction. Gradually a conditioned reflex may be built up, so that artificial stimulation is unnecessary. This is probably a better method than violent purgation, but it may help to give sub-laxative doses of senokot twelve hours before the expected time of rectal evacuation.

Elderly patients with weak abdominal and levator muscles may need the help of a suppository or a small self-administered enema in order to empty the rectum regularly and save themselves the discomforts of impacted faeces.

Spastic or Irritable Colon

AETIOLOGY

There is a strong constitutional, and possible a hereditary, predisposition to this disorder which may persist throughout life, but exacerbations are usually triggered by environmental stresses, such as: (1) Conflict, frustration, and anxiety. (2) Over-fatigue, irregular meals, inadequate sleep, long-distance motoring. (3) Smoking and alcohol. (4) Foodstuffs, commonly onions and nuts. (5) Dysenteric infections.

Motility studies have shown that sufferers develop more intense colonic contractions after a meal, after smoking, and after worrying conversations than do normals, and that ring contractions of circular muscle may build up high intraluminal pressures in isolated zones of the colon. Experimentally it has been shown than cholecystokinin can alter the motility pattern of the sigmoid.

CLINICAL PICTURE

Clinically, spasm of the bowel may be so intense and widespread that the whole of the left colon may be easily felt as a long, hard tube which is tender to the touch.

The symptomatology is extremely variable between patients and between different phases of the sufferer's life. The most constant feature is the story of difficulty in maintaining a normal rhythm of bowel activity, phases of constipation or narrow stools tending to alternate with phases of looseness. On this background, certain symptom complexes can be recognized.

1. Constipation, narrow or pellet stools, pain in the left iliac fossa over a contracted tender colon, excess of bowel wind, and tenderness over a distended caecum. When pain and tenderness in the right iliac fossa, due to the trapping of gas proximal to left-sided spasm, is the main feature, patients are sometimes thought to be suffering from recurrent subacute appendicitis.

2. Cramps in the left iliac fossa associated with irritability of the rectum which produces excessive mucus and usually evacuates itself three or four times in the early hours of the day (used to be known as 'mucous colitis').

3. Severe episodes of cramp-like pain from the transverse or descending colon which may last for hours or days and which tend to culminate, but not always, in a brief attack of diarrhoea.

Patients with an irritable colon are prone to reverse peristalsis higher in the gut which may cause epigastric distress, heartburn, and regurgitation of stomach contents. They may be wakened early in the morning by painful contractions of the bowel, or by reflex effects of these, such as headache and nightmares.

MANAGEMENT

1. Reduce nervous tension by excluding serious disease and making the patient aware of the mechanisms by which his discomforts are caused.

2. Seek modifications in the patient's life to reduce stress.

3. Use regular sedation, e.g., phenobarbitone 30 mg. twice daily if this seems appropriate.

4. Advise curtailment of smoking, abstinence from provocative foods such as onions, and abstinence from haphazard purgation by irritant cathartics. Increase fibre content of faeces by eating whole-meal bread and adding bran to cakes and stews.

5. Bulk up the stools and prevent excessive reabsorption of water by giving methyl cellulose (Celevac) or psyllium seed extract (Isogel granules).

6. Use anticholinergic drugs such as extract of belladonna, or proprietary preparations which contain various combinations of barbiturate and anticholinergic drugs, to treat exacerbations of trouble, and provide the patient who is liable to severe attacks of pain with a quick-acting anticholinergic drug which he can carry with him and take at the first warning of an attack. To relieve pain effectively, dosage must be high enough to cause side-effects such as blurring of vision and dryness of the mouth.

7. Mebeverine, a drug acting directly on smooth muscle, has been shown to alter the abnormal motility patterns in the irritable colon syndrome, and by double-blind therapeutic trial to have a beneficial effect on the symptoms of the irritable colon syndrome. It is given in doses of 100 mg. four times a day. As yet, this drug must still be regarded as under trial.

8. In the case of irritable rectum with mucorrhoea, phenobarbitone 60 mg. at night and codeine phosphate 30 mg. on waking may be helpful in breaking the abnormal habit. Codeine should not be given to patients with a spastic sigmoid.

PROGNOSIS

If patients can adjust their lives to diminish fatigue and stress, and if measures suggested for their relief are reasonably successful, they tend to regain confidence, which in itself has a beneficial effect on the autonomic discord. Attacks of pain become less frequent and phases of irregularity of habit less troublesome. Symptoms may disappear altogether for months or years, but there is always a likelihood of recurrent trouble.

Diverticular Disease of the Colon

AETIOLOGY

Motility and pressure studies have shown that diverticula-bearing zones of colon are prone to strong contractions of the circular muscle which build up extremely high intraluminal pressures; it seems probable that these high pressures are responsible for the herniations of the mucosa through the muscle-coat which become diverticula. The usual position for diverticula is at the mesenteric attachment of the colon, where the entry of blood-vessels weakens the muscle-coat.

Diverticula develop as age advances, and diffuse diverticulosis coli is common in the elderly, the obese, and in diabetics. At an earlier age, localized diverticular disease of the sigmoid region is not uncommon, and possibly this localized form of the disease may have a different aetiology from the often symptomless generalized disease.

Diverticular disease is uncommon in Africa and in south-east Asia where the diet contains more bulk in the form of unrefined carbohydrate, and it has been suggested that the liability of Northern people to diverticular disease is due to their relatively low-residue diet, rather than to genetic factors. The tension or strain on the wall of a hollow organ is related to the pressure within it and to the internal diameter of the organ. Thus if a tube like the colon is habitually of narrow bore then the strain on the wall caused by a build up-of pressure within the lumen will be greater than if the colon was usually distended by faeces. Rats given a low-residue diet will in time develop diverticulosis coli.

PATHOLOGY

It has long been recognized that patients with diverticular disease of the sigmoid have a thickened circular muscle-coat. This thickening of the muscle is probably a true work-hypertrophy. It may antedate the development of diverticula, and minute examination of resected specimens of sigmoid done in patients with the so-called prediverticular syndrome have shown that:

a. The muscle thickening can precede the formation of diverticula.

b. Muscle weight per 100 muscle nuclei is increased.

c. The early stages of diverticular formation can be seen to occur by herniation of the mucosa through gaps in the muscle layer.

Fully developed diverticula have no muscle-coats and therefore cannot empty. Stagnation within them may cause inflammation of the mucosa, blockage of the neck, and the formation of an abscess. Small local or pericolic abscesses may burst into the lumen of the gut or may set up a diffuse inflammation and fibrosis which causes narrowing of the gut. Granulation tissue may bleed profusely. A large pericolic abscess may form, or diffuse peritonitis may be caused when a small diverticular abscess bursts. Pericolic inflammation tends to involve neighbouring organs, so that those become stuck to the diseased bowel, and consequently fistulae may form. Vesicocolic fistulae cause cystitis, pyelitis, and pneumaturia. Ileocolic fistulae will cause contamination of the ileal contents and so malabsorption.

CLINICAL PICTURE AND COMPLICATIONS

Diverticular disease causes no specific symptoms, but sometimes an elderly patient is encountered who has widespread diverticulosis and who suffers from mild chronic diarrhoea. There is a possibility in such a case that the motility of the bowel may have been altered in such a way as to impede the reabsorption of water from the faeces. The colon is unusually inert when examined radiologically.

Sigmoid diverticular disease has symptoms similar to those of the irritable colon syndrome. Left iliac fossa pain and tenderness, irregularities of bowel action, narrow stools, or the passage of mucus may all worry the patient. The thickened colon can often be felt and, on sigmoidoscopy, spasm at the rectosigmoid bend prevents further passage of the instrument.

Diverticulitis may cause symptoms from:

1. *Local inflammation* which may give rise to fibrosis and narrowing of the colon; subacute intestinal obstruction may follow, but there is usually a tender mass to be felt in the left iliac fossa, constipation and narrow stools, and possibly bouts of fever.

2. *Pericolic abscess* usually causes local pain, tenderness, fever, and leucocytosis, and perhaps the development of a mass, but occasionally the local symptoms may be indefinite or masked by obesity and distension, in which case the problem may be one of pyrexia of unknown origin. If an abscess forms in the pelvis there are symptoms of bladder and rectal irritation and a mass may be felt per rectum.

3. *Peritonitis.* Perforation of a diverticular abscess into the peritoneum rarely causes such a dramatic onset of peritonitis as that which follows the perforation of a peptic ulcer, and since many of the patients are old or enfeebled, the local reaction of tenderness and rigidity may be slight. Abdominal pain, shock, tachycardia, and increasing abdominal distension with loss of bowel-sounds are the main features.

4. *Penetration.* Abdominal pain usually precedes the formation of fistulae, but it may not be remarkable. Pain on micturition, haematuria, and pneumaturia occur when a vesicocolic fistula forms, and the urine may contain a brownish sediment full of pus cells and vegetable fibre. The symptoms of an ileocolic fistula are more insidious—diarrhoea, bulky offensive stools, and weight-loss may lead to a fully developed malabsorption state with hypoproteinaemic oedema, sore tongue, and anaemia.

5. *Haemorrhage.* Bleeding from granulations can cause either an abrupt rectal haemorrhage necessitating blood transfusion or an insidious loss which causes iron deficiency. This may be the first symptom of diverticulitis. Brisk bleeding in an elderly patient may cause anxiety, but the condition is not dangerous if blood is available for transfusion.

DIAGNOSIS

The patient with diverticulitis is often first seen by a surgeon after a complication such as peritonitis, but some may complain of long-standing symptoms which point to disease of the sigmoid colon. In making the diagnosis, age, physical constitution, and local signs are evaluated, and a barium enema is done after cleansing of the bowel by wash-outs and purgatives. Diverticula which fill under pressure but do not readily empty may be seen both before and after evacuation of the barium from the colon. Narrowing of a segment of the sigmoid colon with many diverticula above suggests diverticulitis. Pericolic abscesses do not, as a rule, fill with barium; vesicocolic fistulae are difficult to demonstrate, but ileocolic communication can best be shown by this method. Occult or frank blood may be present in the stools, the haemoglobin may be reduced, and the white-cell count elevated. Sigmoidoscopy may reveal spasm or narrowing above the rectum, sometimes mucosal oedema, and occasionally bleeding from above the instrument.

DIFFERENTIAL DIAGNOSIS

The rare diverticulitis of the caecum and ascending colon may cause symptoms indistinguishable from appendicitis, and if an abscess forms in that region it may well be due to the former, perforated carcinoma of the caecum being a third possibility.

Table 22. DIFFERENTIAL DIAGNOSIS OF DIVERTICULAR DISEASE, CROHN'S DISEASE, AND CARCINOMA OF COLON

METHOD	DIVERTICULAR DISEASE	CROHN'S DISEASE	CARCINOMA
Length of history	Long	Months or years	Months
Examination	Tenderness, guarding, perhaps fever	Fever and raised E.S.R. common	Palpable hard mass
Barium examination	Diverticula elsewhere. Longer segment of narrowing. No sharp irregularities. Proximal colon unlikely to be much dilated. *N*-butyl hyoscine i.v. may relax spasm	Spiky outline of barium in colon. Mucosal oedema and possible linear ulcers	May be a few diverticula. May be short zone of narrowing. Irregularities of outline. Proximal colon may be dilated
Sigmoidoscopy	Mucosa of upper rectum may be inflamed	Oedema of rectal mucosa. Granulomatous anal tags	Mucosa normal below, but blood may come from above

The appearances of the sigmoid colon affected by prediverticular disease may sometimes be difficult to distinguish from those of Crohn's disease of the colon, and both may occur in older people. If a segment of colon is narrowed and indistensible it may be due to diverticulitis or to carcinoma.

In some cases it is impossible to tell the two conditions apart, even when the colon is handled at operation. Certain features are helpful in making the correct diagnosis, but any of them may be misleading in a particular case (*Table 22*).

In about 12 per cent of cases of carcinoma, diverticulosis is also present. There is no apparent causal relationship.

TREATMENT

Medical

The indications are mildness of symptoms, absence of complications, or an aged, high-risk patient.

The diet should contain an increased quantity of roughage in the form of fruit and salad, oatmeal, etc., but soft fruits containing pips, pears, fruit-skins, nuts, and currants should be avoided. If costive, a bulk preparation such as Celevac or an emulsion containing agar and liquid paraffin may help to retain water in the stool and keep it soft. Some patients are better suited by liquid paraffin or sub-laxative doses of Senokot, and some need occasional bowel wash-outs. Pain, fever, and tenderness necessitate bed-rest, a fluid diet, gentle purgation, and a course of treatment with parenteral antibiotics, such as streptomycin and penicillin. Morphine and codeine are contra-indicated.

Surgical

The indications are: (1) Severe symptoms with recurrent pericolic inflammation around localized disease in a reasonably young and healthy patient. (2) Onset of complications such as intestinal obstruction, pericolic abscess, peritonitis, fistulae, and haemorrhage.

The type of operation varies according to the localization of disease and the complications, but the primary aim is one-stage removal of the diseased segment with end-to-end anastomosis of the healthy colon above with that below. If complications render this unsafe the distended bowel should be decompressed and the faecal stream diverted away from the diseased area. This means proximal colostomy as the first stage, resection, and reanastomosis at the second, and closure of the colostomy as the third and final stage.

In practice, a patient with an uncomplicated case of localized disease is prepared for operation by correction of anaemia, reduction of obesity, and breathing exercise to improve lung ventilation. Associated conditions are treated, and for 2 days before operation the bowel is cleansed by a fluid diet and bowel wash-outs. Antibiotics are usually reserved for the post-operative phase, but some surgeons recommend insoluble sulphonamides for 7 days or neomycin for 2 days before operation. Some cases of localized sigmoid diverticular disease causing recurrent pain and associated with muscle hypertrophy can be treated by a long division of the muscle-coats (myotomy).

Patients with either intestinal obstruction or matted bowel and fistulae are given a right transverse colostomy in the first place. Later a barium enema is done to determine the extent of the lesion, and in due course when inflammation has subsided the diseased bowel is resected and fistulae closed. Occasionally vesicocolic fistulae can be closed in a one-stage operation.

A pericolic abscess must be drained and if necessary a colostomy made. Generalized peritonitis must be treated by resuscitation and peritoneal toilet followed by a transverse colostomy.

PROGNOSIS

Although the patient with diverticulitis who first comes to medical attention with faecal peritonitis has a 10 per cent chance of dying from this episode, there is good evidence that the life expectancy of most patients diagnosed as suffering from diverticulitis is not much reduced. The prognosis is determined more by the presence or absence of obesity, coronary arterial disease, or diabetes. The patient with complications less serious than faecal peritonitis, such as subacute obstruction or vesicocolic fistulae, can be expected to recover with skilled and experienced surgical treatment. The inexperienced surgeon is well advised to leave such cases to his seniors.

Ischaemic 'Colitis'

The splenic flexure of the colon is at the junction of the blood-supply of the superior and inferior mesenteric systems, and in situations where the blood-flow to this area drops below a critical point infarction of the mucosa may occur while the muscular coat and serosa remain intact. Such an event is only likely to occur in elderly patients with atheromatous disease of the aorta or mesenteric trunks, in those with rheumatoid arteritis and intravascular sludging, or after a severe drop in cardiac output.

The clinical picture produced by such an event is striking; the patient develops violent blood-stained diarrhoea and becomes severely shocked. On sigmoidoscopy blood can be seen coming from above but the rectal mucosa looks normal. If the patient can be tided over by blood and plasma transfusion aided perhaps by low molecular weight dextran, improvement begins within a week, and eventually the patient recovers completely. Subsequent barium enema may show a characteristic sacculation of the colonic wall below the splenic flexure, and an incomplete stricture may develop.

Endometriosis

Ectopic endometrial tissue may be present in the rectovaginal septum or in the rectal wall. The patient, who is usually childless or unmarried, is subject to severe dysmenorrhoea and possible rectal bleeding. Eventually a stricture forms in the rectum or rectosigmoid and intestinal obstruction may follow. Before a stricture develops, the best treatment is an ovari-ectomy or panhysterectomy, but if the whole pelvis is full of fibrous tissue an artificial menopause helps to reduce pain and further damage.

Benign Tumours of Colon

Adenomata

These may be single, but are often multiple, and are found most frequently in the rectosigmoid in males over the age of 40 years. When they are large and polypoid they may cause colicky pains, bouts of diarrhoea, and rectal bleeding. Villous tumours are less common. They produce mucus and provoke diarrhoea which may be severe enough to cause symptoms of hypokalaemia. Adenomatous polyps may be seen with the sigmoidoscope or demonstrated by air–barium contrast after an enema. Surgical treatment is discussed in Chapter 21.

Carcinoma of the Colon

AETIOLOGY

The risk of carcinoma of the colon increases with age, but occasionally it may occur before the age of 40 years. Two conditions predispose to an early onset—ulcerative colitis and polyposis coli. Since simple adenomatous polyps may be found in patients with carcinomata of the colon, it is reasonable to infer not only that adenomata may become carcinomatous, but also that the liability to formation of adenomata is linked to that of carcinoma. The factors responsible are unknown. It is a curious fact that whereas carcinoma of the rectum is commoner in males, carcinoma of the rest of the colon is commoner in females. An explanation for the high incidence of carcinoma coli in Europeans as opposed to Africans might be found in the low residue diet and increased bowel transit time of the former. This might alter the faecal flora and allow carcinogens to remain in contact with the bowel mucosa for a longer period.

PATHOLOGY

It is estimated that about 50 per cent of all colonic carcinomata involve the rectum and rectosigmoid junction, and that 15 per cent involve the sigmoid, 15 per cent the caecum and ascending colon, while the remaining 20 per cent are found in the transverse and descending portions; 85 per cent are adenocarcinomata, the remainder being colloid or undifferentiated. Growths can be graded according to the degree of differentiation, the most poorly differentiated being the most invasive and the most rapidly fatal. The growth may be ulcerous, proliferative and polypoid, or infiltrating and stenotic, but it is the cellular differentiation which determines the prognosis. Spread is most often into mesentery, neighbouring organs, and lymphatic glands, but metastases in the liver occur quite early if the growth is poorly differentiated. Transperitoneal spread occurs less commonly than from carcinoma of the stomach, and metastasis to lungs, brain, and other tissues is uncommon.

CLINICAL PICTURE

The early stages of growth are entirely symptomless, and even large carcinomata may cause remarkably little disturbance of general health.

About 25 per cent of cases are admitted as surgical emergencies, but the rest develop insidiously.

Symptoms are attributable to blood-loss, interference with the colonic rhythm, obstruction of the gut, and spread of the growth to neighbouring tissues causing pain.

Growths in the caecum and ascending colon often cause the following symptoms: Diarrhoea; pain after meals; vomiting; anaemia; loss of weight; tenderness in right iliac fossa.

Growths in the left half of the colon tend to cause: Constipation with phases of diarrhoea; distension; colic; anaemia.

The physical signs and symptoms may be grouped in the following way:

1. Loss of blood in the stools, either noticeable or occult, giving rise to iron-deficiency anaemia.

2. Signs of the carcinoma itself, which may be felt per abdomen or per rectum, but small growths or those in the rectosigmoid region cannot be palpated.

3. Signs of obstruction of the gut. Left-sided obstructing lesions tend to cause flank distension, ballooned caecum, loud borborygmi, colic, pain, and vomiting when the obstruction is nearly complete. Right-sided growths tend to cause bouts of vomiting with distension of the small intestine visible centrally.

4. Signs of secondary infection such as tenderness, fever, and passage of pus in the stools.

5. Signs of penetration and perforation. Vesicocolic and ileocolic fistulae as in diverticulitis (*see* p. 305). Sudden acute peritonitis.

6. Signs of spread and metastasis. A sigmoid or rectal growth may involve nerve-roots, lymphatics, or veins giving symptoms in the legs or perineum. Haemorrhoids may develop. Enlarged para-aortic glands may cause lymphatic obstruction. Ascites may develop and secondaries commonly cause enlargement of the liver, and, less frequently, jaundice.

DIAGNOSIS

All patients who have suffered a rectal haemorrhage or who have noticed a change in bowel habit should be examined abdominally for a carcinoma of the colon. A digital rectal examination is followed by a deep proctoscopy using a sigmoidoscope, and the stools are tested for occult blood on several successive days. After thorough preparation, a barium enema should show any but the smallest carcinomatous lesions provided that barium–air contrast pictures and oblique views of the sigmoid region are obtained. Faecal residue often obscures the mucosal pattern and limits the usefulness of this investigation, and in these circumstances small ulcerous lesions may be missed (*Fig. 71*). In cases of abdominal distension, the gas shadows in a straight radiograph may indicate the site of obstruction. Colonoscopy using a long fibrescope is reserved for cases where radiological studies are unhelpful or confusing. Colonoscopic inspection of the whole colon is very time-consuming and requires experience. One advantage of the method is that intraluminal biopsies can be taken.

Wherever possible a biopsy should be taken through a sigmoidoscope and for this, general anaesthesia, preceded by thorough bowel cleansing, is preferable.

A constantly positive faecal occult blood-test and a history of bowel disturbance are sufficient to warrant an exploratory laparotomy even though sigmoidoscopy and barium enema yield no evidence of neoplasm.

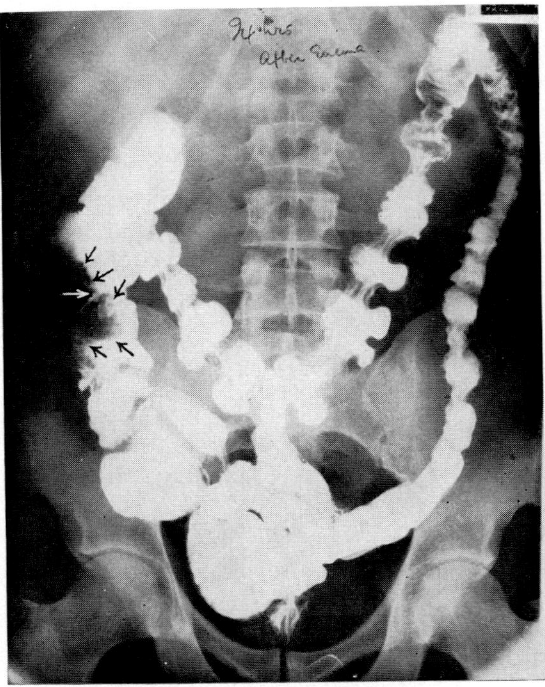

Fig. 71. Carcinoma of ascending colon.

The serum of a proportion of patients with carcinoma coli reacts with antibodies prepared against foetal colon-cell antigen. The diagnostic value of this test is not yet great enough to warrant its widespread use.

DIFFERENTIAL DIAGNOSIS

Strictures caused by diverticulitis, Crohn's disease, ulcerative colitis, and, more rarely, endometriosis and tuberculosis, may cause symptoms and signs readily confused with those of an infiltrating carcinoma. Careful study of the barium films, the sigmoidoscopic appearances, and the results of mucosal biopsy resolve the problem in most cases, but there are inevitable difficulties in the presence of diverticula, pericolic inflammation, and fibrosis, difficulties which often cannot be resolved until the mass is safely in the hands of the pathologist. Polypoid adenomata should be regarded as malignant until biopsy proves them otherwise, and the large ones should be resected with a wide margin. An amoebic granuloma should be suspected if a rectal mass is less than hard, and there is a history of dysentery or residence in the tropics, in which case fresh swabs should be examined and a biopsy taken.

Segmental Crohn's disease or ulcerative colitis may closely resemble a carcinomatous lesion in the mid-colon, and such doubtful lesions should always be explored.

Carcinoma of the caecum may cause pericaecal inflammation or an abscess identical clinically with that caused by retrocaecal appendicitis or diverticulitis. Anaemia and the constant presence of occult blood in the faeces suggest carcinoma, and drainage of such an abscess not only fails to cure but causes a faecal fistula.

TREATMENT AND PROGNOSIS
(*Fig. 72*)

Few cancers are potentially more treatable than carcinoma coli, and none in the gastro-intestinal tract offers the surgeon better results. This optimistic outlook is often spoilt by great delay in diagnosis.

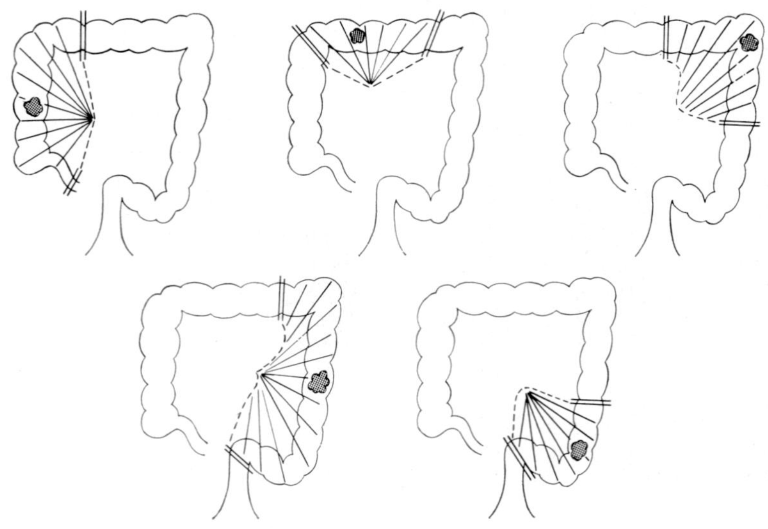

Fig. 72. Operations for carcinoma coli.

Operative mortality is 3 per cent and 5-year survival 30 per cent. About 75 per cent of right-sided and 60 per cent of left-sided growths are resectable when diagnosed.

The principles of treatment are:

1. Repletion of deficiencies, and the building up of general condition and respiratory efficiency prior to operation.

2. Reduction of bowel flora preoperatively by insoluble antibiotics given orally.

3. In uncomplicated cases, resection of the colon bearing the tumour together with the lymphatic drainage area followed by end-to-end anastomosis (*Fig. 72*).

4. In complicated cases, preliminary colostomy is necessary. The faecal stream must be directed away from growths which are secondarily infected, penetrating, or perforated, and grossly distended gut above the lesion must be allowed to shrink. A transverse colostomy is usually chosen, but if the lesion is right-sided, an ileostomy or ileotransverse anastomosis serves the purpose.

5. If secondaries are present the growth should, if possible, be by-passed or a permanent left-sided colostomy established. Permanent caecostomy or transverse colostomy are avoided.

6. If a solitary secondary deposit in the liver is present with a resectable colonic growth both should be excised.

FURTHER READING

Hirschsprung's Disease
BODIAN, M., CARTER, C. O., and WARD, B. C. H. (1951), 'Hirschsprung's Disease', *Lancet*, **1**, 302.
EDITORIAL (1963), *Ibid.*, **1**, 1196.

Irritable Colon
CHAUDHARY, N. A., and TRUELOVE, S. C. (1962), 'Irritable Colon Syndrome', *Q. Jl Med.*, **55**, 307.

Diverticular Disease
ALMY, T. P. (1965), 'Diverticular Disease of the Colon—the New Look', *Gastroenterology*, **49**, 109.
PARKS, T. G. (1968), 'Diverticular Disease', *Post-grad. med. J.*, **44**, 680.

Ischaemic Colitis
MARSTON, A., PHEILS, M. F., LEA THOMAS, M., and MORSON, B. C. (1966), 'Ischaemic Colitis', *Gut*, **7**, 1.

Colonic Carcinoma Antigens
KLEINMAN, M. S., HARWELL, L., and TURNER, M. D. (1971), 'Studies of Colonic Carcinoma Antigens', *Ibid.*, **12**, 1.

Chapter 21

Ulcerative Colitis

THIS DISEASE which used to be known as the 'bloody flux' is now generally called 'ulcerative colitis' (colitis ulcerosa). This name gives a misleading impression because essentially it is not an ulcerative process but rather an inflammatory reaction in the subepithelial zone of the colon. Because more than half the sufferers have only disease in the rectum and sigmoid, the alternative name of 'proctocolitis' is gaining wider acceptance. The essential unity of localized proctitis and generalized colitis is proven by the identity of the early pathological changes and the fact that about 10 per cent of those who start with proctitis only will later develop more extensive colitis.

AETIOLOGY

There is a slight excess of female sufferers, and although the disease may start at any time from infancy to the ninth decade, the maximum incidence is in the third and fourth decades. About 5 per cent of sufferers have a first-degree relative with the disease and several families have been described in which four or more members from three generations have been affected. When related to the known prevalence of ulcerative colitis in the populations studied, this familial incidence is highly significant and suggests a genetic framework within which the disease tends to occur. Such a conception is strengthened by the low incidence of the disease in New Zealand Maoris compared with their compatriots of European origin and the apparent rarity of the disease in the large populations of China, Japan, and south-east Asia. The disease appears to be particularly common in Britain, and also amongst North American Jewish communities. Furthermore, it has been found that ankylosing spondylitis occurs in over 5 per cent of patients with ulcerative colitis, and with significant frequency in their relatives. In the relatives of colitic patients there is also a significantly high prevalence of diseases such as Crohn's disease, eczema, and polyarthritis. All this suggests a hereditary predisposition to a constellation of diseases, the nature and cause of which are as yet undefined.

There are a number of clues which suggest that auto-immunity is the most probable cause of colitis. About 7 per cent of patients with chronic active (auto-immune) hepatitis may later develop ulcerative colitis. It has been shown that lymphocytes from colitic patients will in cell culture kill living colonic cells obtained from other humans. Pretreatment of the lymphocytes from colitic patients with horse serum containing an antithymus factor removes their cytotoxic effect. The serum from colitics has no effect on foetal colon-cell cultures. One hypothesis based on a small body of evidence is that antigens from certain strains of *Esch. coli* may stimulate the production of lymphocytes which are destructive to colonic cells. The demonstration by immunofluorescence of the presence of cell-specific antibodies in the serum of only about 10 per cent of colitics suggest that this phenomenon may be the result rather than the cause of the disease.

Similarly it is now thought that the presence of antibodies to milk proteins in the serum of some colitics may be a secondary feature due to ulceration of the colon which allows the reticulo-endothelial system to be exposed to the allergens. There are, however, occasional cases where this milk allergy becomes the dominant aspect of the clinical picture. In other cases milk intolerance may be due to alactasia caused by the non-specific damage to small-intestine absorptive mechanisms which is often found in severe colitis.

The psychological aspects of ulcerative colitis have excited much controversy and it seems that it is no more than a secondary part in provoking the overt disease. However, there is some evidence that the disease occurs more commonly in people of a particular personality-type, who tend to be conscientious, fastidious, studious, and introverted. Such people may form part of a large group unduly prone to be colitics in the same way that certain races are.

In the present state of our knowledge the most useful concept is that ulcerative colitis is a disease which in common with other diseases occurs in a genetically predisposed group, that the mechanism of cell damage is by lymphocyte-mediated (type IV) hypersensitivity, and that the disease may possibly be triggered off by physical or psychological stress.

PATHOLOGY

Biopsy of the rectal mucosa in early or quiescent ulcerative colitis has shown that infiltration of the lamina propria by round cells is often present without ulceration of the mucosal surface. The earliest change is degeneration of the subepithelial reticulum fibre layer, dilatation of capillaries, and oedema with cellular infiltration in the lamina propria. Exudate, finding its way to the surface through intercellular spaces, consists of eosinophils, polymorphs, and red cells. Such an exudate may be found on the mucosa before there is any ulceration, and the latter takes place as the epithelial cells are destroyed from below. In more active disease this infiltration of the submucosa becomes more intense, and numbers of plasma cells and neutrophil or eosinophil polymorphs can be seen as well as lymphocytes. Collections of polymorphs form and may discharge into the mucosal crypts, and these are known as crypt abscesses.

Ulceration is at first scattered and shallow, but at a later stage the mucosal surface is lost over wide areas, leading to a considerable loss of tissue, serum protein, and blood. Inflammation may spread to involve the muscle layers causing muscular paralysis, and to the serosa rendering perforation imminent. Islands of intact mucosa or granulation tissue may stand out in a sea of erosion, and these may later become epithelized to form pseudopolypi or mucosal bridges.

Whenever colitis becomes active the mast cells within the lamina propria become more numerous; they also lose their granules, which suggests that they are actively liberating the histamine, heparin, serotonin, and proteolytic enzymes which these cells are known to contain. The liberation of such substances could account for some of the observed pathology within the lamina propria.

In ulcerative colitis it is remarkable that destruction is followed by so little fibrosis. For this reason the large gut may, in the acute stage, become very thin and friable and, later, when healing has set in, stricture formation is rare. It is possible for severe ulcerative colitis to heal leaving no visible changes in the mucosa, but usually there is some simplification and flattening of the mucosa with a reduction in the number of crypts. Long-standing ulcerative colitis may lead to a progressive shortening of the whole colon.

In general, it may be said that it is the erosive and destructive aspects of ulcerative colitis, leading to thinning and friability of the colon, which distinguish it from the lymphoedematous, fibrotic, and thickening tendency of Crohn's disease (*Table 23*).

Ischiorectal abscesses and rectovaginal fistulae also are less common in ulcerative colitis than in Crohn's disease. Carcinoma develops in the colonic mucosa disorganized by ulcerative colitis. The risk is related mainly to the extent but also to the duration of the disease. In localized proctitis the risk is not enhanced, whereas in total colitis, whether acute or chronic in onset, the risk approximates 10 per cent after 10 years and may rise by 2 per cent annually thereafter. If the disease starts before the age of 25 this enhances the risk. It is thus mainly those cases which for other reasons such as chronicity and nutritional impairment should have a total colectomy who are most at risk from cancer.

CLINICAL PICTURE

Symptoms vary. In the mildest cases blood may be noticed in the stools though there is no constitutional upset. At the other extreme a violent illness like cholera causes continuous diarrhoea, vomiting, and prostration which may kill a patient within a week. Between these extremes there are many variations of a clinical picture which typically comprises: diarrhoea, abdominal cramp-like pains; tenesmus after defaecation; blood and pus in the stools; fever; tachycardia; loss of appetite; weakness; tenderness over the colon.

Of the really characteristic symptoms, nocturnal diarrhoea is one, and the painful passage of blood without faeces is another.

Investigations reveal: (1) Lowered haemoglobin levels. (2) A rapid E.S.R. (3) Visible or occult blood in the stools, with red blood-cells seen in wet specimens examined microscopically. (4) A characteristic appearance of the rectal mucosa when viewed through a sigmoidoscope or colonoscope. (5) In acute cases, a straight X-ray of the abdomen may show gas-filled loops of colon, particularly in the transverse and descending areas, and the outline of the colonic mucosa may show ulceration. (6) Altered mucosal pattern and outline by barium enema.

At a later stage, or in patients who are deteriorating quickly, the following may be found: (1) Lowered serum albumin. (2) Lowered serum potassium, or sodium with or without dehydration. (3) Gaseous distension of transverse colon seen on straight abdominal radiograph.

Table 23. PATHOLOGICAL FEATURES OF ULCERATIVE COLITIS AND CROHN'S DISEASE OF COLON

	ULCERATIVE COLITIS	CROHN'S DISEASE
Colon	Thin	Thick
Mucosa	Eroded surface; pseudopolypi	Cobblestone appearance; linear ulcers
Microscopic	Cellular infiltration; crypt abscesses; erosion of mucosa and submucosa	Giant cells; eosinophils; sarcoid-like lesions; lymphoedema
Complications	Perforation; haemorrhage; carcinoma	Fistulae; stricture; obstructed gut

Sigmoidoscopic Appearances in Ulcerative Colitis

Compare the normal—Salmon-pink shiny mucosa with submucous vessels readily visible through it.

First stage—Hyperaemia and oedema of the mucosa which render the submucosal vessels invisible and which blur the normal light reflection, thus giving a uniform matt or granular appearance.

Second stage—Increased hyperaemia and granularity. Blood oozes out from wherever the instrument touches the mucosa.

Third stage—Plum-coloured mucosa, bleeding spontaneously from multiple, often invisible ulcers.

Other possible appearances, usually late—Scarring, rigidity, pseudopolypi, and deep ragged isolated ulcers.

Colonoscopy can more accurately determine the extent of the disease than a barium study.

Radiology in Ulcerative Colitis

In fulminant cases of colitis an erect and supine X-ray of the abdomen may show the gas-filled colon and the character of its margin may give some indication as to the degree of mucosal damage.

Barium Enema. With no purgative or enema preparation a small quantity of barium can be run into the colon and evacuated by catheter. Air is then introduced so that air and barium-contrast pictures are obtained. This technique is suitable for acute cases, but where there is faecal retention proximal to an area of proctitis or left-sided colitis, prior purgation may be necessary. The purpose of the examination is to determine the extent and severity of colonic involvement. The findings may be:

1. Early and mild—Outline of barium-filled colon may show fine irregularities. Oedema of the mucosa gives a coarse pattern in the post-evacuation films, the folds retaining barium being widely separated and often running along the length of the colon. There is usually a lack of the muscular haustral pattern. In very mild cases the X-ray changes are so slight that they cannot be distinguished with certainty.

2. Early but acute and severe—Fine irregularities at margin of barium-filled colon. Perhaps evidence of barium seeping below undercut mucosa. Altered appearance of half-empty colon. Increase in space between rectum and sacrum.

3. Late chronic—Shortening and rigidity of colon. Total loss of haustral pattern. Pseudopolypi may displace barium and give a mottled appearance.

DIAGNOSTIC TESTS IN ULCERATIVE COLITIS

Visible or occult blood in stools (invariable).
Raised E.S.R. and low haemoglobin (not invariable).
Low serum albumin if disease extensive.
Abnormal rectal mucosa (95 per cent):
   Stage 1—Hyperaemia and oedema.
   Stage 2—Hyperaemia and stroke-bleeding.
   Stage 3—Ulceration and copious exudation of blood and pus.
   Stage 4—Pseudopolypi, mucosal bridges, thinning, and scarring.
Abnormal barium-enema pattern:
   Post-evacuation film shows coarse pattern.
   Irregularity of edge in barium-filled colon.
   Loss of haustral pattern.
   Barium runs beneath undercut mucosa.
   Pseudopolypi.
   Shortening and narrowing of colon.

COMPLICATIONS AND ACCOMPANIMENTS
(Fig. 73)

Skin lesions are common. Sometimes patients have suffered from eczema or psoriasis before they develop colitis, but sometimes the skin lesions may be an acute manifestation of the general disease. An example of the latter is acute erythema nodosum which sometimes ushers in a first attack or an acute exacerbation of colitis. Atypical nodose erythematous lesions occasionally occur around the ankles and calves and become chronic. A deeper nodose involvement, which sometimes ulcerates and which commonly involves the legs or perineum, is known as 'pyoderma gangrenosum'.

Iritis and episcleritis, and other forms of uveitis occur in about 4 per cent of colitics.

Polyarthritis causing intermittent episodes of synovial effusion in the large joints with little residual deformity occurs in about 10 per cent and the incidence is not intimately related to the severity or duration of the disease. Radiological evidence of sacro-iliitis can be found in 18 per cent and ankylosing spondylitis in 5 per cent.

Ileus and Toxic Megacolon

In acute fulminating cases the abdomen may distend, vomiting occurs, and the picture resembles that of mid-intestinal obstruction with gross toxicity and faint bowel-sounds.

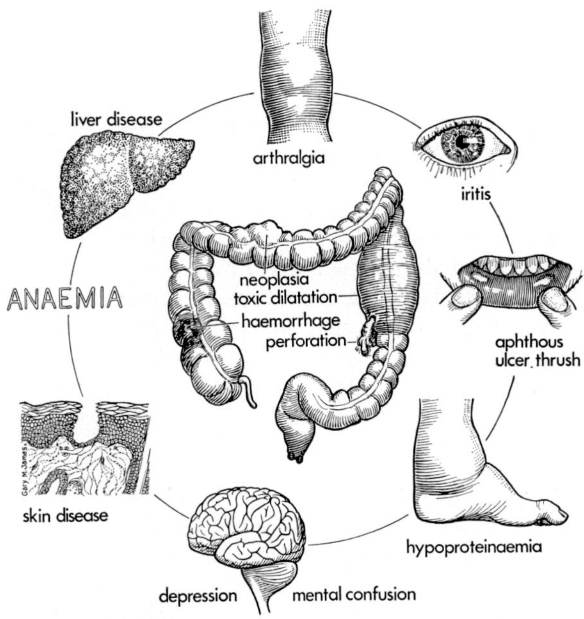

Fig. 73. Some complications of ulcerative colitis.

Perforation

Perforation may occur because the colon distends with gas and ruptures at the flexures. The clinical picture after perforation changes but little, and the only clue is often a sudden increase of pulse-rate and general deterioration. For this reason daily straight radiographs of the abdomen are necessary in acute ulcerative colitis with abdominal distension.

Bleeding

This may be slight and continuous, depleting the iron stores and calling for occasional transfusion; more rarely, it may be sudden and acute; though alarming, it is only very rarely that acute bleeding is serious enough to warrant emergency surgery.

Mental Confusion

This is often associated with extreme toxicity and electrolyte depletion, but may also occur as the most serious complication of corticosteroid therapy.

Mouth Ulcers: Oral and Anal Moniliasis

Ulceration in the mouth and around the anus is not always due to moniliasis, but the latter is more likely if broad-spectrum antibiotics and/or corticosteroids have been given.

Fistulae and Ischiorectal Abscesses

These may occur in acute or chronic forms of the disease.

Liver Disease

Portal bacteriaemia has been found in acute colitis, but its relation to the inflammatory pericholangitis sometimes found in colitics subjected to liver biopsy is uncertain; such patients may have very high levels of serum alkaline phosphatase, but they remain relatively well and their livers can recover. More serious forms of active chronic hepatitis with resulting cirrhosis may occur in about 2 per cent of colitics; the liver disease sometimes antedates the colitis and may continue after colectomy. There is an association between carcinoma of the bile-passages and colitis, and certainly sclerosing cholangitis, which is a rare disease, may occur in colitic patients.

Carcinoma (see p. 316).

DIFFERENTIAL DIAGNOSIS AND ASSESSMENT FOR TREATMENT

Diagnosis must be firmly based on sigmoidoscopic inspection, occult blood in the stools, lowered haemoglobin, and raised E.S.R., with a barium enema whenever possible. It is quite wrong to diagnose ulcerative colitis solely after hearing a history of diarrhoea and blood in the stools, or on the basis of a barium enema. One source of difficulty is the 'featureless' descending colon sometimes seen on barium-enema films. Such an appearance can arise from the continued use of purgatives, or for other reasons. Patients wrongly diagnosed as suffering from colitis may suffer unnecessary mental anguish. Ninety-five per cent of colitics have rectal involvement easily seen with the sigmoidoscope.

In cases where rectal pain and bleeding are the chief features, there is sometimes difficulty in distinguishing Crohn's disease of the rectum. In Crohn's disease, however, there is a more thickened rigid mucosa and more tendency to stricture and fistula formation around the anus which is often surrounded by granulomatous tags. A biopsy may be helpful, but a non-committal report does not exclude Crohn's disease, the typical histological lesion of which may not be represented in the biopsy.

Diverticular disease of the sigmoid or a spreading carcinoma in that region may cause doubt and difficulty even after sigmoidoscopy and radiological studies, but it is more common for ulcerative colitis to masquerade as one of the other two than the reverse.

Rare diseases of the rectum such as schistosomiasis, lymphogranuloma, and the more common amoebiasis sometimes give trouble to the experts who have to distinguish them.

If colitis is segmental and does not involve the rectum (5 per cent of cases) the differential diagnosis of Crohn's disease, carcinoma, and occasionally tuberculosis must be considered.

MANAGEMENT AND TREATMENT

In ulcerative colitis more than in any other condition it is the patient, rather than his disease, who must be treated. There are certain basic principles underlying the management of all cases, but the assessment and understanding of the individual patient determine the details of treatment (*Table 24*).

Table 24. PLAN OF TREATMENT OF ULCERATIVE COLITIS

TYPE	TREATMENT
All cases	Psychological support. Repletion of deficiencies
Proctitis with constipation	Cure constipation. Use stool softeners such as Isogel
Relapsing proctitis	Predsol retention enemata (20 mg. prednisolone-21-phosphate in disposal plastic pack) or Prednesol effervescent tablets (5 mg. prednisolone disodium phosphate) dissolved and injected into the rectum by the patient, Predsol suppositories (5 mg.), or sulphasalazine suppositories
Left-sided colitis	Hydrocortisone or Predsol drip or Predsol-retention enemata
Smouldering colitis	Sulphasalazine
Acute fulminant colitis	Oral corticosteroids plus hydrocortisone drip. Colectomy within 2 weeks if treatment fails or dangerous complications blow up
Long-standing colitis with disorganized mucosa and persistent symptoms or relapses	Advise surgery if symptoms are disabling or duration of disease is longer than 3 years

Basic Principles of Treatment

1. Understanding and sympathy.

2. Removal or amelioration of stress factors which may be physical or emotional.

3. The amelioration of symptoms such as diarrhoea, pain, nausea, vomiting, and sleeplessness.

4. Repletion of physical deficiencies caused by the disease, such as anaemia, protein deficiency, potassium deficiency, or dehydration.

5. 'Specific' treatments to help in bringing about a remission.

6. Control of secondary infection and its complications.

7. Surgical removal of diseased bowel.

All patients will probably need help under the first three headings.

1. The patient needs from his doctor a helpful and sympathetic attitude to his sufferings, and a conception of the disease which is hopeful and not alarming. To explain that 'it is just like a sort of eczema, but in the lining

of the bowel rather than on the skin' may be sufficient to allay masked fears of cancer, internal poisoning, and lifelong invalidism. The doctor's attitude should always be hopeful and buoyant. Gloomy thoughts on prognosis should be kept for the privacy of the side-room. Time should be set aside for getting to know the patient, who is often a shy person, and it is such a person who will not voice his fears until he knows his doctor well.

2. Physical stress factors which may be contributory are food allergies (i.e., to milk), or drug allergies, i.e., to tetracyclines. Other physical stresses such as pregnancy, general infections, and fatigue may be recognized, though they cannot be altered. Emotional stresses concerned with examinations, parental conflict, jealousy, love affairs, sexual failure must be ascertained by the doctor and recognized by the patient, for only then can conflicts be resolved, and the irritant stresses lessened.

3. Nocturnal diarrhoea can be eased by oral codeine phosphate 30–60 mg., Diphenoxylate 5–10 mg., or Mist. Kaolin et Morph. B.N.F. in double the normal dose; and vomiting by injections of a phenothiazine drug. Pethidine 100 mg., though helpful for pain, should be used sparingly with phenothiazines in severe cases. In milder cases a barbiturate at night is sufficient. Chlorpromazine is very useful in alleviating nausea and controlling the tendency to vomit.

4. In chronic or remittent cases iron deficiency indicated by a low mean corpuscular haemoglobin concentration should be treated by oral or parenteral iron. If oral iron seems to cause diarrhoea, then iron dextran complex (Imferon) may be given by deep intramuscular injection in doses of 5 ml. containing 100 mg. of iron, or Iron Sorbitol (Jectofer) may be given in doses of 2 ml. daily. A gramme of iron as Imferon may be given by intravenous infusion in 1 litre of 5 per cent dextrose over 6 hours.

BLOOD

Blood transfusion helps to restore blood-loss and to improve well-being when haemopoiesis is impaired by the acute illness. It will also help to restore protein losses from the bowel. Small repeated transfusions should be given if and when the haemoglobin falls below 11 g. per cent.

WATER AND POTASSIUM

In acute cases, dehydration and potassium deficiency may call for appropriate intravenous therapy, potassium replacement solutions, or glucose saline being used in quantities determined from a reading of the serum electrolyte pattern, the urine output, muscle power, and the height of the T-waves in the electrocardiograph.

5. SPECIFIC TREATMENTS

The following have been shown to have a beneficial effect in ulcerative colitis when subjected to a double-blind therapeutic trial.

Cortisone acetate, 200 mg. daily by mouth.

Corticotrophin gel, 80 units daily by injection.

Hydrocortisone hemisuccinate, 100 mg. dissolved in 120 ml. normal saline and administered by intrarectal drip in 1 hour.

Prednisolone phosphate, 20 mg. in 100 ml. administered by retention enemata.

Salicylazosulfapyridine (sulphasalazine), 3 g. daily by mouth.

It is probable that all corticosteroid drugs are as effective as cortisone acetate. Numerous other remedies which have had their moments of favour in the past 50 years have either never been subjected to therapeutic trial or have failed and passed into the limbo of forgotten treatments.

Specific treatment is sometimes not necessary in ulcerative colitis as the measures listed under headings 1–4, or Mother Nature herself in benign mood, may effect a remission. This occurs in about 15 per cent of acute attacks. With optimum corticosteroid therapy the remission rate may be 50 per cent. Opinions vary as to the best methods of treatment by cortico-steroids and sulphasalazine, but the working basis used by the present authors is given in *Table 24* and below.

a. Acute Disease confined to the Rectum. Prednisolone phosphate (Predsol) retention enema nightly from a prepared plastic bag (20 mg. in 100 ml.). The nozzle of the bag is lubricated, inserted 5 cm. into the rectum while the patient lies on the left side, and the solution is squeezed in. The bag is then discarded and the patient rolls on to his face and stays thus for half an hour, sleeping afterwards. Preparations of Betamethasone (Betnesol) are also available for intrarectal injection. Treatment should be continued for 2–8 weeks. This method is convenient for home care. Prednisolone disodium phosphate (Prednisol) 5 mg. tablets which are effervescent and soluble may be dissolved by the patient, drawn up into a bladder syringe, and injected by catheter into the rectum. Prednisolone suppositories 5 gm. (Predsol) are helpful for disease confined to the anal canal. Acetarsal suppositories are also sometimes used, while sulpha-salazine suppositories are currently under trial.

b. Acute Disease confined to Left Half of Colon. Treatment as above or hydrocortisone hemisuccinate intrarectally given by slow drip. This method is possibly more penetrative and convenient in hospital practice.

c. Stercoral Proctitis. Occasionally rock-like constipation is a factor in the causation of proctitis. In such cases it may only be necessary to clear the bowel by enemata and purgatives, and then to prescribe regular stool-softeners, such as isogel granules, 1 teaspoonful followed by a glass of cold water nightly.

d. Chronic Smouldering Colitis involving All or Most of the Bowel. Sulphasalazine 1 g. t.d.s. seems to be most effective in this type of disease, though it may also be used to supplement local or general corticosteroid therapy. One in ten patients cannot take this drug because of nausea, while the occasional patient may develop haemolytic anaemia. It is an effective drug but the mode of action is unknown. When symptoms have cleared and the disease seems to be inactive, the dose may be reduced and then discontinued, but some patients have to take the drug indefinitely to control their symptoms, or may have to use it intermittently to cure exacerbations.

e. Acute Fulminating Colitis. Great care is necessary in the management and a daily watch must be kept, not only on pulse, temperature, and stool count, but also on serum electrolytes, urine output, haemoglobin, the abdominal measurements, and the bowel-sounds. Daily straight radiographs of the abdomen may be necessary if abdominal distension is marked in order to distinguish toxic megacolon (indication for surgery) and perforation of the bowel, which may be quite silent and undramatic.

Full doses of prednisone 40–60 mg. a day are given by mouth, and hydrocortisone hemisuccinate given by intrarectal drip. Food may be withheld and nutrition given in the form of glucose drinks, intravenous blood, plasma, amino-acid solutions, and fat emulsions, with appropriate electrolyte control. Vitamin-B complex preparations and antibiotics may also be given intravenously through the drip. Hydrocortisone 100 mg. should be given into the drip if vomiting prevents the administration of oral prednisone. Oral steroids may be poorly absorbed if diarrhoea is severe, and for this reason many physicians prefer to give steroids parenterally for the first week, and some will give corticotrophin 80 units daily as the initial treatment. Nights are made easier if codeine phosphate 60 mg. is given at 22.00 hr. or, in the worst cases, 15 mg. of morphine by injection.

If the patient begins to improve after 48 hours, liquid and semi-solid food is given and the dose of steroid or corticotrophin scaled down very gradually. Milk should be given sparingly and not at all if there is any sign of a reaction to the ingestion of milk. Milk-derived protein foods are often well tolerated. Antibiotic cover may be necessary during the early acute stages and intramuscular injections of penicillin and streptomycin are often the most convenient method during the first week. Later, oral sulphonamides may be given. If after a week the pulse, temperature, number of stools, and general condition indicate a remission, surgery is unlikely to be needed. Corticosteroid therapy should not be continued for longer than 2 weeks unless definite improvement occurs. In this event, oral corticosteroids may be tailed off during the ensuing 2 months and sulphasalazine 3 g. daily added to the régime. Local steroid therapy may be continued until the disease appears to be inactive and the patient has resumed a normal life.

Serial measurements of serum albumin and of gamma-globulin are helpful. Falling serum-albumin levels indicate widespread loss of colonic mucosa, and a rising gamma-globulin level is a hopeful sign that a remission will set in. When improvement begins the serum albumin level may not rise for one or two weeks. If the patient's condition is worse or unchanged, or if the gamma-globulin and albumin levels are both falling, a surgeon should be consulted within a week of commencing full medical treatment. The relative risks of immediate proctocolectomy and of continued medical treatment should be evaluated jointly. In the best surgical hands, proctocolectomy during acute ulcerative colitis carries a mortality of around 10 per cent, but if operation is delayed until serum albumin levels are below 2 g. per 100 ml. or until perforation of the colon occurs or is imminent, then the mortality will be higher. Patients who have fulminant total colitis and who show an inadequate response within a week will probably need proctocolectomy, but a policy of brinkmanship can be justified if the physician and surgeon make a daily assessment and are satisfied that an improvement may be expected. The patient's willingness to have a permanent ileostomy is also a factor to be taken into account.

In children or young adults with total colonic improvement surgery may still be necessary even though medical treatment appears to be helping. Having regard to the physical and the psychological aspects of the case, surgical treatment must be correctly timed.

The patient in an acute attack should have his bed next to the lavatory or commode, and should be encouraged to get up as soon as he can. Very ill patients may be incontinent, and have to lie on absorbent pads which are changed frequently.

Colitis in Pregnancy. If an acute attack begins in pregnancy it may be severe, and will get worse in the puerperium. Early treatment is vital, and it should be continued until the patient is safely through the puerperium. In long-standing colitis, pregnancy does not make the disease worse, but the puerperium is a danger period.

6. RADICAL SURGERY IN ULCERATIVE COLITIS

Indications. First, a danger to life, as in acute fulminating disease complicated by toxic megacolon, colonic perforation, severe haemorrhage, or when there is no response to optimal medical treatment. Secondly, in more chronic disease: malnutrition, the discomfort and misery of chronic diarrhoea, strictures, fistulae, and the risk of carcinoma. Continuous whole-colon disease carries the highest risks.

Naturally, some doctors and some patients would opt for surgical treatment in less serious situations than others. More often the doctors may have to persuade the patient to the radical cure. Usually the patients are afterwards grateful for the deed.

Operative Procedures

a. The radical cure is one-stage total proctocolectomy with concurrent ileostomy.

b. Another procedure is subtotal colectomy and ileostomy as the first stage, and abdominoperineal resection of the rectum as a second stage 2–12 months later.

c. Colectomy with ileorectal anastomosis is only indicated in the 5 per cent of patients in whom the rectum is free from disease.

d. Ileostomy without colectomy may be chosen in severely ill patients unfit for the more radical operation, but the advantage of a shorter and safer operation is outweighed by the disadvantage of leaving a septic, protein-oozing colon in situ.

e. Double ileostomy, using the distal opening to irrigate the colon with hydrocortisone, may have a place in the management of the acutely ill, life-endangered patient, who is loath to part with his colon.

Ileostomy Care

a. The ileostomy is placed to the right of the midline, just above or below the level of the umbilicus. It is wise to select the exact site by discussion with the patient prior to operation. When completed by suture of skin and mucosa, the ileostomy should project for 2·5–3·5 cm. An adherent, plastic bag of the Chiron type is applied immediately. This is used for five to seven days, and may be renewed as required. For a few days, the ileal contents discharged into the bag are very fluid, and it is important to correct water and salt loss on the basis of replacement by equal volumes of normal saline. If skin irritation occurs, silicone barrier creams may help to prevent this.

b. When the ileal contents becomes more solid, a change is made to one of the permanent ileostomy appliances, usually one with an adherent flange and a replaceable bag.

c. No specific diet is necessary beyond the need for increased protein.

d. The ileostomy is no bar to normal life and activity, including marriage and pregnancy.

e. In general, the longer a patient has had an ileostomy, the better adapted he becomes to its care. Great help is afforded by the Ileostomy Association, formed by patients and doctors, all of whom do a great deal by personal contact and through their journal.

f. Although stenosis, retraction, or prolapse of the ileostomy may occur, such complications can be prevented by careful construction of the ileostomy at the outset. Intestinal obstruction, however, from adhesions between the terminal ileum and anterior abdominal wall, needs surgical intervention.

PALLIATIVE SURGICAL PROCEDURES

Ischiorectal abscesses are dealt with in an orthodox manner, but associated proctitis should be treated by predsol enemata, and antibiotic cover is often necessary.

Haemorrhoids should not be treated surgically unless the proctitis is first brought under control.

Rectovaginal fistulae rarely heal after surgical attempts at closure if proctitis is active. Rectal strictures can be dilated by bougies while the patient is under general anaesthesia, and kept open by a dilator used by the patient. Systemic corticosteroids may be used to diminish the tendency to inflammatory fibrous reaction while strictures are being dilated.

PROGNOSIS AND MORTALITY

(*Fig. 74*)

There is good evidence for suggesting that mortality is inversely proportional to the care, skill, and experience with which the colitic patient is treated. Probably in most hospitals twenty years ago the mortality of a group of patients ill enough to be admitted to hospital would have been 30 per cent over a 5-year period of observation. Today this figure might be 5–10 per cent. Most of the mortality is from the acute fulminating attacks; 15 per cent of such patients may die.

Surgical mortality in the best centres is as low as 5 per cent for the chronic cases and 10 per cent for the acute cases, but in many areas the mortality for surgery in the acute attack is about 30 per cent.

For those who respond to medical treatment, about 25 per cent return to a normal life, and apparently have normal colons and a normal blood-picture. They are liable to acute relapses which will respond better

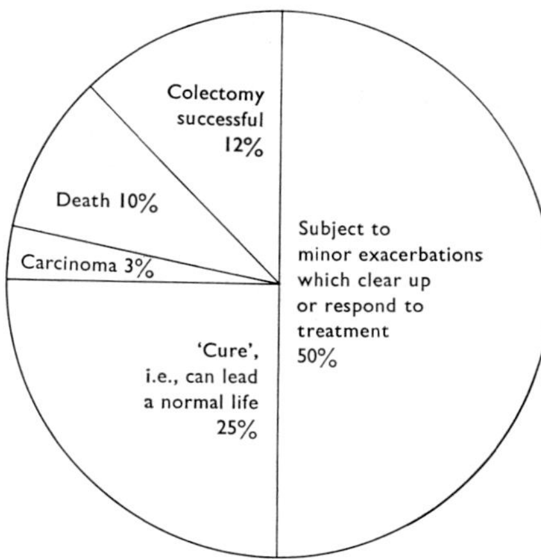

Fig. 74. The outlook in ulcerative colitis.

if treatment is started early. The risk of carcinoma is greatest in those with continuous disease (*see* p. 316) involving the whole colon. Patients with whole-colon disease which does not clear up for long periods also have the highest risk from all other causes of death. In left-sided or remittent disease the risk is much less—probably under 2 per cent in 15 years. About half of all colitics have some disease activity or, rather, frequent minor exacerbations which respond readily to treatment. The remainder do less well, and either prefer to put up with their discomforts or to undergo radical surgery.

FURTHER READING

General
GOLIGHER, J. C., DE DOMBAL, F. T., WATTS, J. M., and WATKINSON, G. (1968), *Ulcerative Colitis.* London: Baillière, Tindall, and Cassell.

Aetiology
SHORTER, R. G., SPENCER, R. J., HUIZENG, K. A., and HALLENBECK, G. A. (1968), 'Inhibition of *in vitro* Cytotoxicity of Lymphocytes from Ulcerative Colitis . . .', *Gastroenterology*, **54**, 227.

Pathology
DONNELLAN, W. C. (1966), 'Early Histological Changes in Ulcerative Colitis', *Ibid.*, **50**, 519.

The Systemic Complications
WATKINSON, G. (1968), 'The Systemic Complications of Ulcerative Colitis', *Post-grad. med. J.*, **44**, 693.

Medical Treatment
TRUELOVE, S. C. (1959), 'Medical Treatment of Ulcerative Colitis', *Post-grad. med. J.*, **35**, 62.

Surgical Treatment
GOLIGHER, J. C. (1961), 'Surgical Treatment of Ulcerative Colitis', *Br. med. J.*, **1**, 151.

Prognosis
EDWARDS, F. C., and TRUELOVE, S. C. (1963), 'The Course and Prognosis of Ulcerative Colitis', *Gut*, **4**, 299.
JALAN, K. N., PRESCOTT, R. J., SIRCUS, W., CARD, W. I., MCMANUS, J. P. A., FALCONER, C. W. A., SMALL, W. P., SMITH, A. N., and BRUCE, J. (1970), 'An Experience of Ulcerative Colitis', *Gastroenterology*, **59**, 589 and 598.
WATTS, J. M., DE DOMBAL, F. T., WATKINSON, G., and GOLIGHER, J. C. (1966), 'The Long-term Prognosis of Ulcerative Colitis', *Br. med. J.*, **1**, 1447.

Urgent Surgery in Ulcerative Colitis
LEADING ARTICLE (1970), *Ibid.*, **4**, 698.

Chapter 22

Anorectal Diseases

By L. R. Celestin

THE RECTUM and anus are the site of some of the commonest diseases known to man. Whilst many of the conditions are entirely local, it is important to remember that some are secondary to disease in other parts of the alimentary canal and elsewhere. From the clinical point of view, direct examination with the eye and the finger usually permits a precise diagnosis in anorectal disorders.

PRELIMINARY CONSIDERATIONS

The general topographical features of the area may be studied in textbooks of anatomy, but the basic facts are shown diagrammatically in *Fig. 75.* Certain items need particular emphasis.

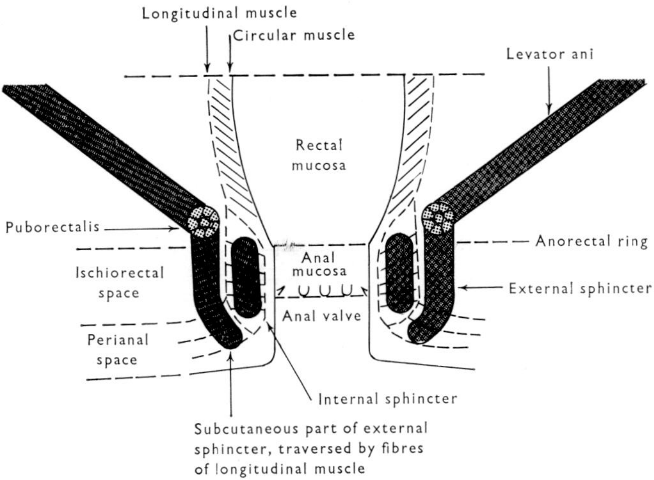

Fig. 75. Basic anatomy of rectum and anus.

1. Embryology of the Anal Canal

The upper part is formed from the cloaca and is endodermal in origin. The lower part, derived from the anal pit, is ectodermal. The junction of these demarcates areas of different blood-supply and lymphatic drainage.

2. The Rectosigmoid Junction

Anatomically, the rectum begins at the level of the third piece of the sacrum, but from the point of view of sigmoidoscopy, it lies approximately 15 cm. from the anal verge. The anorectal junction, of course, is at the level of the pelvic floor.

3. Peritoneal Reflection

The upper part of the rectum has a peritoneal covering on its anterior and lateral aspects. The reflection anteriorly forming the rectovesical or recto-uterine pouch is 8–10 cm. from the anal verge in the male and 6–8 cm. in the female.

4. Anal Sphincters

These are best regarded as two muscular cylinders, one within the other—the internal and external sphincters. The external sphincter descends to a lower level than the internal sphincter and curves inwards below it. During defaecation and under anaesthesia this lower end of the external sphincter retracts and makes the lower end of the internal sphincter more pronounced. The external sphincter, made of striate muscle, is supplied by the inferior haemorrhoidal nerves and the perineal branches of the sacral plexus. The involuntary internal sphincter, however, is innervated from the autonomic system.

5. The Anorectal Ring

This is a functional concept of fundamental importance. It is the junction of the upper borders of both anal sphincters and the puborectalis, and its preservation is essential for continence.

6. Sensation

Whereas colonic sensation is vague and is mediated through the sympathetic nerves, rectal sensation is more precise and is transmitted via the pelvic autonomic plexus (S.2,3). The rectum, especially in the ampulla, can appreciate fullness and can differentiate between faeces and flatus.

7. Anal Intermuscular Glands

Small ducts, arising in the crypts above the anal valves, run outwards through the internal sphincter to end in small tubular or multilocular glands. Their importance is twofold—as an avenue of infection from the anal canal, and as a site for adenocarcinoma.

The significance and the application of these facts will be discussed later in relation to various pathological processes and surgical procedures.

THE DIAGNOSIS OF ANORECTAL DISEASE

The main symptoms that occur are as follows:
1. Bleeding—during defaecation or apart from it.
2. Pain—especially in relation to defaecation.

3. Prolapse—spontaneous or with defaecation.
4. Swelling.
5. Discharge—mucoid or purulent.
6. Alteration of bowel habit.
7. Changes in character of the stools.
8. Pruritus.

In addition, there may be abdominal symptoms, e.g., colic, distension, borborygmi, and general features such as weight-loss and anaemia. Inquiry must be made of previous illnesses, especially tuberculosis and tropical diseases.

After the history has been taken and a general and abdominal examination done, a complete rectal examination is carried out. This involves direct examination of the anus and perianal area, digital examination of the anal canal and rectum, and the use of the proctoscope and sigmoidoscope. During these, a check is made for the presence of occult blood in the stools. A barium enema, or a barium meal with follow-through technique and a chest radiograph are done at this stage of the examination.

Biopsy of the lesion, examination of the faeces for parasites, cysts, ova, etc., and serological tests may be necessary to complete the investigation.

CONGENITAL ABNORMALITIES

The main congenital deformities are usually grouped together and referred to as 'imperforate anus'. Modern classification, however, recognizes two main groups (*Fig. 76*).

1. Low Abnormalities

'Ectopic anus', for example, due to failure of the primitive anus to migrate to its usual site, and 'covered anus', resulting from excessive fusion of the lateral genital folds.

2. High Abnormalities (rectal agenesis or cloacal abnormalities)

In these cases, the bowel ends above the pelvic floor and the anus is absent. The blind end of the bowel may have a fistula connecting it to the posterior vaginal fornix or the prostatic urethra.

Anorectal stenosis is intermediate between these groups. The importance of this classification is seen in the end-result of management. Patients with low abnormalities, although frequently stenotic, usually achieve normal continence. Those with high abnormalities may get some control by 6–7 years of age but are not really continent. In addition, this latter group may have other congenital abnormalities—sacral agenesis with neurological disorder, genito-urinary defects, and oesophageal atresia.

The surgical treatment involves a very specialized programme, and has been presented in an excellent review by Nixon (1961), to which the reader is referred.

Haemorrhoids

Haemorrhoids or 'piles' are very common, and become increasingly so with age. They are more common in men than in women. Essentially they are varicosities of the submucous internal haemorrhoidal veins situated in the upper half of the anal canal. Each haemorrhoid has an arterial branch from the superior haemorrhoidal artery, and the terminal branches

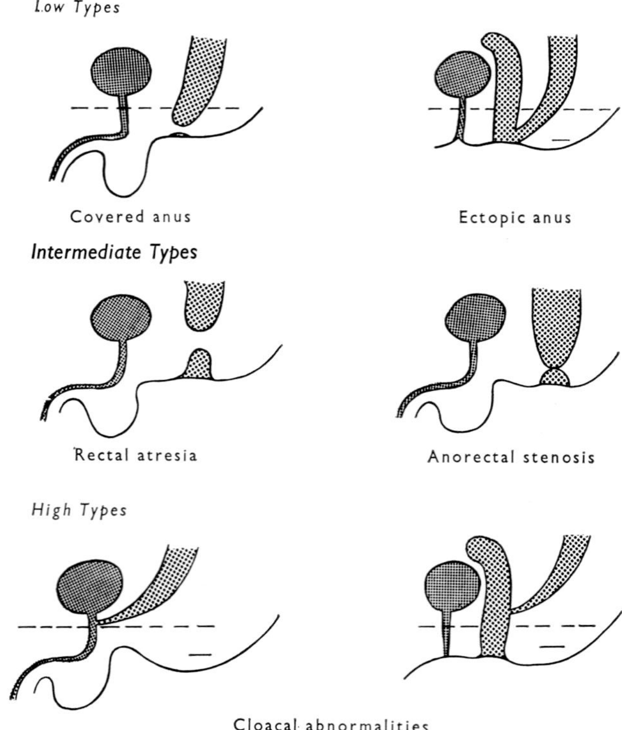

Fig. 76. Varieties of 'imperforate anus'.

of this vessel determine the disposition of the haemorrhoids in the anal canal, i.e., one on the left and two on the right. When viewed in the lithotomy position, they occupy positions corresponding to 3, 7, and 11 o'clock.

In its early stages, each haemorrhoid is a small bulge covered by mucosa, starting above the anal valves. As it progresses it becomes larger, and descends within the anal canal. Eventually it may appear at the anal verge as a bluish mass, the inner surface covered by mucosa, the outer side with skin. This fully developed state is the so-called 'intero-external' haemorrhoid.

The vast majority are 'idiopathic' in origin and dependent on a variety of factors, e.g., hereditary defect in the wall of the veins, the erect posture, and faulty bowel habits which involve straining. Some, however, are secondary to specific causes—portal obstruction, abdominal tumours, pregnancy, and prostatism. In women, it is probable that pregnancy is an important aetiological factor.

SYMPTOMS

The main clinical features are as follows:

1. Bleeding. This occurs at defaecation, but may continue for a time afterwards. Continuous blood-loss may produce anaemia.

2. Prolapse of the haemorrhoids may occur during defaecation or spontaneously in advanced cases. Sometimes reduction occurs spontaneously, but often the haemorrhoids have to be returned with the fingers.

3. Pain occurs with prolapse or with thrombosis.

4. Discharge of mucus is a feature associated with prolapse, and may cause pruritus ani.

It is customary to grade haemorrhoids in the following manner:

1. First degree—bleeding only on defaecation.

2. Second degree—prolapse on defaecation but with spontaneous reduction.

3. Third degree—prolapse but needing digital reduction.

The fully developed intero-external pile may be called fourth degree. Diagnosis depends on the history as well as the findings on direct examination. The most advanced forms may be visible. It is difficult to feel the early haemorrhoids, on digital examination of the anal canal, but they become increasingly easy to feel as they become larger. Proctoscopy reveals the haemorrhoids in full relief. It must be stressed that sigmoidoscopy should be routine in all these cases, especially after the age of 40 years, to exclude coexisting lesions, e.g., carcinoma and ulcerative colitis, both being contra-indications to local treatment of the haemorrhoids. Abdominal examination, of course, is mandatory in view of the important causes of secondary haemorrhoids. At this point, it may be mentioned that when haemorrhoids coexist with severe prostatism, the former should not be treated until prostatectomy has been carried out.

TREATMENT

Palliative

In all patients, a good bowel habit must be encouraged, with the aid of aperients. Senokot is perhaps most suitable for this. Considerable improvement often follows the establishment of the 'night bowel habit', i.e., emptying the bowels before retiring. The traditional local applications are valueless.

Injection Therapy

The standard method is the injection of 5 per cent phenol-in-oil into the submucosa above each haemorrhoid, at the level of the anorectal ring; 3–5 ml. may be used for each site. If the injection is too superficial the mucosa becomes white, and will undergo necrosis; if too deep—into the muscle layer—a red swelling is produced. Correct placing of the injection in the submucosa produces a yellowish bulge in which the vessels can be seen. The appearance resembles the retina, and is called the 'striate' or 'retinal sign'. Injection therapy is indicated particularly for first-degree haemorrhoids, but may be used in other patients who are bleeding but decline surgery, are unfit, or who have to wait a long time for surgery. When used for first-degree haemorrhoids the results of this treatment are excellent. Fibrosis is produced in the submucosa which obliterates the vessels. Occasionally the injections have to be repeated and sometimes complications follow, such as necrosis with ulceration, abscess, and stricture, but these are rare.

The presence of a fissure, or any other anal lesion needing surgery, is a contra-indication to the use of injections. They must also not be used in the presence of thrombosis. Many believe that pregnancy is also a contra-indication, but, in fact, there is a place for injection therapy to control severe bleeding until after parturition when the haemorrhoids resolve.

Surgical Treatment

This is indicated for second-degree or more advanced piles, the standard operation being that of 'ligature and excision' of the haemorrhoids. As already stated, the presence of a fissure with haemorrhoids is best treated surgically.

The régime after operation is usually of the following pattern:

1. On the second evening after operation, liquid paraffin or a mild aperient is given.

2. On the third day, if there is no bowel action, an olive-oil enema is given.

3. The daily drill then becomes—bowel action, bath, and a dressing. The local application for the dressing may be 1:5000 bradosol solution, or Milton, or 1 per cent streptomycin cream, completed with a large pad of cotton-wool and a T bandage.

4. From the seventh day, the daily insertion of a well-lubricated, gloved finger into the anus is worth while for a few days.

This form of postoperative routine applies to most anal procedures.

Thrombosis of Haemorrhoids

This special complication occurs in large second- or third-degree haemorrhoids. Large, very painful, purple masses appear at the anus, skin-covered on their outer surface, but covered by mucosa on the inner side. The patients are in acute distress. Although some resolve spontaneously with rest, sloughing and necrosis of the piles may occur. Portal pyaemia is an additional risk.

With reference to management, it must be stressed that, if resolution occurs, there may be a dramatic improvement in the previous state of the haemorrhoids. Bearing this in mind a conservative attitude is preferable to immediate surgery. Bed-rest, with the foot of the bed raised, is essential.

Local compresses with firm support, supplemented by the use of codeine
or opiates, give great relief. Chemotherapy is not usually necessary.
Resolution usually proceeds with this management, and after an interval
of approximately one month the case should be reviewed. Then, formal
haemorrhoidectomy can, if necessary, be performed with much greater
ease and with more speedy healing. If conservative measures fail, surgery
is indicated.

Acute External Piles

A painful swelling at the anal verge can develop quite quickly when
straining at stool during a bout of constipation. This swelling, which is
exquisitely tender, smooth, and blue, is usually a haematoma caused by
rupture of a vessel in the subcutaneous plexus. Only rarely is it due to
thrombosis.

The majority become painless and are absorbed, especially if treated
by bed-rest, local heat, and the use of mild aperients. If the swelling is
large and the pain persistent, operative treatment affords rapid relief.
The skin over the haematoma may be incised and the clot evacuated. It
is probably safe, however, to excise the lump, leaving a flat wound, for
although healing may take longer, the risk of abscess formation is reduced.

Chronic External Piles—Anal Skin Tags

Anal skin tags, which are common, are of two varieties:
   1. Painless—usually needing no treatment.
   2. Painful—usually associated with a fissure—the 'sentinel pile'.
This is treated at the same time as the fissure.

Anal Fissure

This is a linear ulcer in the lower half of the anal canal. It is a very painful
condition and may occur at any age. In the vast majority of patients the
fissure lies in the midline posteriorly, but occasionally in women the lesion
is on the anterior wall. Situated in the cutaneous part of the anal canal,
it extends from the anal valves to the anal verge over the lower part of
the internal sphincter. With the fissure there may be two associated
features:
   1. An oedematous, tender tag of skin at the lower end of the fissure—
the sentinel pile.
   2. A polyp at the upper end—probably an oedematous valve.

In its primary form, the fissure is probably due to trauma by hard
faeces. Many of these heal quickly, but some become chronic. Secondary
fissures may occur after anal surgery, or in association with proctocolitis,
tuberculosis, carcinoma of the anus, and frequently in Crohn's disease.

SYMPTOMS

The important symptom is pain, which occurs during defaecation and
persists for some time afterwards. Initially, when the fissure develops
during a bout of constipation there may be bleeding. Some discharge

may occur. Occasionally, it is the tender anal tag which is the most irritating feature.

On direct examination with the buttocks gently held apart, the lower end of the fissure is visible. A very characteristic sign is the intense spasm of the sphincter, which often makes full examination with the finger impossible in the acute stage. At some time, preferably when the initial acute phase has settled, sigmoidoscopy is necessary.

TREATMENT

When acute, a palliative régime may be adopted, with which some fissures heal in two to three weeks. The bowel action must be made easy with mild aperients, and an anaesthetic ointment (e.g., nupercainol) should be introduced into the anal canal before defaecation and afterwards. When the fissure is chronic, as indicated by induration, the presence of a large sentinel pile, and persisting spasm, surgical treatment is necessary. Excision of the fissure, with or without immediate skin cover, may be done, but the best treatment is sphincterotomy—i.e., division of the lower part of the internal sphincter with excision of the polyp and sentinel pile. Relief of pain is speedy and healing occurs in two to three weeks. In view of the simplicity of this procedure, injection of the perianal area with anaesthetic agents in oil is outdated. Histological examination of excised tissue is necessary to check the aetiological factors mentioned above. If untreated, a stricture caused by fibrosis in the sphincter may occur. After treatment by sphincterotomy, recurrences develop in 5 per cent of patients, and some 25 per cent may be troubled by soiling or staining of their undergarments.

Anorectal Abscess and Fistula-in-ano

These conditions are considered together, as the first is frequently a precursor of the second.

Anorectal Abscess

Although abscess formation around the anus and rectum is common, a portal of entry of infection is not evident in about 75 per cent of the cases. Abrasions in the anal mucosa may be present, but the probable route is by the anal intermuscular gland system. In the remaining 25 per cent of cases the source of infection may be known, e.g., following injections, via fissures, or after operations. Some are associated with Crohn's disease, tuberculosis, or ulcerative colitis.

The sites of abscess formation are shown in *Fig. 77*. Of these, two are common, the perianal and the ischiorectal, and two are rare, the submucous and pelvirectal.

The perianal abscess is usually obvious as a red, painful swelling close to the anal verge. The pain is aggravated by sitting and often by coughing or straining.

The ischiorectal abscess, being more deeply situated, is not so obvious. There may be only tenderness to one or other side of the anus, but later the area becomes brawny and the mass of the abscess can be felt laterally on rectal examination. It is important to appreciate that an ischiorectal abscess may be a downward extension of a pelvirectal abscess.

The pelvirectal abscess is very insidious; there is little in the way of localizing signs but considerable fever and constitutional upset. Occasionally there is evidence of previous pelvic infection or other predisposing disease. When developed, the abscess may be felt high up on rectal or vaginal examination.

Submucous abscesses cause a dull ache within the rectum and a palpable swelling in the upper anal canal. Most patients, however, are seen when the abscess discharges itself per anum.

The essential treatment is early and free drainage. Overlying skin must be removed to 'de-roof' the cavity, which must be explored to break down septa. The infecting organisms are usually staphylococci,

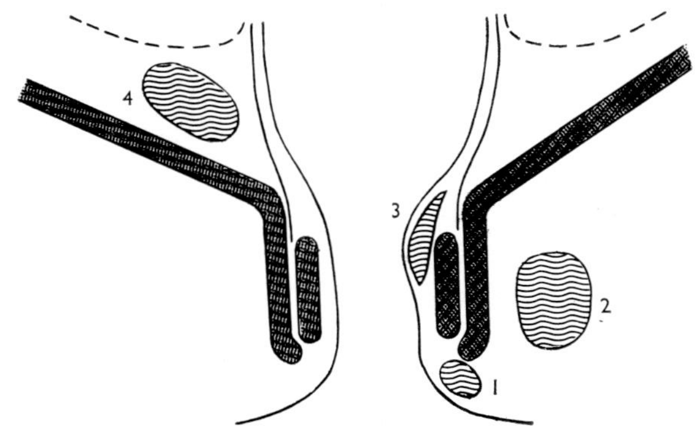

Fig. 77. Sites of anorectal abscess. 1, Perianal; 2, Ischiorectal; 3, Submucous; 4. Pelvirectal.

streptococci, or *Escherichia coli*, but it is important to check as a routine for the presence of tuberculosis. Occasionally, during exploration of the abscess an internal fistulous opening into the anal canal is found. Preliminary drainage is all that is required in the first instance, formal operation for the fistula being deferred for two weeks. Rarely, on exploration of ischiorectal abscesses, it will be found that the primary condition is a pelvirectal abscess. In these, free drainage of the supralevator part of the abscess may be obtained by enlarging the opening through the levator ani.

Fistula-in-ano

A fistula is a chronic granulomatous track between two epithelial surfaces. The track itself is fibrous. In the anal region even those tracks which are really sinuses, having only one opening and a blind end (50 per cent), are included in the grouping of 'fistula-in-ano'.

Some 85 per cent of fistulae follow abscesses which have been allowed to burst spontaneously or have been inadequately drained, or occur after anal fissures or operations. The remaining 15 per cent are of specific aetiology, i.e., tuberculosis, Crohn's disease, ulcerative colitis, and malignant disease. The association of fistula-in-ano and Crohn's disease deserves special mention. If Crohn's disease is localized to the small intestine some 25 per cent of patients develop anal fistulae, whereas if it involves the large bowel the incidence is nearer 75 per cent. The association of diarrhoea and fistula-in-ano should always make one suspect Crohn's disease. Indeed, it can be held that a recurring fistula-in-ano is due to Crohn's disease until proved otherwise.

Though there are many variations in their form, fistulae may be classified in the manner suggested by Milligan and Morgan:

1. Submucous and subcutaneous—5 per cent.

2. Anal—entering the anal canal below the anorectal ring: (*a*) Low—entering canal at or below level of anal valves—75 per cent; (*b*) High—entering above valves—15 per cent.

3. Anorectal or pelvirectal—5 per cent. The track reaches a level above the anorectal ring, but may or may not enter the rectum. The importance of these lies in the fact that some have 'horseshoe' extensions to the opposite side around the anal canal posteriorly. These variations are illustrated in *Fig. 78.*

Clinically, fistula-in-ano presents with recurring abscess formation and recurring discharge from the cutaneous opening. Inspection may reveal this opening, but in quiescent periods it is not always easy to find. The fibrous track may be felt subcutaneously and in the anal canal. The passage of a probe from the skin opening, with the finger in the rectum, enables one to define the type of fistula and to demarcate it with reference to the anorectal ring. Proctoscopy and sigmoidoscopy must be done to observe the state of the mucosa and exclude associated disease. For the same reason, a chest radiograph and a barium enema are done. Occasionally, lipiodol may be introduced to define the fistula, but it is doubtful if this is of any value at all.

Further aid in defining the type of fistula may be obtained from consideration of certain facts:

1. The nearer the external opening to the anal verge, the lower the internal opening will be in the anal canal. In the case of anorectal fistula, the external opening may be some 5 cm. from the anus.

2. Goodsall's rule (*Fig. 79*). Fistulae with external openings anterior to a transverse diameter through the anus run in a radial direction to enter the anal canal in its anterior segment. Fistulae with openings behind this line enter the anus in the midline posteriorly. This rule is generally true except for subcutaneous or low posterior fistulae, which may run radially to the anus.

3. The presence of bowel disturbance, abdominal pain, or weight-loss may indicate that the fistula is secondary to other causes.

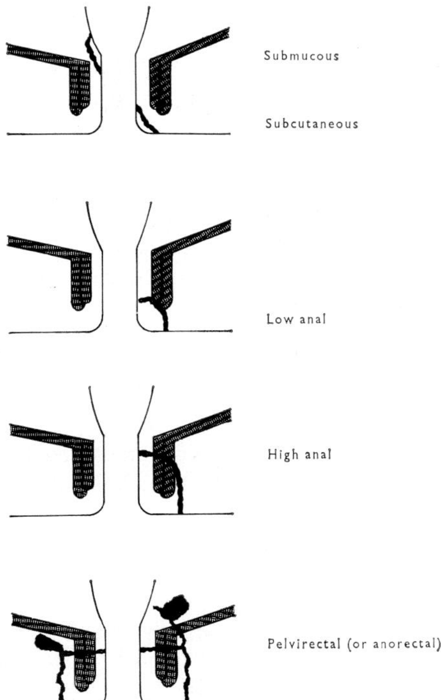

Fig. 78. Various types of fistula-in-ano. *Note:* Any of these may have only one opening and so be incomplete.

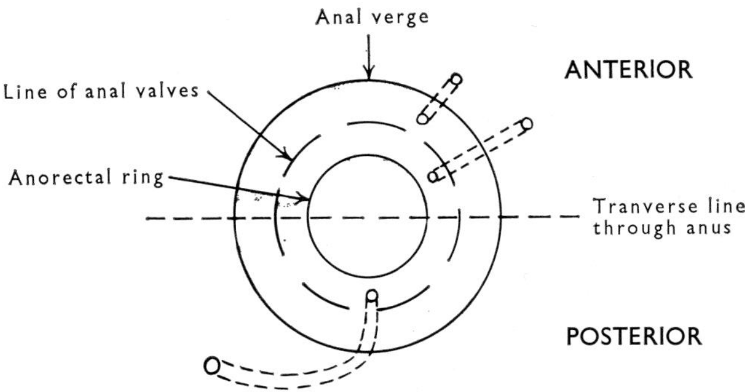

Fig. 79. Goodsall's rule for fistulae.

Urethral fistulae must be differentiated from anterior fistulae, and pilonidal sinus and a sinus from a postanal dermoid from posterior fistulae.

TREATMENT

Before dealing with this trying problem, two facts should be mentioned:

1. Spontaneous cure of fistula-in-ano is extremely rare.

2. Carcinoma may develop in a chronic fistula.

Surgical extirpation, therefore, is essential, a procedure requiring great patience and meticulous care. The traditional operation consists of defining the fistula with a probe, laying open the area, and excising the fibrous tube surrounding the track. Part of both the external and internal sphincters may be divided, but the preservation of the anorectal ring is mandatory. The wound is allowed to heal by granulation. Variations of the operation consist of immediate or delayed skin-graft to the wound, or primary suture. These are applicable to low or superficial fistulae, and necessitate preliminary sterilization of the faeces with antibiotics.

The concept that the fistula has its ancestry in a chronic recurring abscess, the site of which is in the intermuscular glands, demands that this source must also be removed. Strong support for this is afforded by the fact that some 60–70 per cent of fistulae have epithelial lining similar to that found in the anal intermuscular glands.

Rarely, in extremely difficult fistulae, after many operations, recourse may have to be made to a preliminary defunctioning colostomy in the left iliac fossa.

Following operations for fistula, inadequate control of faeces or of flatus may occur in about 10 per cent of patients, and 25 per cent may have soiling of underwear.

With reference to the specific fistula, a modified drill may be necessary. In the case of tuberculous fistulae, standard procedures are safe if the disease is quiescent. If not, simple drainage is followed by antituberculous chemotherapy. In the case of Crohn's disease, the diseased segment of bowel must be excised before the fistula will heal. No local treatment of the fistula is indicated when it is caused by ulcerative colitis, which must first be treated.

Rectal Prolapse

This condition occurs in the young and in the elderly. Generally, classification is as follows:
1. Incomplete or mucosal.
2. Complete when the entire thickness of the rectal wall is extruded.

Rectal Prolapse in Young Children

This is usually mucosal in type, and occurs during the first two years of life, and is rare after 5 years of age. It is more common in boys than in girls. The essential cause is probably a faulty bowel habit, i.e., the child being allowed to sit at stool for very long periods. The absence of the sacral curve in children may be a predisposing factor, but the condition may be aggravated by chronic cough, episodes of diarrhoea, and possibly, though very doubtfully, by wasting. The prolapse must be seen by the doctor, and prolapsing adenoma excluded.

Mucosal prolapse is a self-limiting condition in children, and almost 100 per cent success may be obtained by a conservative régime. This consists of correcting the bowel habits by such agents as syrup of figs or milk of magnesia. A daily enema may be necessary to start regular bowel actions. Prolonged sitting must be forbidden. Support by strapping across the buttocks is useful in babies.

In older children it is more difficult to obtain lasting relief and relapse may occur later in life. In addition to the simple measures discussed above, recourse to other methods of treatment may be necessary, e.g., (*a*) submucosal injections—similar to those described for haemorrhoids to produce fibrosis and fix the mucosa, (*b*) linear cauterization of the mucosa.

Rectal Prolapse in Adults

Mucosal prolapse may occur, but complete prolapse is more common. The mucosal type may be really severe third-degree haemorrhoids, but may occur after fistula operations if the anorectal ring has been divided, with atrophy of the sphincters in the very old, and occasionally in association with disease of the central nervous system. The complete variety occurs most commonly after 60 years of age in women, and may be associated with uterine prolapse. It is really a sliding hernia through the anterior wall of the rectum, the apex starting in depth of the pelvic pouch of peritoneum. It is associated with loss of normal tone of the muscles of the pelvic floor (*Fig. 80*).

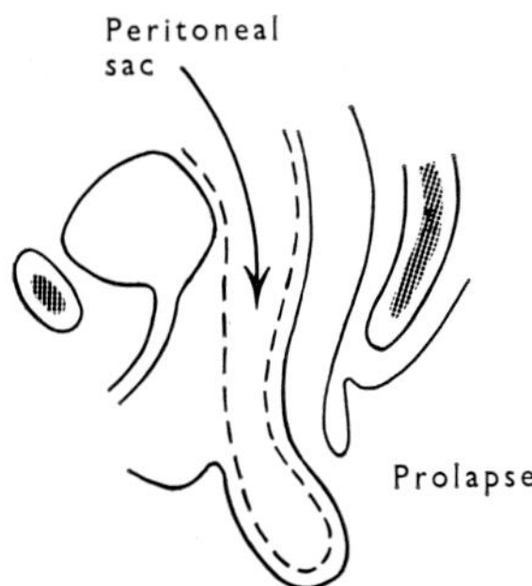

Fig. 80. 'Sliding hernia' in complete rectal prolapse.

Complete prolapse must be suspected if the length of the prolapsed tissue exceeds 5 cm. in length.

The patient may complain of actual prolapse on defaecation or coughing, but soiling from mucus discharge or incontinence may be much more distressing.

TREATMENT

When mucosal, the decision rests on the state of the sphincters. If the sphincters are normal, haemorrhoidectomy is usually sufficient. When they are lax the introduction of a ring of wire, subcutaneously around the anus, may control prolapse.

For the complete variety, some sixty operations have been described—an index of the unsatisfactory results of treatment, a high incidence of recurrence or of incontinence. The basic procedures are suspensory, repair of the pelvic floor, or excision of redundancy. The main operations done are as follows:

1. Amputation of the prolapse from below—rectosigmoidectomy (Miles); 60 per cent recur after this operation and 90 per cent of patients are incontinent.

2. Anterior resection of the rectum (Muir) The bowel adheres to the sacrum at the site of the anastomosis, and the results are good

3. Graham's operation and its modifications. This is probably the best as it aims at removal of the deep rectovesical or recto-uterine pouch, and restoration of the pelvic floor by suture of the puborectales in front of the rectum, after the latter has been drawn up to its correct position.

4. The rectum may be fixed to the front of the sacrum by the use of an Invalon implant, which surrounds some two-thirds or three-quarters of the rectal circumference. There appears to be a risk of sarcomatous change with this, and it should be reserved for the very old.

The abdominal procedures are preferable, but in the very feeble one may have to be satisfied with a simple introduction of wire around the anus.

Proctitis

Proctitis usually causes painful diarrhoea and the passage of blood, mucus, and pus. In its commonest and most important form it is part of ulcerative colitis, which has been described elsewhere (*see Chapter 21*). Another variety is due to prolonged constipation.

There are, however, many other rare forms of proctitis or granulomatous states occurring in the anorectal area. They are often identified by exclusion, and the most important aspect of diagnosis is to be aware of their possible existence. The following list indicates the wide potential range:

1. *Crohn's disease.*

2. *Tuberculous proctitis*—as local lesions, in people with chest tuberculosis.

3. *Actinomycosis.* This may occur in the rectum either as a primary lesion or secondary to a lesion elsewhere in the alimentary canal. The presentation is that of chronic abscesses and fistulae.

4. *Amoebiasis.* Chronic or latent amoebic infection may occur with ulceration and scarring of mucosa, but in addition a large granulomatous mass—the amoeboma—may occur in the rectum. *Entamoeba histolytica* will be found in scrapings or biopsy material more easily than in the stools. It is important to appreciate that even in Britain amoebiasis may occur in patients who have never been abroad.

5. *Schistosomiasis.* This occurs especially in subtropical areas. There is an initial acute phase, followed by a chronic state with pseudo-papillomata, strictures, and fistulae. The diagnosis is established by finding ova (*Schistosoma mansoni*) in the stools or biopsy material.

6. *Gonorrhoeal proctitis and anorectal syphilis.* The importance of the former lies in the fact that there is an apparent increasing incidence.

7. *Lymphogranuloma venereum.* This condition has a world-wide distribution, but is especially found in coloured races, and is due to a virus of the psittacosis group. After the initial acute proctitis, severe stricture formation occurs some 3–5 cm. from the anal verge. The strictures are long and tubular and may resemble a 'hole through a hard turnip' (Rendle Short). The diagnosis is confirmed by the Frei test or a complement-fixation test.

8. *Irradiation proctitis.* This may be seen after radiation for carcinoma of the cervix. There is an early phase of acute proctitis which occurs during treatment, the mucosa being very hyperaemic. Resolution usually occurs, but may be followed some six months later by ulceration, fibrosis, and stricture formation.

9. *Proctitis or ulceration* may occur after the use of some broad-spectrum antibiotics (aureomycin, terramycin), rectal injections, or due to self-inflicted injury. In addition, there is a very rare 'idiopathic ulceration' of the rectum of unknown aetiology.

RECTAL TUMOURS

A general classification is shown in *Table 25.*

Although many different varieties occur in the rectum, the most important one is the adenoma, which may be single or multiple, and the villous papilloma, which is usually single (*Fig. 81*). Their chief significance is their relationship to malignant disease.

Table 25. A CLASSIFICATION OF RECTAL POLYPS AND TUMOURS

A. Benign	1. Neoplasia	
	a. Epithelial	Adenoma
		Villous papilloma
	b. Connective tissue	Benign lymphoma
		Leiomyoma
		Lipoma
	2. Hamartoma	Peutz syndrome
		Haemangioma
	3. Inflammatory	Ulcerative colitis
	granulomata	Crohn's disease
B. Malignant	1. Epithelial	Carcinoid
		Carcinoma
	2. Connective tissue	Lymphosarcoma
		Leiomyosarcoma
	3. Secondary carcinoma from	
	stomach, prostate, cervix	

Notes: 1. All the connective-tissue tumours are rare, the benign ones usually being detected by chance.

    2. Cysts of epithelial origin may also occur—either dermoids or postoperative implantation cysts—again rare.

Rectal Adenoma

This is a smooth or slightly lobulated lesion and occasionally may be pedunculated. Its size is variable but may be as large as a cherry. The mucosa over it is the same colour as that in the rectum. In the majority of cases the adenoma is single; in about 30 per cent of cases there may be several, whilst in 5 per cent of patients they may be very numerous in both the rectum and colon. The term 'polyposis' is applied to this last group.

Histologically, an adenoma consists of closely packed gland tubules of intestinal mucosal type, with a central core of connective tissue and blood-vessels. The degree of differentiation within a particular adenoma

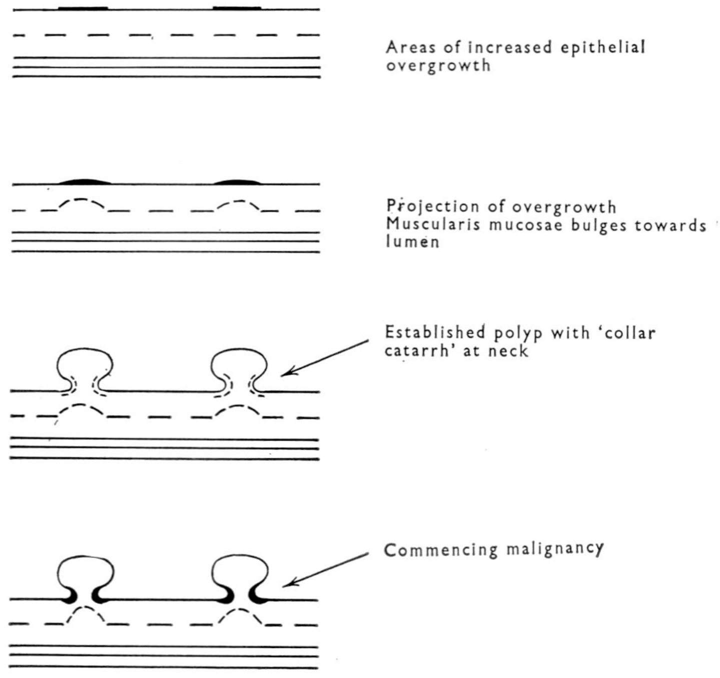

Fig. 81. A concept of polyposis (Dukes).

may vary. Some 15 per cent of carcinoma arise from them, and nearly 50 per cent of carcinomata have satellite adenomata. This association of adenoma and carcinoma, and the fact that the areas of maximal incidence of both are identical, support the contention that adenomata are pre-malignant, either of themselves or as an index of abnormal intestinal mucosa.

Clinically, they may cause bleeding and anaemia. In children a pedunculated adenoma may prolapse through the anus. High lesions may cause intussusception and colic. Diarrhoea and mucus discharge may also occur.

With reference to treatment, they may be removed locally per anum, or fulgurated with diathermy through a sigmoidoscope. For those higher than the level of the peritoneal reflection from the rectum, approach through the abdomen is preferable. The bowel may be opened and the lesions removed, or a segmental resection may be done. Detailed histological examination of each lesion is essential.

The problem of malignancy needs careful consideration, and the following points may help:

1. In children, the adenoma is always benign. The risk of malignancy increases with age.

2. Sinister features are induration at the base, increased vascularity, and ulceration.

3. The presence of a family history of polyps (this is discussed later).

4. Biopsy. Positive histological evidence of malignancy is valuable, but negative evidence is valueless unless the whole lesion is examined. If the lesion is genuinely innocent no further treatment is necessary. If the malignant change is focal and low grade, conservative surgery and a watchful attitude may be adopted. On the other hand, if the malignant change is diffuse, high grade, or invasive, radical surgery is essential.

The Villous Papilloma

This is soft, sessile, single, and has a ragged and ill-defined edge. It may be about 5 cm. in diameter, and is somewhat darker than the surrounding mucosa. It is usually seen in adults and is not nearly as common as the adenoma. The lesion is made up of numerous branches or villi, covered by a layer of columnar cells, with a central core of vascular and connective tissue. It is confined to the rectum and distal sigmoid. It may become malignant after a long time and, like adenomata, the malignant change may be focal.

Typically, the villous papilloma causes profuse mucous diarrhoea, so severe that it may lead to dehydration, hypokalaemia, and electrolyte depletion. Bleeding may occur later. These lesions are within easy reach of the sigmoidoscope. Barium enema is not necessary, as the lesions are usually single.

The management is determined by site. If within easy reach of the finger, and thought to be benign, removal per anum or destruction with diathermy is possible, but if very large or indurated, abdominoperineal resection is done. High lesions, out of reach of the finger, are best treated by anterior resection through the abdomen.

The Problem of Polyposis

Three varieties of polyposis may be recognized, all with a familial or genetic background:

1. Polyposis of rectum and colon—no other abnormality.

2. Polyposis of rectum and colon—with multiple epidermoid cysts, exostoses, fibromata, or other connective-tissue tumours.

3. Peutz syndrome. Although polyps occur in rectum and colon, they are much more numerous in the small intestine, and there is pigmentation of the skin, especially around the lips and buccal mucosa.

In the first two groups, malignant potential is great and prophylactic surgery is essential. The lesions in the Peutz syndrome are hamartomata, and the chance of malignancy is low.

The natural history of familial polyposis may be summarized thus:

a. It is transmitted in Mendelian fashion by a dominant gene. In an afflicted family 50 per cent of the offspring, both male and female, may develop polyposis. Only those who have it, however, can transmit it.

b. The colon and rectum are normal at birth.

c. The polypi develop from puberty onwards.

d. Symptoms, often recurrent diarrhoea, usually start at about 20 years of age.

e. Untreated, carcinoma develops at the age of 35 years, with death at 40 years.

These considerations form the basis of management:

i. A 'family tree' is drawn up to check on affected members.

ii. Routine examination of all members of affected families is started at 10 years of age, and repeated every two years. The majority who have inherited the gene will have polypi before the age of 20 years. If there are no polypi at this age, routine check every five years is continued until 40 years of age. If there are no polypi by this age, then the gene has not been inherited.

iii. No case of carcinoma in polyposis has been recorded before 20 years of age. Therefore, the best time for prophylactic surgery is between leaving school and taking up work.

1. Total colectomy plus excision of rectum with permanent ileostomy.

2. Total colectomy with preservation of the rectum, with ileorectal anastomosis.

This second procedure must be followed by a routine check of the rectum every three months to deal with polyps by diathermy.

MALIGNANT TUMOURS

Carcinoma of Rectum

Some 50 per cent of large bowel cancers occur in the rectum and recto-sigmoid junction. Of the carcinomata in the rectum proper, about half occur above the level of the peritoneal reflection and half below. Carcinoma of the rectum is more common in men than in women (3:2); 50 per cent occur after the age of 60 years, but may occur earlier in women than in men. In particular, it occurs earlier if it follows ulcerative colitis or polyposis.

The tumour starts as a local nodule in the mucosa or in a pre-existing adenoma or papilloma. As it progresses, it may take one of several forms: (1) Polypoid—without much infiltration of the rectal wall. (2) Ulcerative—infiltrating the wall. (3) Annular. (4) Diffusely infiltrating. (5) Colloid carcinoma—highly malignant.

The ulcerative and annular types are commonest, but the polypoid variety may be seen in the ampulla. Multiple tumours occur in 3 per cent of patients, and some 30 per cent have associated adenomata in the rectum. In general, the polypoid type is made up of more differentiated cells than is the ulcerative variety, but all the tumours are graded by the pathologist on the basis of the type of cells in the tumour, i.e., low-grade, average, or high-grade malignancy.

Once initiated, the spread of the carcinoma may occur in several directions, the more anaplastic the tumour the greater the spread.

1. Direct spread in the rectal wall. The whole circumference may be involved in about two years from the onset.

2. Lymphatic spread (*Fig. 82*). This is important and is seen in 50 per cent of cases at operation. It occurs particularly in an upward direction along the superior haemorrhoidal vessels to the glands around the inferior mesenteric vessels, and so to the para-aortic glands. Lateral spread may occur to the side wall of the pelvis and the glands on the internal iliac vessels. This lateral spread is probably more important in tumours lying below the peritoneal reflection than in those above it. Downward spread is not common.

3. Blood-stream metastases. Secondary deposits in the liver from portal venous spread are seen in about 10 per cent of patients at operation. Occasionally, the lungs and bones may be involved.

4. Invasion of the peritoneal cavity may occur.

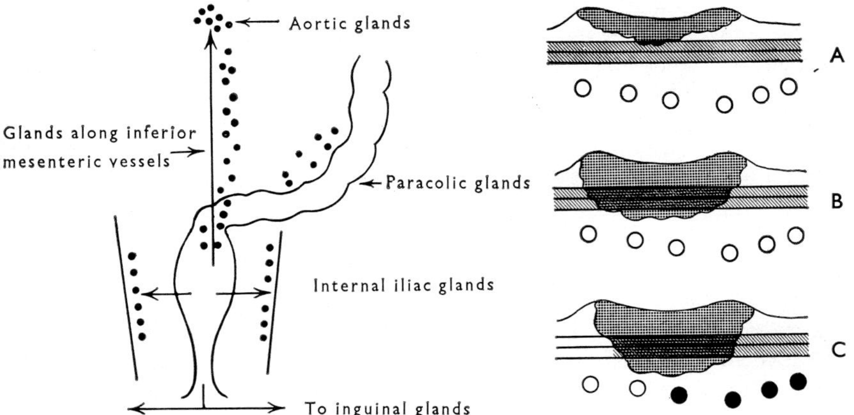

Fig. 82. Lymphatic drainage from rectum and anus.

Fig. 83. Dukes's stages (A, B, and C) in carcinoma of the rectum.

5. Mucosal implantation.

In addition to histological grading mentioned already, the gross spread may be classified into various stages (Dukes):

A. 15 per cent. The tumour is confined to the rectal wall.

B. 35 per cent. Spread to extrarectal tissues but no lymphatic metastases.

C. 50 per cent. Lymphatic metastases present.

These stages are illustrated in *Fig. 83*. Stage C tumours may be further subdivided into C.1 and C.2; in the former the highest glands in the excised tissue are free from tumour, whilst in the latter they are involved.

SYMPTOMS

Although many patients may be free from symptoms for a period, rectal bleeding and altered bowel habit are the cardinal features. Cancer of the rectum must be the first possibility if a change of bowel habit occurs after the age of 40 years. There may be increasing constipation or diarrhoea, or these may alternate. Spurious diarrhoea—the passage of mucus, blood, and flatus without much faeces, is common. These frequent, ineffectual calls to stool occur with greatest frequency during the morning. Occasionally there may be abdominal distension, colic, weight-loss, and anaemia. Pain tends to be late and may be sacral in site. Some cases present with obstruction and perforation of the gut causing peritonitis.

The diagnosis is made from the history, rectal examination, and endo-scopy. Some 75 per cent of rectal cancers are within the reach of the finger, and the size, site, and mobility of the tumour must be noted. The raised edge and induration are typical features, and biopsy should always be done. Barium enema does not help.

TREATMENT

This is essentially surgical, and is possible in some 90 per cent of patients after preliminary cleansing of the bowel by sulphathalidine and strepto-mycin, or neomycin. Blood transfusion is valuable and usually necessary. The standard operation is the abdominoperineal resection, performed either by one surgeon or by two, one working in the perineum and the other in the abdomen. The extent of the resection is shown in *Fig. 84*, which illustrates the principle of mono-block removal of the tumour and its lymphatic drainage area. The upper limit of resection is determined by ligation of the inferior mesenteric vessels either at the level of the bifurcation of the aorta or at the higher level near its origin opposite the lower border of the duodenum. Although high ligation is not universally accepted, its effect is to reduce the number of cases which would be classi-fied as Stage C.2 by about 10 per cent.

The operation is done in about 75 per cent of patients coming to surgery, and of course leaves them with a permanent colostomy. In approximately 25 per cent of patients it is possible, by preserving the lower rectum and anal sphincteric mechanism, to do a direct anastomosis after resection as shown in *Fig. 84*. It will be seen that in this 'anterior resection of the rectum' the dissection of the upward spread of the tumour is identical with that of the abdominoperineal operation.

The justification for this alternative lies in the fact that downward spread of rectal carcinoma is not common unless the tumour is anaplastic, and apart from these, only about 2 per cent show a downward spread of more than 2 cm. The operation is done for high tumours of the recto-sigmoid or intra-peritoneal part of the rectum which are more than 10 cm. from the anal verge. It is contra-indicated in low tumours, in the young, and when the tumour is anaplastic. If the tumour is within easy reach of the finger, it is too low for anterior resection. Section of the rectum at operation is done 5 cm. (2 in.) below the tumour.

RESULTS

The operative mortality is about 5 per cent; survival-rate based on staging is approximately as follows: Stage A, 80 per cent; Stage B, 60 per cent; Stage C, 30 per cent.

Comparison of results of the two operations described is difficult because, as will be appreciated, anterior resection is done primarily for the more favourable type of tumour. However, if correction is made for

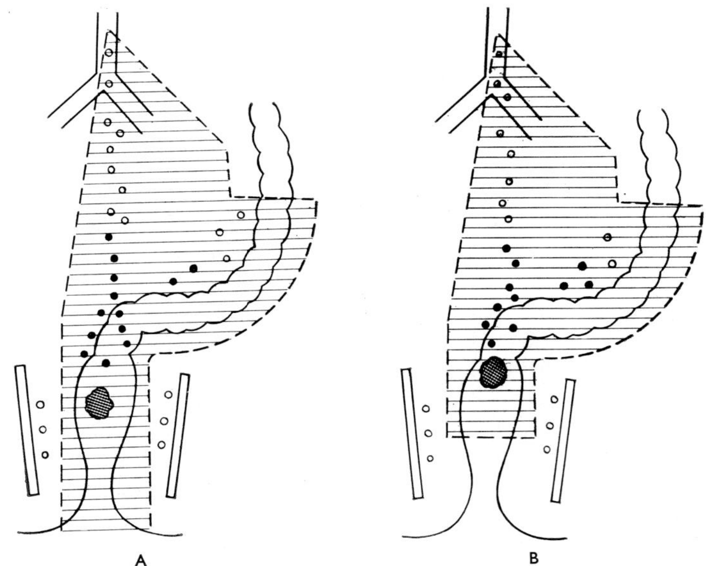

Fig. 84. Amount resected in two operations for carcinoma of the rectum.
A, Abdominoperineal resection; B, Anterior resection.

this, a 5-year survival-rate of 78 per cent for the abdominoperineal resection and 76 per cent for anterior resection has been obtained. Recurrences in the perineum occur in about 10 per cent of patients.

Apart from these results related to the nature of the disease, there are some special sequelae of rectal excision worthy of mention:

1. Intestinal obstruction may occur, through the pelvic floor peritoneum early after the operation, or in the left paracolic gutter between the colostomy and the parietes. The gutter should be obliterated by suture at operation.

2. Perineal hernia. This is not common, but may occur in women if hysterectomy is done in addition to rectal excision.

3. Bladder dysfunction. Decompression of the bladder is a routine for five postoperative days, but even after that residual urine after micturition must be checked. Injury to the nerve-supply to the bladder and backward

tilting of the organ may interfere with emptying. In men, prostatic obstruction may be brought into relief, and either prostatectomy or transurethral resection may be necessary.

4. Impotence. This occurs in about 30 per cent of men, but recovery can be expected up to three years after operation.

NOTE ON COLOSTOMY MANAGEMENT

It is very important to start on this problem before operation. The reasons for the colostomy must be explained to the patient, and he or she must be reassured that a colostomy is not a bar to a full and active life. Great help can be given by introducing to the patient someone who has already had a colostomy for some time.

At the end of the operation the construction of the colostomy is completed by suture of the colonic mucosa to skin. Thereafter, a plastic adherent bag of the Chiron type is applied over the colostomy opening. This kind of appliance may be used for ten to fourteen days, changing it as often as required. At the end of two weeks it is customary to change to the standard colostomy belt.

From the point of view of function, it must be remembered that in a colostomy there is neither adequate sensation nor a sphincter mechanism. Nevertheless, good regular control can be achieved. The aim is to make the colostomy act at a regular and convenient time each day. In a large number of patients this occurs with surprising ease, but if necessary, help can be obtained by the use of diet, drugs, or colon wash-out.

In the early days after operation flatus is passed first and then faeces, which may be soft and frequent. A constipating diet, free from fresh greens and fruit and based on porridge, meat, bread, and potatoes, is valuable. Following this, the diet is increased by adding further items singly. In this way, any food liable to disturb the colostomy actions is eliminated. Methyl cellulose can be added if the faeces continue to be too frequent. If a regular action is still not obtained, a wash-out may be given at the same time each day to train the colostomy.

The majority of patients aim to have the colostomy action in the morning, on rising or after breakfast, but it may be more convenient after the evening meal. After the action the opening and surrounding skin are washed and then thoroughly dried. A pad of cellulose wadding is then applied and the colostomy belt put on. In the early weeks after operation, the skin around the colostomy may benefit from a little zinc oxide or other protective cream.

Sarcoma of Rectum

This is rare, but may be a cause of large tumours in the young. The commonest type is lymphosarcoma, and is usually single, unlike its counterpart in the small intestine where it is multiple. In addition, the rectum is the commonest site for sarcoma occurring in the large intestine. Although it responds to radiotherapy, this rectal tumour is best treated by abdominoperineal resection.

MALIGNANT TUMOURS OF ANUS AND ANAL CANAL

Four varieties of tumour may be recognized in this area:
1. Adenocarcinoma of the rectum spreading downwards.
2. Squamous-cell carcinoma of anus and anal canal.
3. Basal-cell carcinoma.
4. Malignant melanoma.

When a growth projects at the anus there is a fifty-fifty chance that it is of rectal origin. If treated by abdominoperineal resection it is important to note that the inguinal glands may need extirpation also.

With reference to the squamous-cell carcinomata, it is important to distinguish between carcinoma of the anus and carcinoma of the anal canal, the former being much more common in men, whilst the latter are commoner in women. In addition, carcinoma of the anal canal is the more serious disease. On the basis of histological grading two-thirds of the carcinomata of the anus have a well-differentiated cellular structure, the remainder being anaplastic. The reverse is true for anal canal tumours, the majority showing an anaplastic structure.

Pruritus, leucoplakia, and simple papillomata of the anal skin very rarely undergo malignant change, but a chronic fistula may do so.

The lesion may present as an ulcer or as a papilliferous tumour. Direct inspection and rectal examination with a finger indicate the site of origin of the tumour and biopsy confirms the diagnosis. Inguinal glands, especially the medial group, may be enlarged, either by inflammatory or malignant change. The latter is present in approximately 25 per cent of cases. Occasionally further lymphatic extension involves the external iliac glands.

In treatment, surgery has largely replaced radiotherapy in view of the risk of radiation proctitis. For carcinoma of the anus, since the majority are slow-growing, local diathermy excision is the treatment of choice. For very large lesions and those showing an anaplastic structure, abdominoperineal resection may be necessary. Carcinoma of the anal canal is treated by abdominoperineal resection too, although simple perineal excision with left iliac colostomy is occasionally done for frail subjects.

When the inguinal glands are involved an interval of a month is allowed for inflammatory reaction to subside and then a gland clearance is made. If the inguinal glands are not involved careful regular supervision must be enforced to be certain they remain free. In general, gland involvement signifies that lasting cure is not possible.

For inoperable cases, especially if anaplastic, radiotherapy may be of use. Otherwise, sacral epidural injections of oily Percaine may help to relieve pain.

RESULTS

Overall 5-year survival, 40–45 per cent. For carcinoma of anus, 50–60 per cent. For carcinoma of canal, 35–40 per cent.

Basal-cell Carcinoma and Malignant Melanoma

These are both rare. The former is recognized by its rolled edge and is treated by simple excision. The melanoma may present as a small polyp or an ulcer. In view of its very malignant nature treatment consists of abdominoperineal resection with high ligation of the inferior mesenteric vessels, together with inguinal gland clearance.

At this point it may be pointed out that there is no relationship between malignant melanoma and the condition known as melanosis coli. This state is found in patients taking purges such as aloes and cascara over a period of many years. The mucosa may have a pavement-like appearance and the pigment is contained in monocytic cells in the submucosa. The condition has no real significance.

Anal Warts

This condition is seen in young men. There are numerous papillomatous lesions, either sessile or pedunculated. If the perineum is very moist they may be white in colour. It is probable that they are due to virus infection, but they must be differentiated from the condylomata of secondary syphilis which are usually larger. They may be treated by the local application of podophyllin (25 per cent in liquid paraffin), and any remnants remaining after this can be excised.

Stricture of the Rectum

It is opportune to recapitulate at this stage some of the causes of rectal stricture that have been described earlier in this chapter:

1. Congenital deformities.
2. Spasm associated with chronic fissure and subsequent fibrosis of the anal sphincter. Goligher has indicated that similar features may follow the habitual use of purges or liquid paraffin.
3. Following inflammatory conditions—ulcerative colitis, Crohn's disease, and, rarely, lymphogranuloma, schistosomiasis, and gonorrhoeal proctitis.
4. Following surgery—for imperforate anus, fissure, haemorrhoids, abdomino-anal resection, rectosigmoidectomy, and diathermy excision of large polyps. Excessive use of sclerosing injections for haemorrhoids carry this risk also.
5. Trauma—injury in warfare, by instrumentation, or foreign bodies.
6. Irradiation.
7. Malignant disease.

The common causes in this country are probably congenital lesions, ulcerative colitis, and carcinoma. In children, the cause is almost certainly congenital. If the stricture is in the anal canal a chronic fissure or carcinoma is a likely cause. If the patient has had a Whitehead's operation for haemorrhoids many years ago this may be the cause of stricture. In the rectum proper the possibilities include carcinoma, ulcerative colitis, irradiation damage, lymphogranuloma, or, rarely, infiltration by carcinoma of the prostate. Sigmoidoscopy will identify carcinoma and ulcerative colitis, but if these are excluded a Frei test should be done. The treatment of stricture is that of the particular cause, but when fully established may involve any of the following procedures: dilators, simple division, proctoplasty, excision, colostomy, or even abdominoperineal resection or resection with a sphincter-saving operation (abdomino-anal or abdomino-sacral).

Anal Incontinence

Normal continence is maintained by reflex tonic activity of the muscles of the pelvic floor and the sphincters. This involves a spinal reflex and the mechanism operates like a stretch reflex. Initially, increase of pressure within the rectum augments the tonic contraction of the muscles. Defaecation necessitates inhibition of the reflex, which can happen voluntarily. The importance of rectal sensation has already been pointed out, and in sphincter-preserving operations sufficient rectum must be conserved to retain this sensation. Incontinence may follow loss of such sensation, damage, or other abnormality of the sphincter mechanism, as well as the interruption of any part of the reflex mechanism of control.

It is customary to summarize the causes of incontinence in the following manner:

1. Congenital—this includes not only congenital abnormalities of the anorectal region but also cerebral and spinal defects, e.g., spina bifida and birth injury.

2. Injury to the sphincters by (*a*) accidental trauma, (*b*) perineal tears during delivery.

3. Postoperative—especially if the anorectal ring is divided in fistula operations or if sensation is lost after sphincter-preserving operations. It may follow irradiation.

4. Local disease—prolapse, large haemorrhoids, carcinoma of anus, impaction of faeces, and occasionally with proctitis.

5. Neurological disorders—tabes, spinal tumours, and injury.

6. Incontinence is seen most commonly in debilitated old people, usually with impaction of faeces.

The treatment is not easy. Prevention plays a major part, especially with reference to operations and the use of radiotherapy. Perineorrhaphy is done in the obstetrical group, but repair of sphincters by suture or by plastic procedures is not satisfactory. Particular care is required for the elderly, especially if confined to bed, to get the bowel emptied regularly by aperients and enemata, beginning if necessary with digital removal of hard faecal masses. If there is mucosal prolapse in these old folk, perianal wire introduction (Thiersch) helps to reduce discharge.

Pruritus Ani

Although this is not strictly a gastro-enterological condition, patients suffering from it are frequently referred to rectal clinics. It is a symptom rather than a disease entity and it is particularly trying, not only for the patient but also for anyone who has to find the cause and advise on treatment. Nevertheless, several groups of patients may be recognized:

1. *Those in whom no real cause can be found.* Unfortunately this seems to include the majority. Some are obese and perspire freely. Poor perineal hygiene and coarse underwear may be factors, but this is not certain. Others are exceptionally clean but suffer equally badly.

2. *Those in whom there is a local anorectal* (fissure, fistula, or piles) *or gynaecological lesion* with discharge. Such conditions may start the pruritus and the treatment must be directed to this local cause.

3. *Those in whom there is an infective or parasitic cause.* Several conditions may occur in this group—*Candida albicans* infection following antibiotic therapy, mycotic infection from the toes, and the presence of threadworms or pediculosis pubis. There are specific remedies in this group: (*a*) *C. albicans* infection: nystatin ointment locally and tablets of nystatin (500,000 units) orally. (*b*) Mycotic infection: Castellani's paint. (*c*) Threadworms: piperazine syrup or tablets orally.

4. *Those in whom the pruritus is due to a general disease*, e.g., diabetes, liver disease (even without jaundice), and the reticuloses.

5. Finally, it must be borne in mind that any generalized skin disorder with itching may start in or be confined to the perianal area, e.g., psoriasis, eczema, scabies, neurodermatitis.

The management consists primarily of a diligent search for a cause. If this is found, and it will be only in a minority of patients, then the specific treatment can be given. For the remainder, general palliative measures are applied. These include the following:

1. A daily complete evacuation of the bowel, assisted if necessary by mild aperients, e.g., senokot.

2. Attention to anal hygiene by washing the area night and morning, and especially after defaecation. Water in plenty is essential; excessive use of soap makes the area too dry.

3. Light, porous underwear should be worn.

4. Local applications. Simple talc or dusting powder may be used, but the best preparation is either St. Mark's lotion or 1 per cent hydrocortisone in a silicone barrier cream, applied as often as necessary.

5. Sedation at night with phenobarbitone, possibly with antihistamine in addition.

6. Occasionally, a sacral epidural injection of local anaesthetic helps, even for very long periods, long after the anaesthetic effect has worn off.

If the perianal skin shows no gross macroscopic change these measures may give some relief, even if only for short periods, but perseverance and change of items used are essential. On the other hand, if the skin is thick, excoriated, and fissured, with subcutaneous infection and fibrosis, relief will be minimal. In the past, other procedures have been used, e.g., injection of alcohol (40 per cent) under the perianal skin, and undercutting the perianal skin, but without any impressive benefit. Radiotherapy has also been used, but should be avoided.

Proctalgia Fugax

This is not uncommon, and consists of severe episodic rectal pain of short duration, probably occurring most frequently at night. No abnormality can be detected and it is not related to constipation. It is probably due to spasm of the striated muscles of the anus. It occurs usually in tense, apprehensive patients. Some relief in an attack may be given by a hot bath, the insertion of a lubricated digit into the rectum, or by the use of quinine bisulphate, but it is always doubtful if any of these will be effective.

FURTHER READING

GOLIGHER, J. C. (1961), *Surgery of Anus, Rectum and Colon*. London: Cassell.
NIXON, H. H. (1961), 'Imperforate Anus', in *British Surgical Practice: Surgical Progress* (ed. SIR ERNEST ROCKE CARLING and SIR JAMES PATERSON ROSS), p. 1. London: Butterworth.

Chapter 23

Diseases of the Peritoneum and Related Structures

Peritonitis

INFLAMMATION OF the peritoneum causes exudation of serum or pus. The inflammatory reaction may be localized to one area or generalized. If it is the result of organisms spread by the blood-stream from a focus outside, such as pneumococci from the lungs in pneumonia, the resulting peritonitis is known as primary, but usually it is secondary to inflammation or perforation of an abdominal viscus. Chemical peritonitis can be caused by instillation of chemicals and disinfectants into the peritoneal cavity, in which case the exudate is sterile. Leakage of blood or bile into the peritoneal cavity also produces a sterile peritonitis, but often the peritoneum is infected by direct soiling or by bacterial invasion from adjacent gut.

Peritonitis may result: (1) From penetrating abdominal wounds; (2) By spread of infection from abdominal organs, e.g., salpingitis, appendicitis; (3) From rupture of the alimentary tract, or leakage from it after operation; (4) By blood spread.

PATHOLOGY

Acute inflammation of the peritoneum, both parietal and visceral, leads to exudation and gluing together of bowel and omentum around the inflammatory focus. The omentum is able to seal off and limit the spread of the inflammation. The exudate, at first serous, may then become purulent due to bacterial invasion, and so abscesses may form in such parts of the peritoneal cavity as the subphrenic space or the pelvis.

Localized peritonitis causes dilatation and paralysis of neighbouring loops of small bowel. In diffuse peritonitis most of the small bowel is affected by this paralytic ileus.

CLINICAL FEATURES

Initial symptoms depend on the nature of the primary lesion, sudden after a perforation of the gut or peritoneal bleeding, but more insidious in the peritonitis which follows appendicitis.

If the disorder is generalized the patient complains of severe and diffuse abdominal pain accompanied by vomiting which becomes effortless and faecal in nature. Physical signs include pyrexia, abdominal rigidity, and retraction with tenderness on palpation and reduced or absent bowel-sounds.

Peripheral vascular failure leads to hypotension, tachycardia, sweating, and slight cyanosis. Dyspnoea may occur, and the tongue and sub-cutaneous tissues witness the presence of dehydration.

As ileus increases the patient's abdomen distends and becomes tym-panitic to percussion. The patient's general condition deteriorates and death from toxaemia and vasomotor failure may occur. In favourable cases localization of infection takes place, an abscess forms, and abdominal rigidity disappears.

Patients taking corticosteroids who perforate a viscus or develop peritonitis may show little evidence either of abdominal tenderness and rigidity or of systemic infection. Perforation of the gut is particularly liable to occur in those patients with severe ulcerative colitis who are given systemic corticosteroids, and it is most important for the clinician to remember that there are few signs and symptoms of this potentially fatal occurrence.

TREATMENT

A decision must be made as to whether operation is advisable. As a rule, this is necessary in order to identify and to treat the cause of the peritonitis, but poor-risk patients ill for more than forty-eight hours, or those with resolving and localized peritonitis, may be treated conservatively.

The principles of conservative, preoperative, and postoperative treat-ment are the same—rest in Fowler's position, a suitable antibiotic régime, drainage of the alimentary tract by an intragastric or intrajejunal tube, and intravenous repletion of fluid and electrolyte losses, so as to maintain the constancy of the internal environment and a daily urine output of 700 ml. or more. Dangerous hypotension may be countered by mephine intramuscularly at intervals, by infusions of noradrenaline by catheter into a larger vein, or by intravenous hydrocortisone, the choice depending on the circumstances.

SPECIAL TYPES OF PERITONITIS

Pneumococcal Peritonitis

This occasionally occurs by blood-stream infection in patients with pneumococcal pneumonia or in female children from an ascending genital tract infection. Pneumococcal peritonitis used to be more common in patients with a nephrotic syndrome and is still important in the alcoholic cirrhotic.

Patients with hepatic cirrhosis may develop an infection of ascitic fluid usually due to *Esch. coli.*

Biliary Peritonitis

The leakage of bile into the abdominal cavity following the surgical treatment of biliary disease, needle biopsy of the liver, and, more rarely, trauma, produces a severe and often fatal reaction. During operations on the obstructed biliary tree raised pressure in the biliary apparatus encourages extravasation of bile, and occasionally spontaneous rupture of a gangrenous gall-bladder is responsible.

The reason for the severe reaction to biliary soiling of the peritoneum is unknown. The constituents of bile may themselves be irritant; certainly there is gross extravasation of fluid into the peritoneum.

Severe abdominal pain and shock are of rapid onset. The signs are of peripheral circulatory failure, abdominal tenderness and guarding, which are soon followed by progressive abdominal distension and profound vomiting. The severity of the shock points to bile as the cause of the peritonitis. In patients with hepatocellular disease jaundice may be present, or may appear later owing to absorption of bile from the peritoneum, in which case it is always mild. The treatment is surgical. The biliary leak must be stopped, free bile aspirated, and the peritoneal cavity must be irrigated and drained. Treatment for shock, and antibiotics to combat secondary infection, should be given. The mortality is of the order of 50 per cent.

Tuberculous Peritonitis

This is an important disease which is often forgotten by the clinician because of its comparative rarity, and, as a result, diagnosis is often delayed.

AETIOLOGY

Tuberculous infection of the peritoneum may be part of a miliary dissemination of tubercle bacilli, or may be secondary to infection from caseous abdominal lymph-glands, infected bowel, or Fallopian tubes.

Because of the importance of the female genital tract as a source of infection, the disease is more common in females than in males. It is usually seen in patients of the third to fifth decades. Being common in alcoholics, it may complicate alcoholic cirrhosis. It is also common in certain coloured populations which are susceptible to all forms of tuberculous disease.

CLINICAL PICTURE

Where there is an adhesive type of reaction which binds together loops of bowel and omentum the symptomatology differs from that where there is a considerable outpouring of free fluid into the abdominal cavity. Colicky abdominal pain tends to be more common in the former and abdominal discomfort with distension in the latter, but in neither are these symptoms wholly characteristic. Loss of weight, pyrexia, and deterioration of general health are seen in both types. Tuberculous disease elsewhere may cause other symptoms, such as cough with sputum from pulmonary involvement, and in women there may be a history of pelvic pain, menstrual irregularities, and sterility.

On clinical examination loss of weight is usually obvious, and in patients with ascites the protuberant abdomen contrasts markedly with the wasting elsewhere. Signs of free fluid in the abdomen may be elicited, but are not usually so pronounced as in ascites from other causes such as cirrhosis or neoplasia. In the plastic form of the disease the diagnosis is more difficult, for abdominal rigidity, vague abdominal masses, and a 'doughy' abdomen are physical signs which are easily misinterpreted. Indeed, it is not unusual for the condition to be diagnosed only at laparotomy.

The differential diagnosis includes typhoid fever, intra-abdominal neoplasms, and reticuloses. The important association with alcoholic cirrhosis must not be forgotten, for in these cases the liver may be palpable and the ascites wrongly attributed to hepatic causes. Sustained fever is, however, diagnostic of tuberculosis.

The following investigations are helpful:

1. A family history of tuberculous disease.

2. A chest film may show evidence of tuberculous infection (30 per cent). either localized or miliary.

3. The Mantoux reaction may be positive or negative and therefore alone is not helpful, unless the nature of the reaction was previously known and had changed.

4. In the ascitic variety aspiration of some of the abdominal fluid with a 20-ml. syringe may be of value. The fluid is usually yellow and turbid, of high specific gravity (greater than 1015) and protein content (greater than 2·5 g. per cent). Isolation of tubercle bacilli is infrequent, and microscopical examination and guinea-pig inoculation, though of importance, are often negative. The ascitic white-cell count is usually 250 per c.mm. and may be as high as 10,000 per c.mm.

5. Blood examination may show a mild anaemia. The total white-cell count is usually normal.

6. Examination of the sputum may reveal tubercle bacilli.

Since it is so difficult to isolate the tubercle bacillus from the ascitic fluid, or to find in all cases conclusive evidence of tuberculous disease, diagnosis may be based on clinical suspicion and the effects of a therapeutic trial of antituberculous drugs. Laparotomy or peritoneoscopy to clinch the diagnosis should not be undertaken without antituberculous cover, because of the risk of dissemination of bacteria to brain, meninges, and other organs

TREATMENT AND OUTCOME

The patient is fully treated with antituberculous drugs. If the organism has been isolated, its sensitivity should be assessed and the appropriate combination of two antituberculous drugs given. If, as is the rule, no organism is found, streptomycin, PAS, and isoniazid are administered together. Chemotherapy is usually maintained for eighteen months.

A nutritious diet throughout, with early correction of deficiencies, is important, and the patient is usually kept in bed for the first two months of treatment.

Pseudomyxoma Peritonei

Rupture of a mucocele of the appendix or of a pseudomucinous cyst of the ovary may lead to a chronic mucinous infiltration of the peritoneum, obliteration of the peritoneal space, and thickening of the abdominal viscera. The syndrome is also seen as a complication of mucus-secreting carcinoma of the bowel. Presumably, extruded epithelial cells continue to produce mucus after reaching the peritoneal cavity. The symptoms are variable and depend on the cause, but usually there is increasing abdominal girth and occasional attacks of abdominal pain. If the history is of recurrent attacks of right iliac fossa pain, this symptom, taken in conjunction with the enlargement of the abdomen, should suggest the possibility of this disorder arising from an appendiceal mucocele. Pain can also result from intestinal obstruction, and hypoglycaemia may occur.

On examination, the abdomen is distended, there is often a fluid thrill, and sometimes shifting dullness. Abdominal masses may be palpable and rectal examination may reveal pelvic involvement. The abdomen can on occasion become enormous, but in contrast to the abdominal distension of ascites from liver disease or malignant neoplasms, there is little evidence of tissue wasting unless the condition is secondary to a mucus-secreting neoplasm. The diagnosis may be aided by attempted paracentesis. Though the material is often too sticky to be aspirated, careful examination of the contents of the needle may be helpful, and the inability to obtain clear fluid is in itself diagnostic of pseudomyxoma.

Laparotomy confirms the diagnosis, but the treatment is difficult. Where paracentesis is possible this may suffice to keep a patient comfortable. Otherwise, as much mucinous material as possible must be resected, and perhaps radioactive colloidal gold or cytotoxic drugs may be left in the peritoneum to reduce the spread of growth.

Periodic Disease (Familial Mediterranean Fever; Periodic Polyserositis)

This disease of unknown aetiology occurs particularly in patients of Mediterranean stock. Most are Jewish, but cases are recorded in Armenians, Arabs, Turks, Greeks, and Italians. The disease is often familial and is characterized by recurrent bouts of pyrexia, often beginning in young adult life and lasting for several months at a time. With the pyrexia there is intense abdominal pain and signs of peritoneal irritation such as direct and rebound tenderness. Chest pain of a pleuritic type and arthralgia of the large joints may also occur. Various types of skin disorder, such as urticaria and erythema, may develop and other features include psychosomatic aberrations, nausea, vomiting, and diarrhoea. Occasionally, hepatosplenomegaly and retinal spots or colloid material are found.

There is a tendency for some patients to develop amyloidosis which, if it affects the kidney, causes death from renal failure.

Many of these patients have had recurrent abdominal operations. The only effective treatment of this disorder seems to be intermittent courses of corticosteroids. Apart from those with amyloidosis the prognosis is good. The nature of the disease is unknown. If it is allergic, the allergen is unknown.

Retroperitoneal Tumours

Though primary retroperitoneal tumours are rare they are of importance because of the diagnostic difficulties they cause. The retroperitoneal space is bounded anteriorly by the posterior layer of the parietal peritoneum and the bare area of the liver and extends from the diaphragm to the pelvis. The posterior wall is framed by muscles and the space extends into the mesenteries. The contents of the retroperitoneal space include the aorta and vena cava, the duodenum, pancreas, kidneys, and ureters as well as the major branches of the aorta, the sympathetic chains, the lumbar nerves, and lymph-glands.

PATHOLOGY

Tumours may arise from a variety of retroperitoneal structures and may be either benign or malignant. The commonest malignant tumours are lymphosarcomata or lymphadenoma (Hodgkin's disease), fibrosarcomata, liposarcomata, and rhabdomyosarcomata. Malignant tumours of neural origin, including neuroblastoma and ganglioneuroma, are rarer.

Benign tumours include fibroma, lipoma, and a variety of cysts derived from primitive renal tissue (urogenital ridge) and from lymphatic tissue, from the gut (enterogenous cysts) as well as teratomata.

CLINICAL PICTURE

Retroperitoneal tumours may grow to a large size without causing symptoms. However, after a time, enlargement of the abdomen, abdominal discomfort, and backache may be noticed. Direct pressure on neighbouring structures may produce other symptoms, such as vomiting and constipation from pressure on the bowel. Haematuria and loin pain result from renal or ureteric compression, while pressure on nerves causes pain in specific dermatomes. Patients with large tumours may be breathless from impairment of diaphragmatic action. Attacks of hypoglycaemia occasionally occur and pyrexia is sometimes a striking feature. It is difficult to make the diagnosis from the physical signs. If an abdominal tumour is palpable, little evidence of its origin can be obtained from physical signs. Cystic tumours can be confused with those in the mesentery. Retroperitoneal lipomata and liposarcomata grow to such an enormous size that this is in itself characteristic.

Pressure on adjacent structures may cause other signs such as ascites from portal vein compression or leg oedema from pressure on the vena cava. Loss of weight, anorexia, and pyrexia are features particularly of retroperitoneal Hodgkin's disease. Other tumours may have their own characteristics. Phaeochromocytomata in the retroperitoneal space give rise to attacks of paroxysmal hypertension, or occasionally there is sustained hypertension and mild diabetes. Neuroblastomata occurring only in young children often metastasize to the orbit or they may cause urinary symptoms. A careful search for metastases and enlarged glands in the groins or axillae may help in the diagnosis of a retroperitoneal tumour.

16

The following tests may also be of help:

1. Barium-meal or barium-enema studies will not only exclude an intrinsic tumour of the bowel but show displacement of the bowel. Films taken in the anteroposterior or lateral projections are valuable.

2. A film of the abdomen may show a soft-tissue mass or obliteration of the psoas shadow. Occasionally calcification may be seen.

3. Pneumoperitoneum or presacral insufflation of carbon dioxide may be helpful.

ASSESSMENT AND TREATMENT

The ideal treatment is surgical excision of the tumour as soon as diagnosis is made, but this is only possible in 20 per cent of cases. Where resection is impossible radiotherapy may palliate and in some tumours, e.g., giant follicular lymphoma and Hodgkin's disease, radiotherapy may produce a dramatic, though temporary, improvement. If these conditions are of multicentric origin cytotoxic therapy may be preferable.

Radiotherapy is recommended as an adjuvant to surgical treatment of malignant tumours, e.g., neuroblastoma.

Malignant Ascites

The seeding of multiple malignant deposits over the peritoneal surface may result in the accumulation of ascites. Peritoneal deposits usually originate from a carcinoma of the alimentary tract (stomach, colon, or pancreas) but sometimes from primary growths outside the alimentary tract such as the breast, ovary, or bronchus.

The patient complains of abdominal distension, but cachexia and signs of the primary lesion accompany those of ascites. There are no signs of liver failure and portal hypertension. The diagnosis (*Table 26*) is made as follows:

1. After careful history and physical examination of the patient.

2. After chest radiograph, barium meal or enema to show the primary.

3. If cirrhosis is excluded, paracentesis abdominis may help by allowing palpation of abdominal viscera and tumours.

4. Examination of the ascitic fluid may reveal a blood-stained fluid with a high protein content greater than 3 g. per cent, perhaps showing malignant cells.

5. Peritoneoscopy, needle biopsy of peritoneum, laparotomy, and biopsy of tumour deposits may be required.

TREATMENT

Analgesics are given to relieve pain and paracentesis may lessen the abdominal discomfort. If the patient is in reasonable health, intraperitoneal cytotoxic drugs (nitrogen mustard or ThioTEPA) or radioactive colloidal gold may be given.

Peritoneal Adhesions

'People are divided into two groups: those who form adhesions and those who do not' (Rendle-Short).

Peritoneal adhesions may be congenital (2 per cent), inflammatory (20 per cent), or postoperative (nearly 80 per cent) in origin. Occasionally they may follow radiotherapy to the abdomen. Infection, excessive trauma at operation, or the inadvertent introduction of powder particles into the peritoneum may all play a part. The usual concept of adhesion formation is as follows. An exudate of fibrin occurs where the serosa is inflamed or damaged, and leads to the development of fibrinous adhesions. If the serosa is intact, the fibrinous exudate may be reabsorbed; if the

Table 26. CAUSES OF ASCITES

| | ASCITIC FLUID | | | |
CAUSE	*Protein*	*Cells*	FEVER	OTHER FEATURES
Tuberculous peritonitis	Greater than 2·5 g. per cent	+ + +	+ +	Chest radiograph helpful in 30 per cent
Cirrhosis (unless complicated by hepatoma)	Usually less than 2·5 g. per cent	+	±	Jaundice; splenomegaly; cutaneous signs
Hypoproteinaemia, e.g., nephrotic syndrome, protein-losing enteropathy	Less than 2·5 g. per cent	+	−	Generalized oedema; heavy proteinuria (nephrosis)
Cardiac disease; tricuspid disease; cardiac constriction; severe heart failure	Less than 2·5 g. per cent	+	−	Liver pulsatile; J.V.P. ↑ + +
Hepatic vein thrombosis (Budd-Chiari syndrome)	Greater than 3 g. per cent	+	+	Liver large and tender
Malignancy	Greater than 3 g. per cent (may be bloody)	+ + (may show malignant cells)	±	Large nodular liver or other masses palpable; rectal mass; lymphadenopathy

serosa is not intact, the fibrin is invaded by fibroblasts with the formation of firm adhesions. In other words, adhesions are scars produced by the healing of peritoneum.

Recent work by Ellis (1962) has cast doubt on this traditional belief. Following the observations that large peritoneal defects heal without adhesion formation, he has shown by animal experiments that adhesions develop as a reaction to the presence of ischaemic tissue.

Clinically, adhesions may cause no symptoms at all. On the other hand, there may be recurring episodes of abdominal pain, or even frank intestinal obstruction by bands, kinks, or torsion secondary to the adhesions. Some 30 per cent of cases with obstruction are from adhesions. If the obstruction is incomplete, varying degrees of malabsorption may develop.

In the prevention of adhesions, a little can be done by attention to detail:

1. Exercising extreme gentleness when handling tissues at operation.
2. Eliminating particles of powder from outside of gloves.

3. Avoiding use of too hot packs.

4. Avoiding strangulating sutures in anastomoses and repairs, etc., so that no ischaemic tissue is left in the peritoneum.

Heparin and cortisone have been used, but without success. Fibrinolysin is under trial in animals. There has been some success in controlling adhesion formation, but there is risk of haemorrhage and spread of latent infection.

If surgical intervention becomes necessary for the adhesions, treatment consists of simple division, but occasionally plication of the gut or resection may be necessary (Capper, 1959). By-pass procedures should be avoided as they may lead to a blind loop syndrome. In general, the more localized the adhesions the easier the treatment, whereas diffuse adhesions may present an almost insuperable problem.

Retroperitoneal Fibrosis

This is a rare disease of unknown cause characterized by dense retro-peritoneal fibrosis which obstructs and distorts surrounding structures. Though one cause is the use of antiserotonin agents (methysergide) in the treatment of severe migraine most cases are thought to be due either to an immunological defect, possibly genetically determined, or to an unusual reaction to drugs such as amphetamines. It is of interest that retroperi-toneal fibrosis may occur in association with other disorders associated with abnormal fibrosis such as Riedel's thyroiditis, sclerosing cholangitis (*see* p. 225), mediastinal fibrosis, and pseudotumour of the orbit. One rare form is a reaction to diffusely spreading carcinoma.

The diagnosis is often delayed because of the non-specific and highly variable manifestations. The commonest are due to constriction of the ureters (loin and back pain—chronic renal failure), whilst obstruction of major veins may cause oedema and varicosities in the legs and even portal hypertension.

Fibrosis obstructing the colon and duodenum and oesophagus may cause dyspeptic symptoms and fibrosis in the lung and myocardium may cause dyspnoea, heart failure, and cardiac dysrhythmias. Unfortunately there are no helpful haematological or immunological tests but the E.S.R. is usually raised and the most helpful information is obtained by intra-venous or retrograde urography. Mid-ureteric narrowing and medial deviation are the classic signs and when both ureters are involved the obstruction is usually at about the same level in each though there may be multiple strictures. Surgery is indicated to confirm the diagnosis, to exclude malignancy, and to free the ureters (ureterolysis) where there is impairment with ureteric flow or renal damage. The operative findings are typical dense vascular fibrous tissues spreading across the retro-peritoneal space and are usually maximal at the pelvic brim. Providing the diagnosis is made and ureteric obstruction prevented the prognosis is reasonable and survival for many years is usual. Hypertension, renal failure, and heart failure are possible hazards, but it seems that after a time the disease remits and the E.S.R. falls.

FURTHER READING

Peritonitis
MENZIES, T. (1961), in *Modern Trends in Gastroenterology*, Vol. 3 (ed. CAIRD, W.). London: Butterworths.

Tuberculous Peritonitis
BURACK, W. R., and HOLLISTER, R. M. (1960), 'Tuberculous Peritonitis—A Study of 47 Proved Cases encountered by a General Medical Unit in 25 Years', *Am. J. Med.*, **28**, 510.
JOHNSTON, F. F., and SANDFORD, J. P. (1961), 'Tuberculous Peritonitis', *Ann. intern. Med.*, **54**, 1125.

Periodic Disease
EHRENFELD, E. N., ELIAKIM, M., and RACHMULEWITZ, M. (1961), 'Recurrent Polyserositis (Familial Mediterranean Fever—Periodic Disease)', *Am. J. Med.*, **31**, 107.
REIMANN, H. A. (1951), 'Periodic Disease', *Medicine, Baltimore*, **30**, 219.

Retroperitoneal Tumours
PACK, G. T., and TABAH, E. J. (1954), 'Primary Retroperitoneal Tumours', *Int. Abstr. Surg.*, **99**, 209.

Peritoneal Adhesions
CAPPER, W. M. (1959), 'The Surgery of Peritoneal Adhesions', *Gastroenterologia, Basel*, **92**, 173.
ELLIS, H. (1962), 'The Aetiology of Post-operative Adhesions', *Br. J. Surg.*, **50**, 10.

Retroperitoneal Fibrosis
SAXTON, H. M., KILPATRICK, F. R., KINDER, C. H., LESSOF, M. H., MCHARDY YOUNG, S., and WARDLE, D. F. H. (1969), 'Retroperitoneal Fibrosis. A Radiological and Follow-up Study of 14 Cases', *Q. Jl Med.*, **28**, 159.
WEBB, A. J., and DAWSON-EDWARDS, P. (1967), 'Non-malignant Retroperitoneal Fibrosis', *Br. J. Surg.*, **54**, 508.

Chapter 24

Some Symptoms

THE APPRAISAL of symptoms calls for a review of possible causes and a shrewd judgement of probabilities. Above all the clinician's assessment of his patient's constitution and emotional bias will teach him how much weight to give to these symptoms. Eddy Palmer has written: 'The most seasoned clinician must continuously wonder how organic lesions of the same location, size and nature can provoke symptoms of such differing intensity . . . in different patients.'

Because of this inherent difficulty it is worth while considering certain important symptoms which may arise as a result of gastro-intestinal disease, but which may equally well arise from disease elsewhere or from emotional discord.

ABDOMINAL PAIN

Pain is felt in the abdomen not only when disease attacks the abdominal organs but also when the vertebral column, retroperitoneal muscles, and abdominal wall are damaged. Abdominal pain can, therefore, be considered under two headings: (1) Somatic pain; (2) Visceral pain.

SOMATIC PAIN

The mechanisms of pain referral and causation differ in no way from those in a limb or any other part of the body. The sensation of pain may arise from superficial and epicritic nerve-fibres in the skin of the abdominal wall or from deeper, less percipient pain receptors in muscles, arteries, and bone.

Conveniently, the somatic causes of abdominal pain can be classified:
1. From disease of skin and subcutaneous tissues.
2. From disease of muscles.
3. From disease of vertebral column and ribs and pelvis.
4. From disease of blood-vessels.
5. From irritation of nerve-roots.

Some of the more important conditions which cause somatic abdominal pain are epidemic myalgia (Bornholm disease), herpes zoster, osteomyelitis of the lower dorsal spine, pathological crush fractures of vertebrae, pressure and leakage effects of abdominal aneurysms, and many conditions which cause pressure on lower intercostal nerve-roots, ranging from small simple tumours to multiple leukaemic deposits.

VISCERAL PAIN

This may be subdivided into three main types, depending on the tissue reaction. The character and distribution of the pain, together with the accompanying signs, may to a certain extent enable the physician to know which type of pain is being experienced. The three types are:

1. Visceral colic due to violent contraction of smooth muscle.
2. Visceral tissue ischaemia, tension, or necrosis.
3. Peritoneal inflammation.

1. An example is the fleeting but severe pains of laboured intestinal peristalsis such as may occur with partial intestinal obstruction or enteritis. Such a pain is ill-localized but felt towards the centre of the abdomen. It waxes and wanes, and the patient draws up his knees in search of relief. Uterine peristaltic pain is felt lower in the abdomen and ureteric pain to one or other loin with radiation to the groin. Biliary colic tends to be more prolonged, high in the abdomen or low in the chest, and to radiate to the back.

2. The viscera are not sensitive to artificial stimuli such as cutting or cauterization during the course of operations, but sustained tissue tension or permanent damage to them causes a deeply felt, severe, and not very well-localized type of pain. Typical examples are the pain of myocardial infarction which may spread from the chest to the abdomen, the pain of a gastric ulcer surrounded by inflammatory oedema, the pain caused by the haemorrhages and exudates of allergic purpura or the necrosis of polyarteritis, and the early phases of pain from acute appendicitis. It seems clear that visceral pain of this type is not felt until a fairly high threshold is passed, and in some patients the threshold is abnormally high; this would account for the painlessness of peptic ulceration and myocardial infarction in some people.

3. Peritoneal pain is really viscerosomatic and thus the sensation is well localized to the affected area, is continuous and graded in severity, and is accompanied by tenderness and rigidity of overlying tissues.

NAUSEA AND QUEASINESS

It is a cardinal rule of diagnosis that nausea without abdominal pain may just as well be due to disease outside as to disease inside the abdominal cavity. Emotional distress, endocrine and biochemical disequilibrium, drugs, and disease of the head, nervous system, and special sense organs are all important causes of nausea. When the trouble lies within the abdomen nausea is usually accompanied by pain, but this is not always so, and particularly not if the patient is of the sensitive type who throughout life has been prone to vomit easily. Certain conditions are especially liable to cause nausea with minimal pain, namely, hepatitis, alcoholic gastritis, gastric carcinoma, and pyloric stenosis.

Experimentally, nausea can be induced by distension of the first part of the duodenum. When a migrainous or any other patient suffering from nausea is observed by radiological screening with barium, the stomach is inactive and the first part of the duodenum is contracted.

Emotionally, nausea is often provoked by horror or disgust and is often accompanied by anorexia.

There are a number of other abdominal sensations akin to nausea which patients find difficulty in describing, but usually call 'indigestion', 'fullness', 'bloating', or 'distension'. The distension is, in fact, subjective, and the physician rarely finds it.

There is unfortunately no way of deducing from the description the cause of such symptoms. Frequently, their occurrence suggests functional rather than organic disease, but carcinoma, hepatitis, cholecystitis, and idiopathic steatorrhoea may cause little pain in certain people but only the rather vague manifestations of abdominal distress.

VOMITING

A convenient subdivision is into:
1. Pain-induced vomiting.
2. Obstructive vomiting.
3. Reflex vomiting.
4. Habit vomiting.

1. PAIN-INDUCED VOMITING

This, such as occurs in uncomplicated peptic ulceration or acute appendicitis, is dominated by the pain. Thus, in the presence of severe pain, vomiting may have little significance: it is simply a reaction to stress. Some people will vomit from the pain of a severe bruise or a septic finger, but usually it is the deep visceral pain caused by disease of the abdominal and thoracic organs which most readily provokes vomiting.

2. OBSTRUCTIVE VOMITING

This can usually be recognized by an appraisal of the circumstances and an inspection of the vomitus. Vomiting from oesophageal obstruction tends to occur while eating, the vomitus being alkaline; the vomitus of gastric retention is copious, brownish, and acid, whereas intestinal obstruction causes faecal vomiting.

3. REFLEX VOMITING

If vomiting is neither accompanied by abdominal pain nor obstruction, then it occurs as a reflex in response to a whole variety of stimuli. Diseases of the brain, its meninges, and the special sense organs are important sources of such stimuli, but fever or disruption of the biochemical equilibrium by uraemia, ketosis, or hypercalcaemia are equally important causes.

4. HABIT VOMITING

In Chapter 1 some mention was made of vomiting as a manifestation of some inward disgust. The tendency to vomit may, by gaining the solicitude of others, serve the patient's subconscious motives, and thus becomes a habit. Weight-loss may be only slight.

GLOBUS

The feeling of a 'lump in the throat' is frequently experienced, and is readily conceded by most people to be an emotional response. However, in some the discomfort becomes so intense that they may cough and attempt to vomit. Worry about the symptom and fears of cancer frequently coexist. There is no interference with the muscular mechanics of swallowing as observed radiologically, and the patients do not lose weight.

Because the symptom may be caused by tumours outside but in contact with the pharynx, or by tumours of the lower oesophagus and cardia, it is necessary to do barium studies and endoscopy on all such patients.

REGURGITATION AND RUMINATION

A normal response after a meal may be the regurgitation of a small amount of gastric juice, after a premonition of heartburn. This order of events suggests that it is an oesophagogastric motility disturbance which causes both the heartburn and the regurgitation. Unless the latter is constantly provoked by lying flat or by stooping it is not likely to be due to sphincter incompetence at the cardia, but rather to disordered peristaltic behaviour of the stomach and oesophagus.

Rumination in the adult is a perverted habit and is rarely complained of by the patient. Others may send him to the doctor.

BELCHING AND AEROPHAGY

The gas which is usually present in the stomach is composed of 15 per cent oxygen, 4–8 per cent carbon dioxide, and the rest nitrogen. If air is instilled into the stomach its composition soon changes as a result of absorption or usage of oxygen and release of carbon dioxide.

Gas is replenished by the swallowing of air with the saliva. Some patients feel discomfort from the gas bubble in the stomach, and a sense of relief and satisfaction from belching it up. After belching they swallow more air, and the cycle repeats itself. At a subconscious level the oral satisfactions of belching may compensate for the left hypochondrial discomfort, or, alternatively, the symptom may be the result of a bad habit which might be corrected voluntarily. It is useless to palliate the habit by prescribing so-called carminatives. Upward flatulence developing for the first time in a middle-aged patient may be the first symptom of some serious disease but usually other symptoms and signs are present.

FLATUS DISCOMFORTS

Flatus consists of 40 per cent nitrogen, 40 per cent carbon dioxide, and 20 per cent methane, hydrogen sulphide, and other fermentation products. The formation of bowel gas is normal, but it may give offence to others and worry to its generator. To a certain extent constipation with a spastic colon favours bowel gas formation, but there may be no correlation with either organic or functional disease. If the flatus is trapped as a circular bubble in the splenic flexure it may cause left-sided pain or discomfort, or, if in the hepatic flexure, a feeling of discomfort in the area of the gall-bladder. This so-called *splenic flexure syndrome* is frequently diagnosed in the U.S.A., but much less so in Britain. Increased physical exercise and *Lactobacillus acidophilus* preparations such as Enpac are frequently advised for such patients.

HEARTBURN

It has been shown by experiments on volunteers that a number of different stimuli to the lower oesophagus are interpreted as heartburn. Distension by balloons, heating, cooling, and strong acid infusions may all cause heartburn. The sensation almost certainly stems from dyssynergic contractions of the lower oesophageal musculature.

The sensation itself hardly needs defining as most humans have at some time experienced the sense of pressure and burning beneath the lower sternum. As a symptom it is sometimes accompanied by nausea or excessive salivation. Temporary relief can be gained by belching up a small bubble of gas or by drinking fluid. Many patients rely on antacids, Sodium bicarbonate which releases CO_2 in the stomach may ease heartburn by allowing the patient to belch. Also, gastrin release occurring as the gastric contents are alkalinized tightens the lower oesophageal sphincter.

Heartburn is frequently associated with pregnancy, cholelithiasis, hiatus hernia, duodenal ulcer, irritable colon syndrome, and overpurgation. It can occur in those whose gastric acid secretion has been reduced by surgery to very low levels, and is thought to be provoked in such cases by backwash of bile and tryptic enzymes into the lower oesophagus. The evidence for this is from radiological studies and the aspiration of alkaline bile-stained fluid from the oesophagus. It seems probable, however, that all stimuli of this sort cause heartburn by provoking abnormal muscular contractions in the lower oesophagus.

A feeling of acid taste in the mouth, though sometimes associated with heartburn, is a separate sensation which may occur alone. It is nearly always due to anxiety.

DIARRHOEA

The patient interprets either frequency of bowel action or looseness of the stools as diarrhoea. The physician must by inquiry separate these two elements, and having done so, decide whether the symptoms are but a variation of normal function, or whether they indicate disease of the mind or body.

Generally speaking, frequency of bowel action with normal or near-normal stools is a variation of function, and this is certainly so if defaecation occurs mainly in the morning or after meals. Permanently loose unformed stools are more likely to indicate disease.

MECHANISMS OF DIARRHOEA

It is becoming increasingly obvious that the symptom complex of diarrhoea can be produced by a large number of different mechanisms. Further, the diarrhoea of several alterations of bowel function may contribute to any single disease process. The following is a short synopsis of those mechanisms which are currently recognized, but much remains to be solved.

a. Infective Diarrhoea. The cause of the fluid loss in acute infective diarrhoea is unknown and mucosal ulceration alone seems unlikely. Studies of patients with one form—cholera—have demonstrated mucosal oversecretion with intact absorption and it is possible that this effect which is due to a toxin is also causative in other infective diarrhoeas. The discovery of this lesion in cholera has led to the institution of an oral glucose electrolyte régime which utilizes the intact absorptive mechanism. In cholera there is a direct effect of the toxin on the tissue cyclic 3′5′-AMP system via adenyl cyclase. Increased adenyl cyclase results in increased AMP and thus of electrolyte secretion.

b. Stagnant Loop Syndrome. Bacterial deconjugation of bile-salts is an important mechanism of the diarrhoea (steatorrhoea) that complicates this disorder. A depletion of bile-salts results and it is possible, too, that unconjugated bile-salts have a toxic effect on the small-bowel mucosa.

c. Humoral agents seem directly responsible for diarrhoea in the Zollinger-Ellison syndrome (acid inactivation of lipase and bile-salts), in pancreatic pseudocholera (secretin overproduction in pancreatic non-insulin secreting tumours), the carcinoid syndrome (direct effect of serotonin on small-bowel mobility), and the diarrhoea complicating medullary carcinoma of the thyroid (prostaglandin stimulation of intestinal smooth muscle).

d. Osmotic diarrhoea is seen in patients with disaccharidase deficiency (brush-border disease) where failure to absorb luminal fluid results from impaired action of the sodium-dependent intestinal pump, and there is also accumulation of excessive disaccharide-containing fluid in the gut lumen. This results in osmotic diarrhoea and a shortened intestinal transit time.

e. Disorders of gut mobility are thought to play a part in the diarrhoea of ulcerative colitis where there is diminished intestinal motility in the large bowel (i.e., reduced colonic resistance), and possibly in Crohn's disease and the diarrhoeal form of spastic colon. In thyrotoxicosis it seems likely that diminished intestinal transit rate accounts at least partly for the diarrhoea.

In coeliac disease diarrhoea is explainable on a number of factors, e.g., loss of mucosal surface, impaired carbohydrate absorption with osmotic diarrhoea, and loss of the sodium pump (impaired fluid absorption).

In trying to reach a diagnosis, if not of the precise cause, at least of the category of disease which is provoking chronic looseness of stools, it is essential in the first place to know certain facts. These are the findings on digital and visual rectal examination, the results of faecal occult-blood tests, the haemoglobin level, and the E.S.R. Barium studies of the colon are also usually necessary (*Table 27*). Culture of stools is only valuable in patients with a short history. By plotting the results of these simple screening tests against the five main groups of diseases which cause diarrhoea it is usually possible to make a provisional diagnosis.

The five main groups of causes are:
1. Functional, i.e., emotional, endocrine, biochemical, reflex, etc.
2. Malabsorptive.
3. Infective or parasitic.
4. Inflammatory or allergic.
5. Neoplastic.

The functional group includes diarrhoea from endocrine and metabolic disease as well as the more common nervous type. Thyrotoxic and carcinoid diarrhoeas are probably due to direct stimulation of peristalsis. Diabetic diarrhoea is more difficult to explain. It is probably due to an autonomic neuropathy which may also cause steatorrhoea.

If diarrhoea from emotional, endocrine, or metabolic causes seems unlikely, and if neoplasia, ulcerative colitis, Crohn's disease, and amoebic dysentery have been excluded by the examinations and tests described, a

Table 27. TESTS IN DIAGNOSIS OF DIARRHOEA

TYPE OF DIARRHOEA	Hb	E.S.R.	FAECAL OCCULT BLOOD	RECTAL EXAMINATION (DIGITAL AND VISUAL)	BARIUM ENEMA
Functional	N	N	—	N	—
Malabsorptive	L	N	—	N	—
Infective	?L	?H	+ —	? ulcers or exudate seen	—
Inflammatory	L	H	+	Abnormal mucosa visible	Changes in colon or terminal ileum
Neoplastic	L	?H	+	Mass palpable or visible in 50 per cent	Lesion localized

Hb—Haemoglobin   N—Normal   H—High   L—Low

group of ill-defined diarrhoeal conditions remains. Loose stools, often with mild steatorrhoea and creatorrhoea, may persist for months or years, usually after some acute dysenteric or viral infection. Specific organisms cannot be isolated though the bacterial flora may have altered. The rectal mucosa may look hyperaemic, but there are no gross histological abnormalities. In such cases *Giardia lamblia* may be found in the stools, but its pathogenic role is uncertain. Studies of colonic motility have not shown any characteristic pattern in this type of diarrhoea. In some cases it seems to be due to an abnormal sensitivity to drugs, notably the tetracyclines, but usually it is an acute infective enteritis which sets off the reaction. Nothing is known of the basic pathology, but the known provocative factors suggest an allergic rather than an infective basis.

Empirically, low-fat and low-residue diets have been found to diminish the intensity of symptoms, and recolonization of the bowel by the eating of yoghurt or a dried preparation of *Lactobacilli* is sometimes successful in alleviating the symptoms or shortening their duration.

Equally puzzling cases of chronic diarrhoea occur in elderly people, many of whom have diverticulosis coli. It is not known whether the diverticula play any part in the causation of the diarrhoea and it is not as a rule responsive to antibiotics.

After the investigation of many cases of chronic diarrhoea there will always remain some unsolved problems. For convenience, such un-diagnosed cases may be given the label of nervous or functional diarrhoea, but such a label may be misleading or a cloak for ignorance. The flow of fluid into the lumen of the small intestine and back into the blood-stream from a lower part of the gut is normally very great, and it only needs minor changes in intestinal cell function to influence the balance of these fluxes. At present little is known of the control mechanism and it may well be that cases presently labelled as functional diarrhoea may ultimately prove to have some cell-function defect.

THE SYMPTOMATIC TREATMENT OF DIARRHOEA

Diarrhoea from emotional causes may take the form of: (1) A variant of the spastic colon syndrome causing excess production of bowel mucus, variations in stool consistency, and bowel pain. This is best treated by sedatives such as amylobarbitone or phenobarbitone and antispasmodics such as extract of belladonna or by a drug acting directly on the smooth muscle, e.g., mebeverine hydrochloride. Methyl cellulose can be useful in mopping up water and maintaining stool consistency. (2) An intensifica-tion of the gastrocolic reflex giving postprandial and early morning loose stools, often with tenesmus, urgency, and post-defaecation pain. Codeine phosphate 30 mg. last thing at night and phenobarbitone 30 mg. twice a day may help. Propantheline 15 mg. can be useful.

In cases of post-infective 'allergic' enteritis with watery or fatty stools, codeine phosphate 30 mg. three times a day slows down the rate of transit; diphenoxylate 5 mg. three times daily may be more effective in a few patients. A low-fat diet, with adequate protein and carbohydrate, often makes the patient more comfortable. Cellulose-containing foods should be severely cut, and starch should be taken in the form of cornflour and arrowroot rather than bread and potatoes.

All patients with intestinal hurry tend to improve when given a low-residue diet, but the conventional example of this diet excludes meat and many other items both necessary and pleasant. A low-residue diet should exclude only coarse root vegetables, nuts, raisins, raw salad, soft fruits and pears, and it should include *purée* of green vegetables, cooked apple, fruit juices, and tomato juice.

CONSTIPATION

Constipation is difficult to define because of the extreme variation in normal habits, but the difficulty with the passage of constantly hard stools can be accepted as the meaning of the word.

The attitude of the patient is very often at variance with that of the doctor. The latter is aware that gross alterations of bowel habit are com-patible with continued health, and that the body's physiological processes are rarely disturbed by long delay in the evacuation of the bowel. He is also aware of the harmful effects of purgatives both in causing abdominal discomforts and in leading to addiction which can cause dehydration and hypokalaemia. The obsessive attitude of many bowel-conscious patients is also a sore trial to many harassed physicians.

None the less, constipation, the awareness of constipation, and the fear of constipation do cause symptoms which are unpleasant and difficult to bear, and thus the physician, while trying to educate his patients, must at the same time try to appreciate their miseries and help them to a measure of comfort in their daily life.

In the first place, constipation may cause symptoms of a mechanical nature:

1. Splitting of anal mucosa.

2. Prolapse of haemorrhoids and subsequent thrombosis.

3. Distension of rectum may produce local discomfort and reflex effects such as headache and nausea.

4. Impaction of faeces in rectum may cause spurious diarrhoea and urinary retention with overflow.

5. In elderly people, the colon easily dilates and faecal retention with mental confusion or rectal impaction with urinary and faecal incontinence may cause serious disability.

Secondly, constipation may be caused by spasm of the colon which is in itself a painful condition which leads to a variety of reflex disturbances such as heartburn, epigastric discomfort, right iliac fossa pain, and attacks of severe colic.

Thirdly, constipation may cause considerable predefaecatory pain which is felt both in the abdomen and rectum.

Lastly, the inability to empty the bowel at regular intervals may worry the patient so much that he develops symptoms of anxiety and depression, or, alternatively, the obsessional person may make a hobby of his bowels.

The proper assessment and management of a patient complaining of constipation depend firstly on the correct diagnosis and treatment of such organic disease as may be causative, and secondly, if organic causes are excluded, on knowledge of the functional derangement responsible for the symptoms.

CONSTIPATION CAUSED BY ORGANIC DISEASE

1. General Diseases—Diabetes mellitus. Myxoedema. Uraemia. Fever.

2. Local Diseases—Pyloric stenosis. Other obstructing lesions of small bowel. Carcinoma of colon. Diverticulitis coli and stricture. Other strictures of colon and rectum. Anal fissure and stricture. Congenital megacolon.

CONSTIPATION CAUSED BY FUNCTIONAL DISORDERS

Prolonged recumbency. Constipating drugs. Mental deficiency. Conflicts of childhood. Abnormal diet or fluid intake. Spastic colon. Abnormal anxiety about bowels. Lazy rectum.

The organic general diseases causing constipation are not difficult to recognize if the clinical interrogation and examination are properly done. Local diseases can usually be suspected from the history, but radiological and other investigations are nearly always necessary to make a precise diagnosis.

In the absence of organic disease, the next step is to decide whether the constipation is a variation of the normal habit blown up by an obsessional and worried person into a major problem, or whether there is some recurring error of function of part or whole of the bowel. For example, the lazy rectum situation, which can be expected in young women from disorganized households, is easily diagnosed by history and rectal examination. The spastic colon syndrome common in tense, migrainous, and often middle-aged people can be recognized by the history of pain, narrow stools, excess mucus, and palpability of a tender colon in the left iliac fossa. In other people, habitual purgation may have already caused atony of the whole colon, though a barium enema may show apparently narrow areas.

Treatment of the individual patient must depend on his personality and background, on the length of history, the degree of addiction to purgatives, and the relative importance of the dietary, the spastic, and the atonic factors. In general, it is best to concentrate on a reorganized diet, on habit-conditioning, and suppositories to re-educate the lazy rectum; to use antispasmodics, sedatives, and stool softeners for those with spastic colon; and the regular nightly dose of standardized senna preparations for the elderly and habituated patient with the inactive colon.

Patients with a lazy rectum should avoid intermittent violent purgation as this only upsets their whole gastro-intestinal tract, and patients with a spastic colon are also better without purgatives. Elderly patients with flabby colons should not overload themselves with a diet of bran, brown bread, fruit, and nuts which they propel caudally by a weekly purge. If an elderly patient is found to have faecal retention with rectal impaction, manual removal of faeces, followed by bowel wash-outs and a steady régime of purgation will often lead to a remarkable improvement of general condition, a clearing of confusion and restoration of continence.

It is often astounding to find what gross insults patients will inflict on their own gastro-intestinal tract, what elementary errors are made, and what simple remedies are ignored.

Suppositories of glycerin are nearly as effective as those of biscodyl 10 mg., though the latter does cause direct stimulation of the rectal wall.

Of the anthracene purgatives, standardized senna as sennakot tablets or granules is the least likely to cause pain and spasm.

Stool softeners composed of psyllium seed extract (Isogel) or methyl cellulose are useful if the stools are desiccated and narrow; emulsion of agar and liquid paraffin can be useful, particularly in elderly patients who have difficulty in expelling a hard stool.

Some patients become addicted to strong purgatives and may in consequence develop hypokalaemia which can cause muscle weakness, paralysis, or tetany. A barium enema done on a patient addicted to purgatives will show a featureless colon lacking in normal tone.

TENESMUS

This is a sensation of pain and discomfort in the rectum which either follows defaecation or provokes false calls to stool. It is usually associated with organic disease.

PROCTALGIA FUGAX

This is a severe pain in the posterior pelvis caused, it is thought, by a cramp-like spasm of the levator ani. Some relief can be gained by firm finger pressure on the coccyx and posterior anal margin. Though severe and sometimes recurrent it is associated more with nervous stress than organic disease.

PRURITUS ANI

This condition which is more common in men than women is frequently linked with sexual maladaptation, often occult, and may perhaps reach its severest forms in the obsessive bachelor sons of dominant mothers. It is characteristic of such patients that they indulge in self-treatment so that the damage caused by astringent lotions is added to that caused by scratching; eczematization occurs and a vicious circle is set up. Hydro-cortisone $\frac{1}{2}$ per cent ointment is helpful in lessening secondary effects, but basically the treatment should be guided by a psychiatrist.

FURTHER READING

COOKE, W. T. (1971), 'Laxatives and Purgatives', *Practitioner*, **206**, 64.
LAW-BEER, T. S., and READ, A. E. (1971),'Diarrhoea Mechanisms and Treatment', *Gut*, **12**, 1021.
READ, A. E. (1971), 'Anti-diarrhoeal Agents', *Practitioner*, **206**, 69.

Chapter 25

Radiology of the Gastro-intestinal Tract

By K. T. EVANS

A CAREFULLY CONDUCTED radiological examination is a vital step in the elucidation of many disease processes in the gastro-intestinal tract. However, inconclusive findings in the presence of symptoms such as bleeding, weight-loss, or alteration of bowel habit may indicate that a lesion has not developed sufficiently to be recognizable on a radiograph. In such patients re-examination at intervals is important and investigation by endoscopy and other methods where appropriate is advisable. On the other hand, an abnormality discovered by radiological methods should not be disregarded. It is important to relate the radiological to the clinical findings.

It should be emphasized that considerable thought should be given to the correct sequence of radiological investigations. If examinations of the vascular system, biliary or renal tracts are likely to be required these should be carried out before barium is given as barium residue in the bowel may delay additional examinations with contrast medium.

PLAIN FILM EXAMINATION

Gas within the gastro-intestinal tract provides a natural contrast medium of great help in diagnosis. Gas is normally found in the stomach, but only small collections of gas are usually present in the small intestine except in nervous patients who may swallow large quantities of air. Gas in the colon may be present throughout but more commonly appears as localized collection intermixed with faecal material.

FLUID LEVELS

A fluid level is normally present high in the stomach and occasionally fluid levels are seen in the gastric antrum or first part of the duodenum. A fluid level may also be shown in the caecum.

In the presence of intestinal obstruction there is absence of gas distal to the site of obstruction whereas the proximal bowel becomes dilated by fluid and gas. Characteristic gas fluid levels are seen in radiographs of such patients taken with the patient erect (*Fig. 85*). Diverticula of the small intestine or abscess cavities may also give fluid levels on erect films.

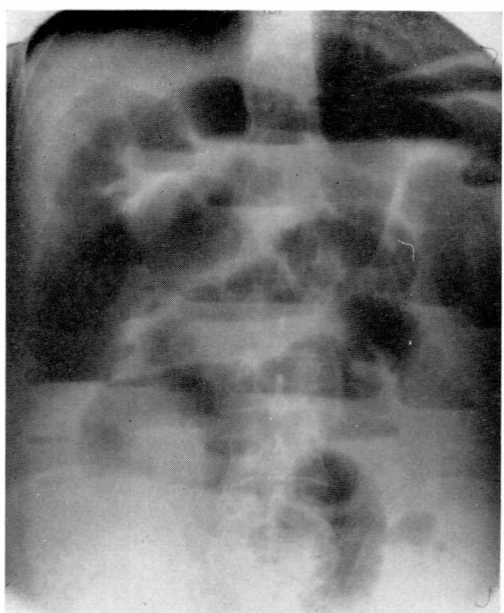

Fig. 85. Patient with small intestinal obstruction showing multiple gas fluid levels.

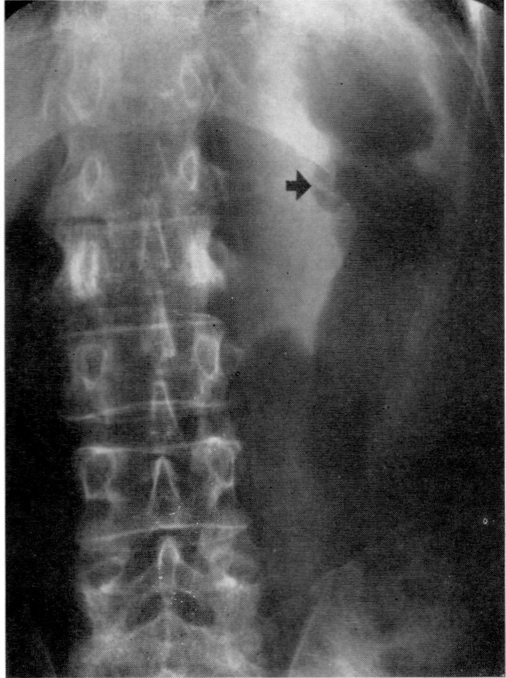

Fig. 86. Gastric ulcer on the lesser curvature of the stomach outlined with gas.

Each portion of the gastro-intestinal tract outlined with gas has a characteristic position, shape, and mucosal appearance. Lesions may be identified by an alteration in these appearances. For example, the presence of a persistent pocket of gas connected to or outside the gas-filled bowel may indicate an ulcer or abscess cavity (*Fig. 86*). Gas-filled cysts (pneumatosis cystoides intestinalis) lying subserosally in the small intestine or colon may be shown on plain films (*Fig. 87*). Narrowing or irregularity of the lumen commonly occurs in malignant infiltration (*Fig. 88*). The presence or absence of gas in the biliary or portal systems should be established.

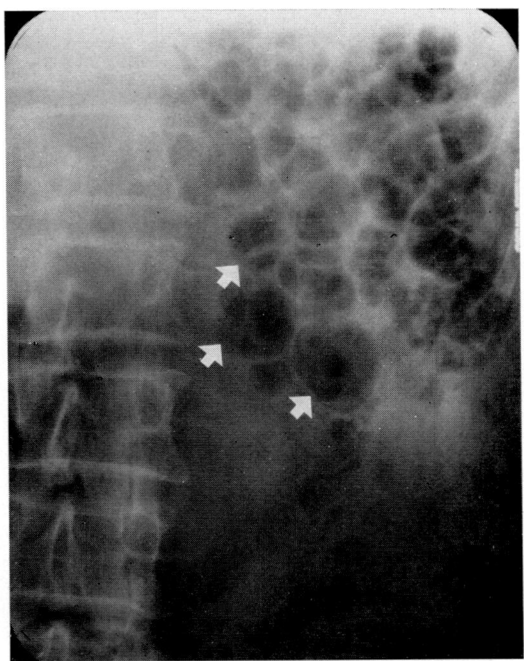

Fig. 87. Multiple subserosal gas-filled cysts in the colon
(pneumatosis cystoides intestinalis).

In patients with ulcerative colitis complicated by toxic megacolon dilatation of a segment of colon with mucosal islands projecting into the gas-distended colon provides a readily recognizable picture (*Fig. 89*).

SOFT-TISSUE DENSITIES

Enlargement of the liver, spleen, or kidney can often be demonstrated. Soft-tissue masses due to collections of fluid in the fundus of the stomach or duodenal cap should not be mistakenly diagnosed as abnormalities. If in doubt, contrast studies would confirm.

PERFORATION OF AN ABDOMINAL VISCUS

A radiograph taken with the patient erect or in the lateral decubitus position showing free gas in the peritoneal cavity is valuable evidence of

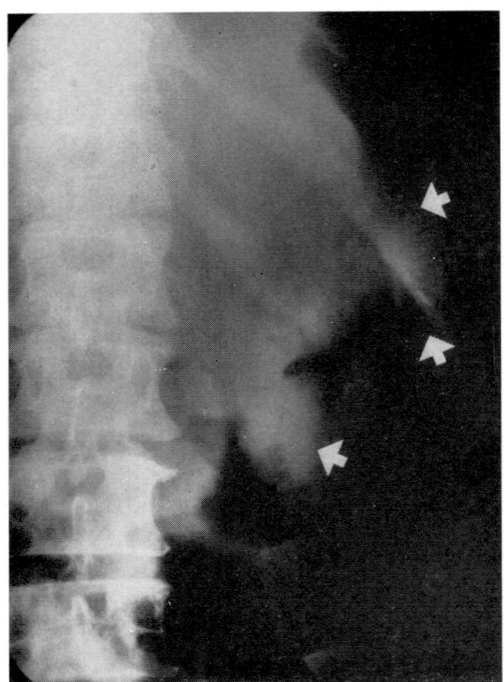

Fig. 88. Extensive carcinoma of the stomach showing distortion of the gas-filled outline.

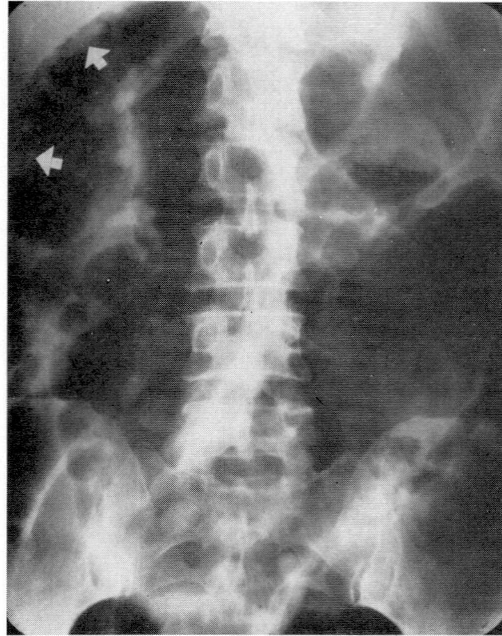

Fig. 89. Ulcerative colitis showing toxic dilatation of the colon. The mucosal islands are a characteristic feature.

a perforation. Its absence, however, does not exclude this diagnosis. The differential diagnosis includes subphrenic abscess or air remaining after a recent laparotomy.

CONTRAST MEDIUM EXAMINATION

Barium sulphate is the most widely used contrast agent in the study of the alimentary tract. Barium, which is inert and non-toxic, has a high atomic number and is therefore opaque to X-rays. Proprietary preparations of barium (e.g., Micropaque) are available and these have the advantage of being stable suspensions of uniform consistency.

RADIOLOGICAL APPARATUS

Sophisticated fluoroscopic tables having a wide variety of movements are now available. Image intensification and television are essential as not only is the accuracy of the examination increased but the radiation exposure to the patient and operator is greatly reduced by their use. Seventy-mm. radiography is being increasingly employed and this has the advantage of providing further reduction in the radiation exposure as well as reducing the cost of the examination.

THE OESOPHAGUS

In patients with obstructive lesions of the oesophagus where there is a danger of inhalation a contrast medium used for bronchography (Dionosil) should be substituted for barium.

It is unwise to investigate an infant with suspected oesophageal atresia with contrast media as there is a danger of aspiration into the lungs. In such cases the site of the obstruction can be determined by passing a radio-opaque tube into the upper oesophagus and taking a radiograph.

The course of the swallowed contrast medium is observed on the television monitor. It is difficult to obtain satisfactory radiographs of the upper oesophagus because of the rapid passage of barium. Cine-radiography is of great value in examining this portion of the oesophagus.

The normal oesophagus is indented by the arch of the aorta and also where it is crossed by the left main bronchus. Abnormal impressions on the lumen of the oesophagus may result from enlargement of the heart or aorta, or by miscellaneous abnormalities in the mediastinum.

Dysphagia

Difficulty in swallowing is a common symptom and can result from a variety of lesions. It is not uncommon for patients to have symptoms referred to the throat when the lesion is situated in the lower oesophagus or upper part of the stomach. In all such cases a full examination of the stomach and duodenum is required.

Diverticula

Pulsion diverticula are most commonly seen in the upper oesophagus. Occasionally the enlargement is such that they extend into the superior mediastinum.

Traction diverticula arise as a result of adhesions from an adjacent inflammatory lesion in hilar glands.

Irregularity of Outline

This may be seen in carcinoma or oesophagitis. The differentiation between the two may be impossible radiologically. Endoscopy is essential in such cases.

The normal mucosal folds of the oesophagus run longitudinally. Distortion and irregularity may be noted in the presence of oesophageal varices (*Fig. 90*).

Hiatus Hernia

A hiatus hernia may appear when the patient lies down, but some method of raising the intra-abdominal pressure such as coughing or manual compression of the abdomen by the operator may be necessary for its demonstration. The presence or absence of associated gastro-oesophageal

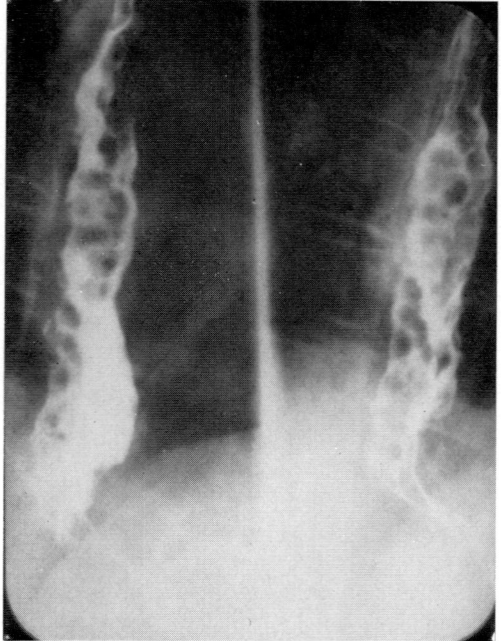

Fig. 90. Dilatation of the oesophagus with gross irregularity due to oesophageal varices.

reflux is more important than the actual demonstration of the hernia. Long-standing gastro-oesophageal reflux may produce oesophagitis with stricture formation.

THE STOMACH AND DUODENUM

It is important that patients should fast for at least 6 hours before a barium-meal examination. The presence of fluid in the stomach dilutes the contrast medium and causes it to flocculate. Furthermore, particles of food in the stomach can be confusing as they may simulate disease. For the same reason it is an advantage to wash out the stomach of a patient with clinically obvious gastric retention before examination.

A barium-meal examination consists of two complementary parts—observation of oesophageal, gastric, and intestinal movements on the television monitor and subsequent examination of films taken during the examination.

Mucosal Pattern Study

A careful fluoroscopic examination of the gastric mucosa supplemented by radiographs in the erect and supine posture is of the utmost importance. Barium penetrates between the gastric folds throwing them into relief. It is necessary to position the patient so that adequate coating of the mucosa is achieved. The presence of food or fluid residue in the stomach prevents adequate demonstration.

Convergence of Rugae

Gastric ulcers frequently show convergence of the rugae towards the ulcer and this convergence persists after the ulcer has healed. Although such convergence is commonly seen in benign ulcers it is sometimes present in malignant ulceration (*Fig. 91*).

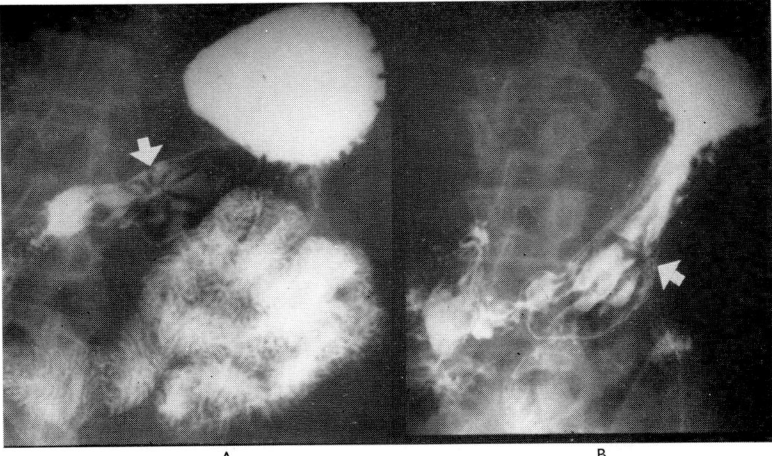

Fig. 91. **A,** Convergence of mucosal folds due to ulcer in the antrum of the stomach. A virtually identical appearance is shown in **B.** This ulcer was in fact malignant.

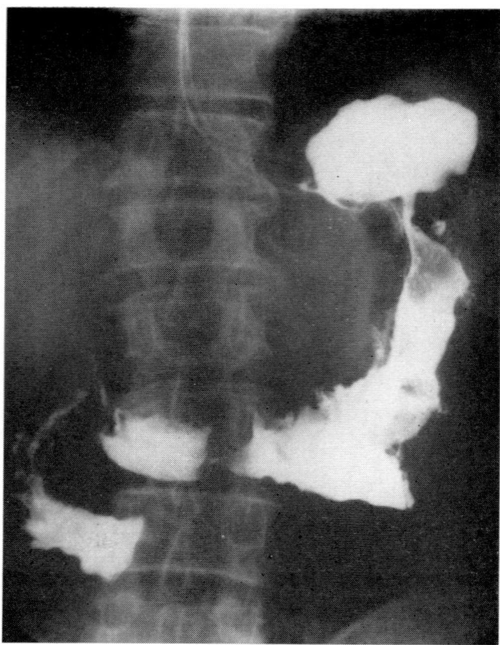

Fig. 92. Extensive destruction of the mucosa in gastric carcinoma.

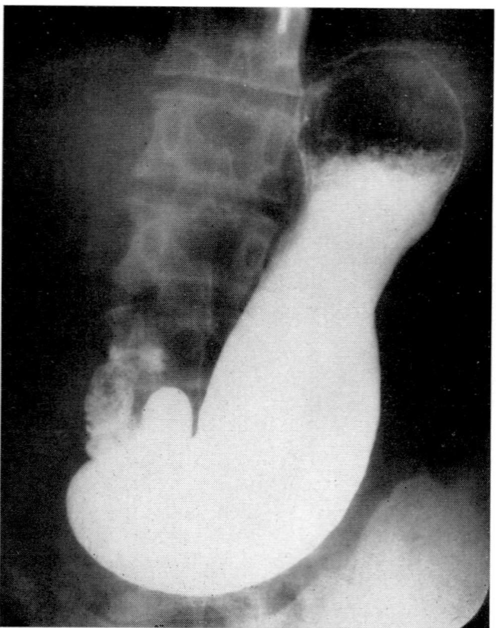

Fig. 93. Patient with atrophic gastritis. Note absence of mucosal fold impressions
over the fundus and greater curvature.

Destruction of Rugae

This is an extremely important sign of gastric carcinoma as a localized or generalized finding (*Fig. 92*). It is difficult to evaluate in patients with gastric retention.

Large Gastric Folds

These are usually a manifestation of an increased acid output and are particularly prominent in patients with the Zollinger-Ellison syndrome. In the rare Menetrier's disease huge mucosal folds are present, particularly in the body of the stomach. The aetiology of this condition is unknown. A similar appearance may be seen in reticulosis. Large gastric varices may simulate a neoplasm.

Small Gastric Folds

Patients with atrophic gastritis may show absence of mucosal fold impressions over the fundus and greater curvature of the stomach (*Fig. 93*).

Displacement of Folds

An extrinsic mass such as an enlarged left lobe of the liver displaces the normal folds and may obliterate the normal convoluted appearances. Localized displacement can occur with an intrinsic tumour such as leiomyoma (*Fig. 94*).

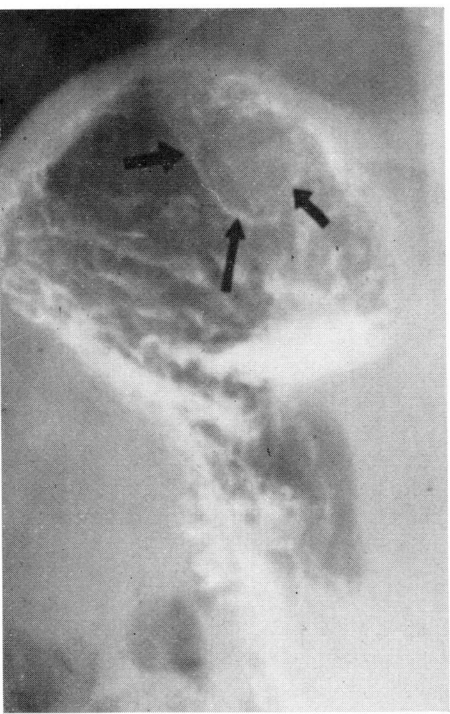

Fig. 94. Leiomyoma of the fundus of the stomach displacing mucosal folds.

The Distended Stomach

Peristalsis

Peristaltic waves normally start in the middle third of the stomach passing downwards to the pylorus. Usually there are three to four such waves at any one time. Increase in the amplitude of the peristalsis is seen in patients with pyloric obstruction.

Peristaltic activity is frequently absent if the stomach is infiltrated by malignant disease.

The Lesser Curvature

This portion of the stomach below the cardia is usually smooth so that irregularities in outline are very suggestive of a disease process. Benign gastric ulcers project beyond the line of the lesser curvature and are frequently conical in shape. Giant ulcers are occasionally found but despite their size are usually benign (*Fig. 95*). It is often difficult radiologically to differentiate a benign from a malignant ulcer. If the ulcer is within the outline of the stomach and is relatively shallow with a broad base it is more likely to be malignant. Interference with peristalsis and localized mucosal destruction would confirm the diagnosis. Endoscopic examination is of great importance in cases where there is doubt as to whether an ulcer is benign.

The Greater Curvature

This is usually irregular due to mucosal fold impressions so that the presence or absence of ulceration is much more difficult to determine in this area. However, few ulcers occur on the greater curvature. They are more likely to be malignant than those on the lesser curvature but as previously stated the characteristics of the ulcer are much more important than its site. An intrinsic impression is common in patients with spleno-megaly.

The Gastric Fundus

Carcinoma in this site is likely to be relatively silent until it produces oesophageal obstruction. Early signs are best detected with erect films where a double contrast produced by air and barium may show a small soft-tissue mass or a double outline to the fundus by a plaque-like tumour (*Fig. 96*). Extrinsic defects due to the spleen may mimic a fundal carcinoma. A pneumoperitoneum may assist in the elucidation of such a mass. Increase of the space between the fundus of the stomach and left dome of the diaphragm may occur in malignancy or subphrenic abscess. The distance is, however, very variable and on its own is not a very useful sign.

The Gastric Antrum

Lesions in the gastric antrum are notoriously difficult to diagnose. Mucosal diaphragms are occasionally seen and may present with vomiting in the elderly patient. Hypertrophic pyloric stenosis in the adult may be very

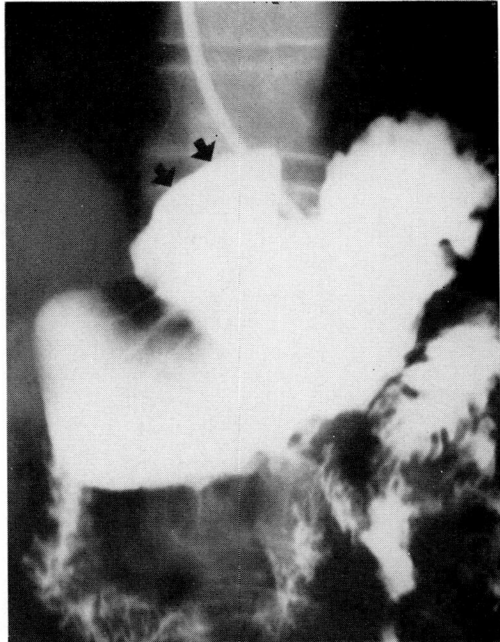

Fig. 95. Large benign gastric ulcer on the lesser curvature of the stomach.

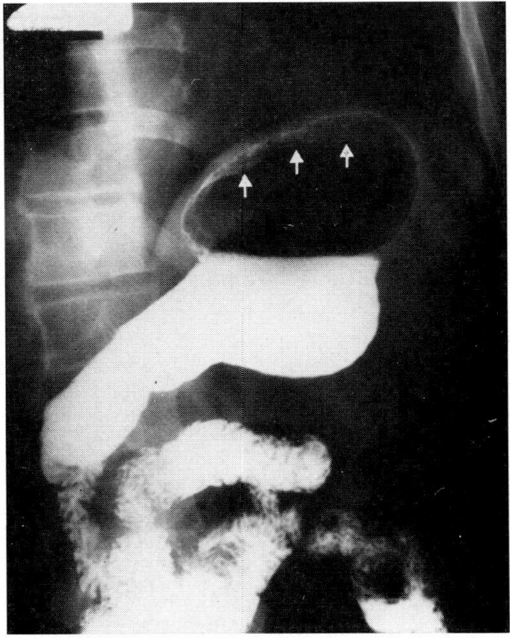

Fig. 96. Carcinoma of the fundus of the stomach showing slight increase in thickness of the stomach wall.

difficult to differentiate from carcinoma. Gastroscopy or laparotomy may be necessary in some cases to differentiate.

The Duodenal Cap

Ulcers in the duodenum occur in the great majority of patients in the first part of the duodenum. Acute ulcers produce no deformity and may only be shown with double-air contrast studies produced by lying the patient on his left side (*Fig. 97*). Chronic ulceration results in deformity of the

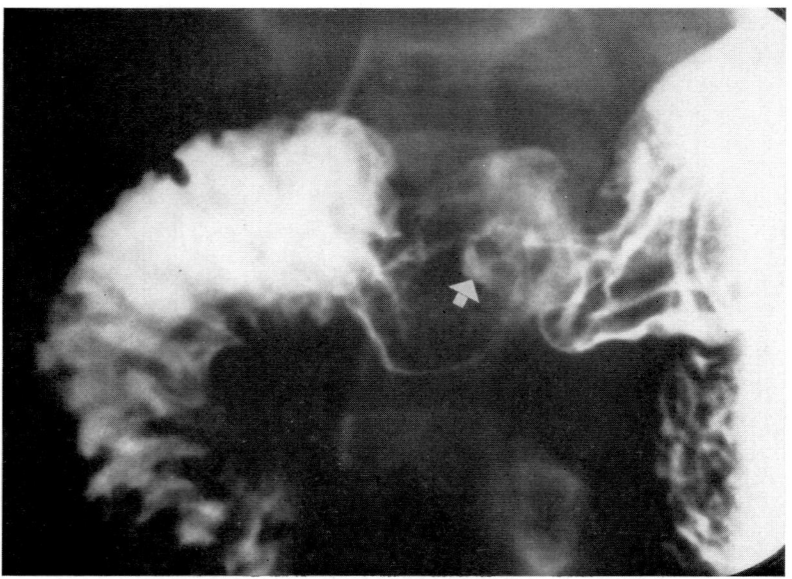

Fig. 97. Duodenal ulcer shown in air-distended duodenal cap.

cap, resembling a clover leaf in appearance (*Fig. 98*). Deformity without ulceration is not uncommonly seen in patients with coarse mucosal folds. These folds may extend into the second portion of the duodenum or upper jejunum. The appearances have been shown to be the result of hypersecretion of gastric acid. It is important to realize that these patients have the same symptoms as those with an established ulcer. Extreme examples are found in patients with the Zollinger-Ellison syndrome. Inflammatory changes with gastric type mucosa have been found histologically in the second part of the duodenum.

THE SMALL INTESTINE

Radiological examination of the small intestine plays an important part in the investigation of many diseases involving this portion of the alimentary tract.

Barium Studies

Most radiologists give 3–4 oz. of undiluted Micropaque by mouth and then lie the patient on the right side to ensure quick and constant gastric emptying. Alternatively, passing a tube to the duodenojejunal flexure allows a small quantity of barium to be used. Hastening agents such as Maxolon (metoclopramide) reduce the time it takes to complete the examination. In all cases it is necessary to take frequent films supplemented by fluoroscopic examination.

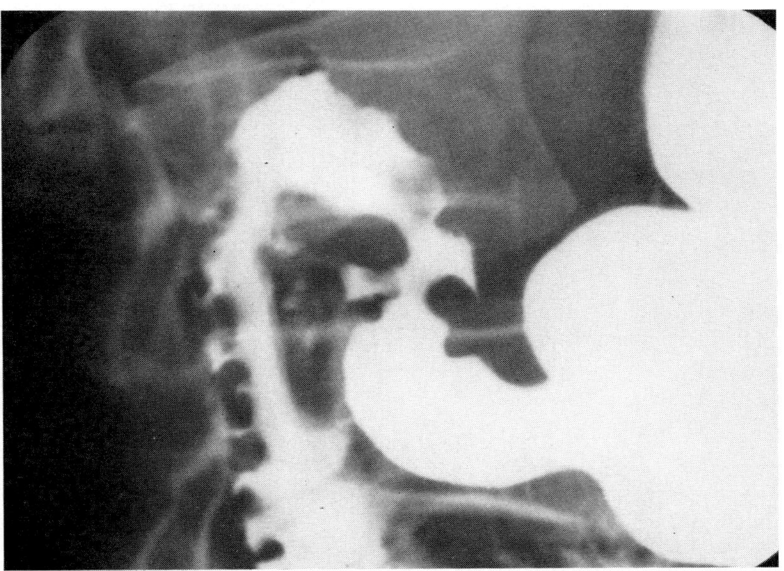

Fig. 98. Marked deformity of the duodenal cap due to chronic ulceration. The coarse folds in the second part of the duodenum suggest a raised acid output.

Normal Appearances of Small Intestine

The transit time to the caecum is very variable and times from 1 to 6 hours can be regarded as normal. In the normal jejunum the barium is finely dispersed and a feathery pattern is produced (*Fig. 99*).

Malabsorption

The radiological appearances of the small intestine in patients with coeliac disease are non-specific. In mild cases or those in remission the follow-through examination may be completely normal. Frequently the calibre of the bowel is increased in width, the mucosal folds are coarse, and flocculation of barium occurs (*Fig. 100*).

Radiological studies are of particular value in patients with structural abnormalities such as diverticulosis, strictures, or blind loops. In such

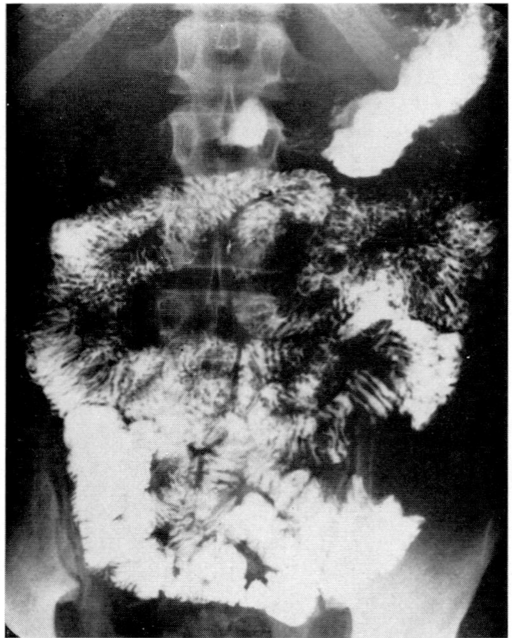

Fig. 99. Normal small bowel pattern.

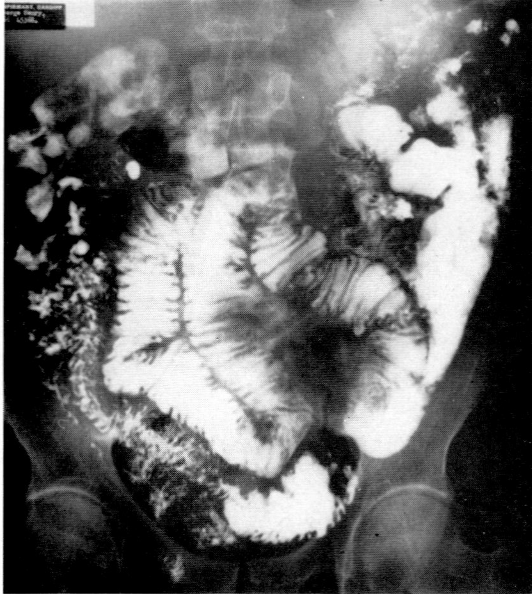

Fig. 100. Dilatation of the small intestine with coarse mucosal folds in a patient with coeliac disease.

patients stagnation of intestinal contents promotes the growth of intestinal flora. Examples are given in *Figs. 101* and *102*.

Disaccharidase Deficiency

Enzyme deficiency of lactase, maltase, or sucrase may result in diarrhoea when the appropriate disaccharide is ingested. Lactase deficiency is the commonest and the diagnosis can be made radiologically by giving a mixture of 25 g. lactose and barium. There is dilution of the contrast medium in the small intestine due to the osmotic effect of the unabsorbed sugar and evidence of intestinal hurry.

THE COLON

A carefully conducted barium enema is a highly accurate examination. The patient must be thoroughly prepared by the use of laxatives, cleansing enemas, or a combination of the two. It is undesirable to perform a barium enema on the same day as a sigmoidoscopic examination and a delay of at least 7 days should occur if a biopsy has been carried out in order to avoid the danger of perforation at the site of the biopsy. It must be stressed that both the preparation and performance of a barium enema may be very taxing in old and debilitated patients.

Tannic Acid

In recent years there has been considerable controversy regarding the use of tannic acid in the barium sulphate suspension. It has the property of precipitating mucus and stimulating contraction of the bowel so that good mucosal pattern films could be obtained after evacuation of barium. However, deaths due to hepatic necrosis have been reported after repeated tannic acid enemata and enemata with a concentration of 2 per cent tannic acid. This complication is excessively rare and is probably related to the concentration of tannic acid used. There is apparently no proof that a tannic acid concentration of 0·25–0·5 per cent ever produced liver damage. Many radiologists have therefore continued its use. It would seem wise to avoid repetitive enemata and to avoid using tannic acid in patients with inflammatory diseases of the colon or those with evidence of liver disease.

Technique of Examination

The use of self-retaining balloon catheters is potentially dangerous as perforation of the rectum has been reported.

Fluoroscopic examination is essential and image intensification with television is preferable. The radiologist observes the column of barium as it passes through the colon. If the patient experiences pain or discomfort the flow of barium is temporarily stopped. There is enormous variation in the position of loops of colon particularly in its pelvic portion. It is important to rotate the patient into the optimum position to unravel these loops. In patients with diverticular disease or carcinoma of the pelvic colon there is often an interruption in the flow of barium. Such 'spasm'

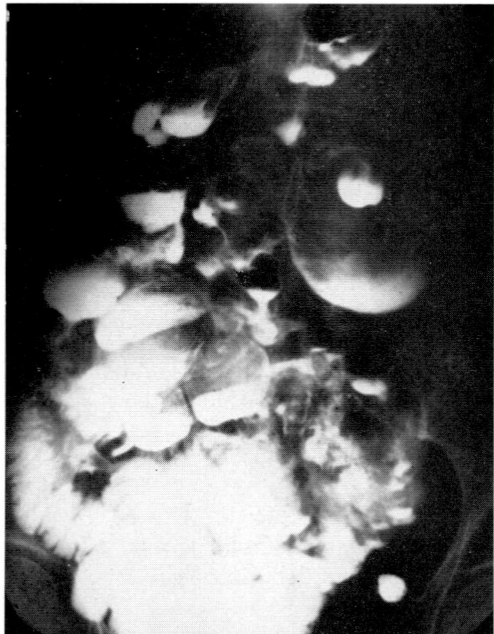

Fig. 101. Diverticulosis of the small intestine.

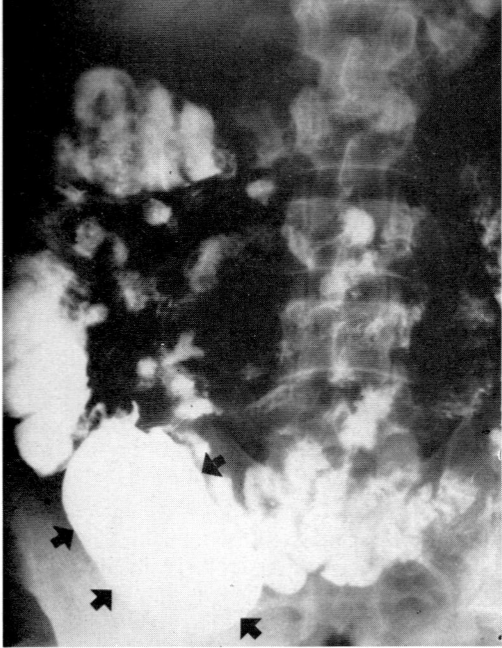

Fig. 102. Large blind loop in the right iliac fossa.

can often be relieved by an intravenous injection of Pro-Banthine. It is
sometimes dificult to know when the caecum has been completely filled
unless the appendix has been outlined with barium or there has been
reflux into the terminal ileum. When the whole colon has been filled
appropriate radiographs are taken with varying degrees of rotation. The
patient is then allowed to evacuate the barium and further films are taken
of the mucosal pattern and of the distended colon after air insufflation.
The latter should be avoided in patients with diverticular disease.

The Filled Colon

Indentations on the outline of the filled colon are due to haustra. They are
particularly well developed in the ascending and transverse portions of
the colon. The descending and pelvic portions of the colon are frequently
devoid of haustra in the normal.

Filling Defects

These may be the result of carcinoma (*Fig. 103*), the appearances remaining
constant in all films including air replacement. Faecal masses may simulate
malignant disease but usually the masses are inconstant in position. In
some cases it may be necessary to repeat the examination for confirmation.

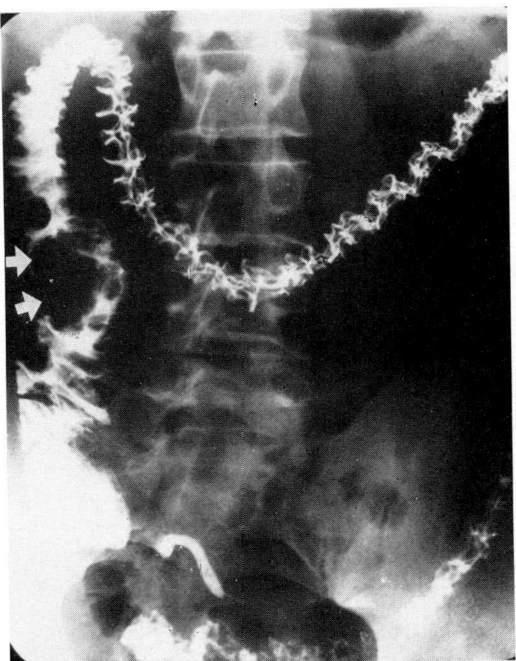

Fig. 103. Carcinoma of the ascending colon showing a filling defect within the
lumen of the bowel.

17

Absent Haustra

These may completely disappear locally or throughout the colon in patients with advanced ulcerative colitis or Crohn's disease and suggests that the disease process has extended into the wall of the bowel (*Fig. 104*). Absence of haustra also occurs in malignant infiltration, systemic sclerosis, or purgative addiction.

Fine Irregularity in Outline

A fine serrated appearance is not uncommonly found in the normal colon, particularly in the pelvic colon. This appearance is attributed to filling of mucous glands.

Diverticula

Diverticular disease of the colon is common after middle age. In this condition, small flask-like projections are most often found in the pelvic colon (*Fig. 105*). Pseudodiverticula are sometimes present in systemic sclerosis.

Ulceration

In *ulcerative colitis* the outline is hazy due to excess mucus and ulceration. Later a serrated border may be seen and undermining of the mucosa may produce a double contour. In Crohn's disease the ulcers are sometimes longitudinal and deep penetrating ulcers and internal fistulae or sinus tracts may develop. It is often difficult to differentiate the two diseases.

Large Crescentic Defects

These may occur in advanced ulcerative colitis where oedematous mucosa between areas of ulceration produces an appearance termed 'pseudo-polyposis' (*Fig. 106*). The differential diagnosis includes ischaemic colitis (*Fig. 107*), pneumatosis cystoides intestinalis, and familial polyposis.

Stricture

Inflammatory strictures are common in patients with Crohn's disease. If a stricture occurs in ulcerative colitis it should be assumed to be malignant until proved otherwise. Rarer causes include lymphogranuloma inguinale, schistosomiasis, and amoebic colitis.

Mucosal Changes

The normal colonic mucosa has an irregular transverse pattern. Localized destruction may occur in carcinoma and extensive destruction in ulcerative colitis or Crohn's disease. Polyps of the colon may be diagnosed by displacement of the mucosal folds.

Air Replacement

This part of the examination is particularly valuable to assess the constancy or otherwise of suspected strictures, and for the diagnosis of colonic polyps.

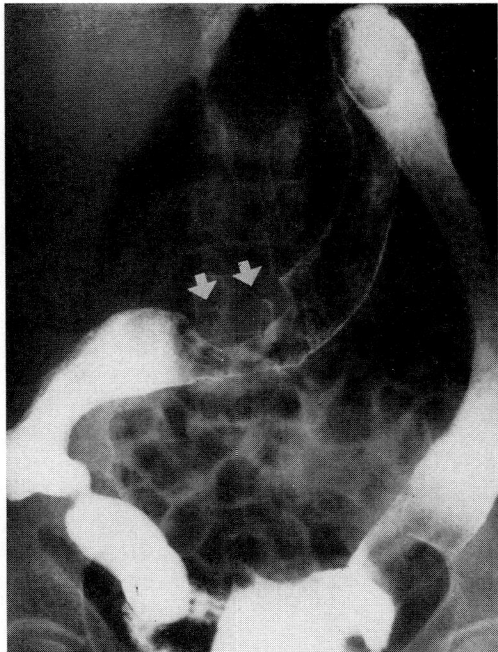

Fig. 104. Complete absence of haustral markings in a patient with advanced ulcerative colitis. Note a filling defect in the transverse colon indicating a carcinoma.

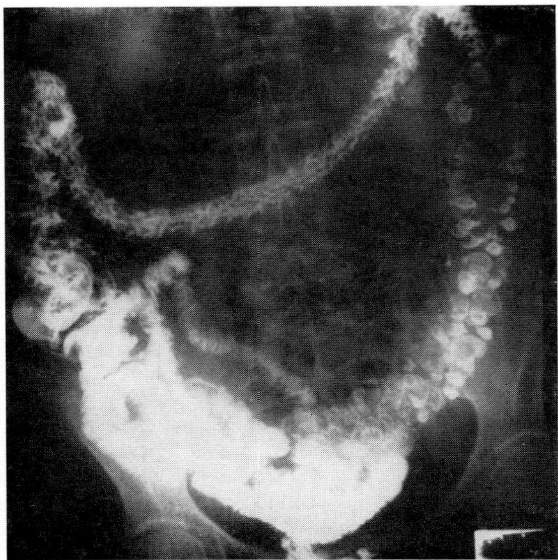

Fig. 105. Extensive diverticula in the descending and pelvic portions of the colon.

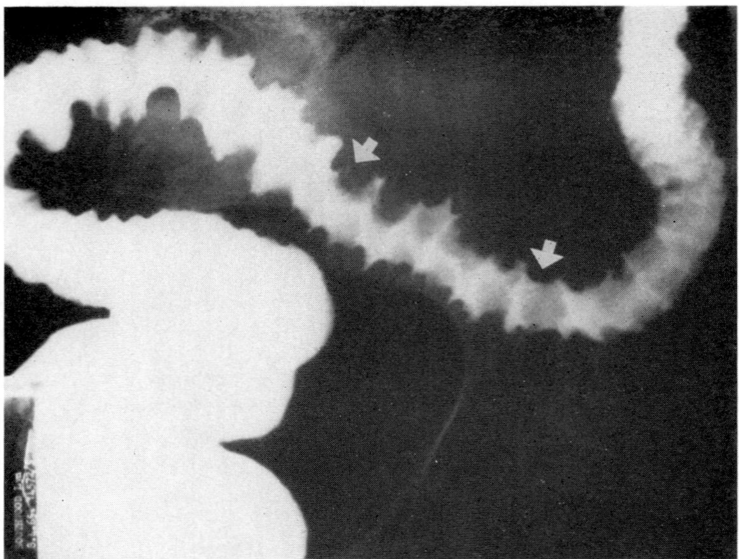

Fig. 106. Ulcerative colitis showing multiple filling defects in the pelvic colon due to pseudopolypi.

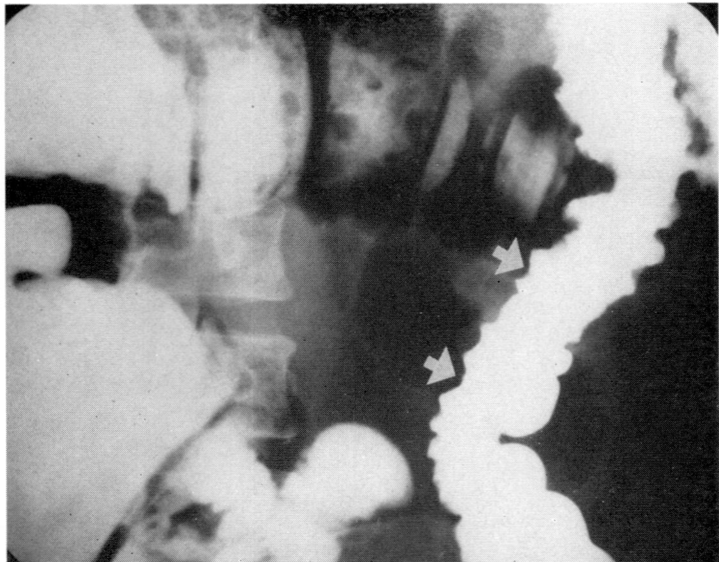

Fig. 107. Irregular outline in the descending colon producing 'thumb-print' defects in a patient with ischaemic colitis.

VARIATIONS OF RADIOLOGICAL TECHNIQUE

Double-contrast Enema

In this examination the colon is filled with barium just beyond the splenic flexure. The patient evacuates the barium and this is followed by air replacement. It is essential to obtain good even coating of the bowel walls. Water can be used instead of air for this examination. It is claimed that the examination is more satisfactory than the normal air-replacement study.

Silicone Foam Enema

Examination of the rectum and sigmoid can be carried out using a silicone foam enema, containing barium sulphate or a water-soluble contrast medium. This forms a mould within the colon and after evacuation normal and abnormal impressions produced by the colon are recorded. It is possible to wash directly any areas under suspicion and obtain cells for cytological examination.

Arteriography

Selective arteriography of the inferior mesenteric artery has been employed for the detection of the site of bleeding and would clearly be of value in the demonstration of vascular tumours. Differentiation of diverticulitis from carcinoma has also been claimed to be possible with this method.

THE PANCREAS

This organ is one of the most difficult to examine by radiological methods as its duct system cannot be demonstrated by any contrast medium ingested or injected systemically. Calcification in the gland sometimes occurs in acute and chronic pancreatitis. It has also been reported in the walls of cysts and in about 10 per cent of cystadenocarcinomata. Very occasionally calcification has been found in adenocarcinoma and islet-cell tumours.

Masses within the Pancreas

Barium studies are conventionally employed as an initial investigation. Cysts displace the adjacent portion of the stomach and duodenum sometimes to a considerable degree. Carcinoma may invade the stomach and if arising in the body may displace the stomach forwards. In the head of the pancreas it may produce widening and displacement of the duodenal loop. Invasion of the medial aspect of the second part of the duodenum above and below the ampulla of Vater gives a characteristic appearance. Barium studies are, however, inaccurate in the diagnosis of masses within the pancreas and it is unlikely that more than 50 per cent of these lesions are diagnosed. Retroperitoneal injection of carbon dioxide combined with tomography has been used in some centres to show the size of the pancreas.

Hypotonic Duodenography

Further information regarding the possible involvement of the second part of the duodenum in patients with suspected carcinoma of the pancreas can be obtained in some cases by performing hypotonic duodenography. In this investigation a double-contrast examination with air and barium is obtained after paralysis of the smooth muscle with Buscopan. Subsequent dilatation of the duodenum may show early rigidity or infiltration not recognizable by conventional barium studies (*Fig. 108*).

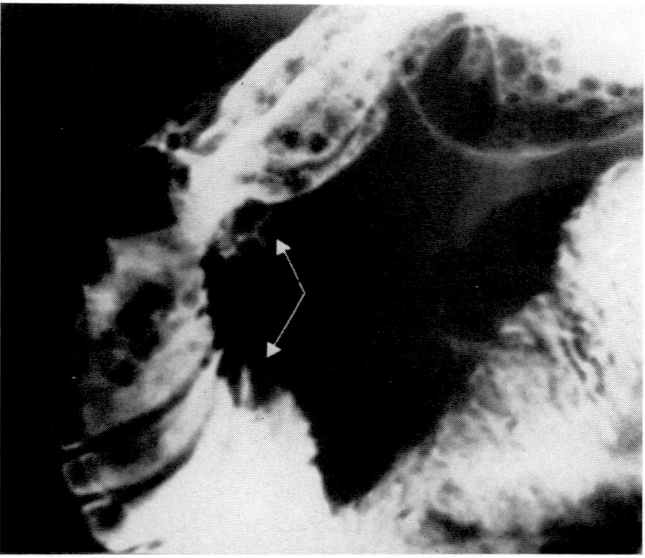

Fig. 108. Hypotonic duodenogram showing irregularity of the medial portion of the duodenum secondary to a carcinoma of the head of the pancreas.

Arteriography

Selective arteriography of the coeliac axis and superior mesenteric arteries has been used extensively in the investigation of pancreatic carcinoma. Unfortunately there is wide variation in the blood-supply and the arteriograms are difficult to interpret. The technique has not gained widespread acceptance in the investigation of suspected pancreatic carcinoma but is, however, of proven value in the demonstration of insulinomas and islet-cell tumours.

THE BILIARY SYSTEM

Plain radiographs of the right upper quadrant of the abdomen may be very helpful in patients with suspected disease of the biliary tract. Opaque gall-stones or the shadow of an enlarged gall-bladder may be shown. Gas in the biliary tree may indicate a fistulous connexion with the gastro-intestinal tract arising spontaneously or following surgical by-pass procedures.

Contrast-medium Studies

Certain iodine-containing compounds are selectively excreted by the liver
and this fact led investigators to the discovery of cholecystography. Contrast media can be given either orally or intravenously.

Oral Cholecystography

A number of proprietary iodine-containing contrast media have been used
in recent years (Pheniodol, Telepaque, Biloptin). Absorption takes place
from the intestine, is excreted with the bile from the liver, and concentrated
in the gall-bladder.

Radiographs of the gall-bladder in the prone and erect positions are
taken 12–15 hours after administration depending on the preparation used.
As most biliary calculi are not opaque to X-rays they produce radiolucent
defects within the gall-bladder shadow (*Fig. 109*). Overlying gas shadows
may simulate calculi, but further films taken with various degrees of
rotation or tomographic examination will be helpful in these cases. The
normal gall-bladder usually contracts after giving a fatty meal, but failure
to observe this function does not necessarily indicate biliary disease.

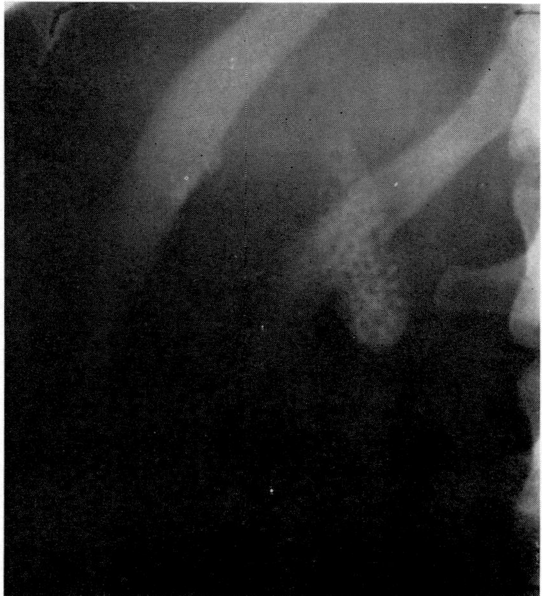

Fig. 109. Oral cholecystogram showing multiple radiolucent gall-stones.

Non-functioning Gall-bladder

In the great majority of patients non-function indicates gall-bladder
disease. It is important to know that the patient has taken the contrast
medium. Failure to absorb as in pyloric stenosis, impaired liver function,

or jaundice are further important causes of failure to demonstrate the gall-bladder. The latter conditions are contra-indications to the examination.

Cholesterol Polyps

These produce irregular translucent defects of varying size on the margin of the gall-bladder. They can be differentiated from calculi within the gall-bladder as they remain in the same position despite changes in the position of the patient.

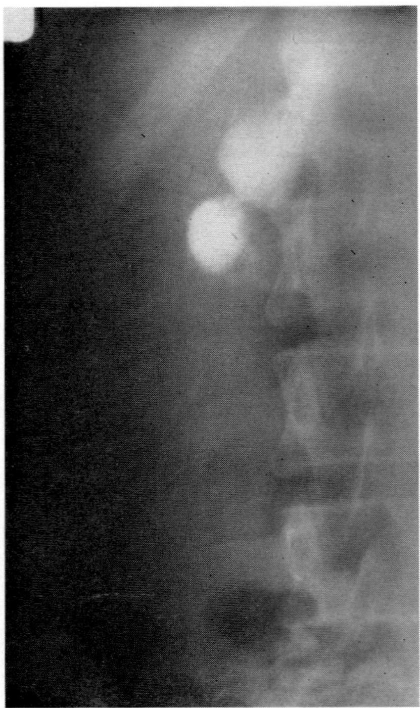

Fig. 110. Marked irregularity of the gall-bladder in adenomyomatosis. Dilated Rokitansky–Aschoff sinuses are shown.

Adenomyomatosis

This is a hyperplastic condition of the wall of the gall-bladder and epithelial lining. It may be associated with cholecystitis or stone formation.

Collections of contrast medium may occur in dilated Rokitansky-Aschoff sinuses around the gall-bladder. Strictures, filling defects, or septa may be present. Usually concentration of the contrast medium is not impaired (*Fig. 110*).

The 4-day technique whereby an oral cholecystographic agent is given for 4 consecutive days occasionally demonstrates calculi not previously shown. In such cases the contrast medium is absorbed by the periphery of radiolucent stones.

Multiple doses of contrast media should be avoided in patients with evidence of hepatic or renal disease as severe toxic effects on the kidney have been reported.

Intravenous Cholangiography

Intravenous injection of iodipamide (Biligrafin) is followed by active excretion by the liver cells. It also has a marked choleretic action so that high concentration in the liver bile is obtained within a few minutes of

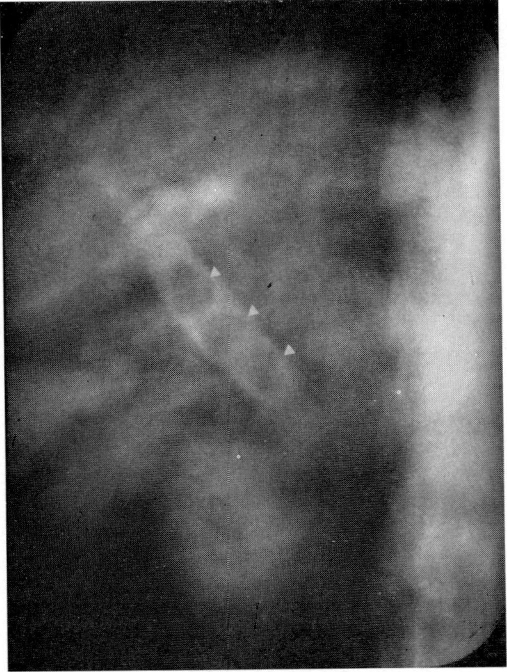

Fig. 111. Intravenous cholangiogram showing dilated common bile-duct with gall-stones.

injection. Usually the maximum concentration is seen in the bile-ducts after 20–30 minutes, but in the presence of obstruction the density of the contrast medium may slowly increase for several hours. In most patients there is relatively poor contrast between the opacified biliary-ducts and the surrounding tissues. Tomography, by eliminating the overlying structures, is an essential part of the examination. Calculi show as translucencies within the common bile-duct (*Fig. 111*).

Indications

The examination is of particular value in patients with symptoms of biliary-tract obstruction in whom the gall-bladder has been removed. It is important to stress that toxic reactions to iodipamide are not uncommon. These can be avoided by injecting the drug slowly.

High-dose Cholangiography

Until recently intravenous cholangiography was of little value in patients if the serum bilirubin was above 2 mg. per cent. Intravenous infusion of 50 ml. of Biligrafin forte given in 150 ml. of saline over a period of 1 hour has been shown to produce fewer side-effects and enables the ducts to be demonstrated with a higher serum bilirubin level.

Transhepatic Cholangiography

This investigation is of value in patients with jaundice in whom the oral or intravenous methods of examination cannot be utilized. The differential diagnosis between obstructive and parenchymal jaundice is frequently difficult on clinical grounds.

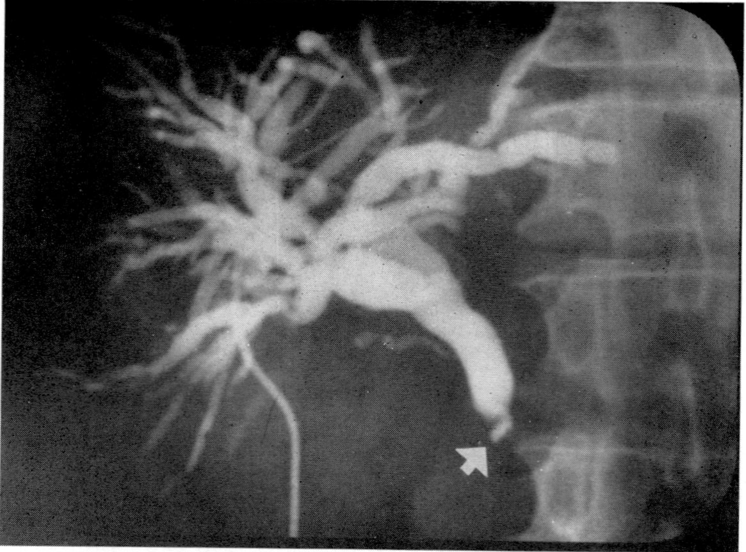

Fig. 112. Transhepatic cholangiogram showing gross dilatation of the common bile-duct and its intrahepatic branches. Note a stricture at the lower end of the common bile-duct due to involvement from carcinoma of the head of the pancreas.

A needle, 15–20 cm. in length, with a tightly fitting sheath of polythene tubing, is introduced into the substance of the liver. The needle is removed and the polythene catheter slowly withdrawn. In patients with obstructive jaundice the bile-ducts are dilated and as the tip of the catheter enters one of the dilated biliary radicles bile is readily aspirated. A water-soluble contrast medium is then injected and its distribution observed by fluoroscopic examination. When the ducts have been adequately shown appropriate radiographs are taken (*Fig. 112*). In the presence of obstructive jaundice it is advisable to leave the tube in situ to allow free bile drainage.

This procedure is not without danger and should only be performed on patients prepared for laparotomy as in patients with obstructive jaundice there is a danger of leakage of bile from the liver. Failure to enter a biliary radicle suggests that the jaundice is not due to extrahepatic obstruction.

Operative Cholangiography

This investigation is imperative in all patients undergoing cholecystectomy in whom there has been a previous history of jaundice or gall-stone colic.

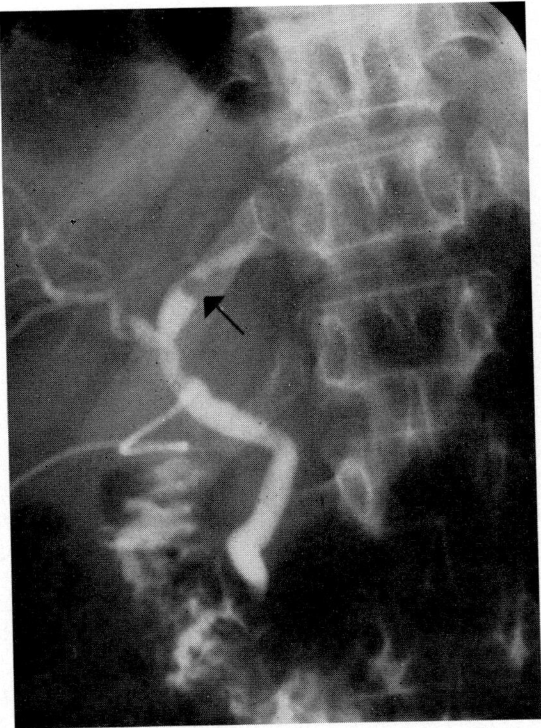

Fig. 113. T-tube cholangiogram showing gall-stone in the left hepatic duct.

It is also of great help in determining the site and cause of an obstructive lesion in the biliary tract. It may be impossible to detect calculi in the common bile-duct by palpation. The finding of a duct of normal size does not exclude the presence of calculi within.

A carefully conducted examination can be of great value to the surgeon as it avoids needless exploration of the common bile-duct in those with normal cholangiograms.

Similarly in the postoperative period gall-stones remaining in the hepatic or common bile-ducts may be identified by injection of contrast medium through a T-tube inserted into the common bile-duct at laparotomy (*Fig. 113*).

Transduodenal Cholangiography (*see* p. 432)

Splenoportal Venography

This procedure can demonstrate the anatomy of the portal venous system and is valuable in the investigation of patients with portal hypertension. It is an essential investigation to assess patency of the portal vein before a portacaval shunt operation is contemplated. Due to the risk of haemorrhage the examination is contra-indicated in the presence of jaundice or if the prothrombin index is low.

A fine-bore needle is inserted into the spleen and an injection of aqueous contrast medium is given. In normal cases the contrast medium is seen to pool in the splenic pulp, and then passes into the splenic and portal vein, subsequently dividing into its intrahepatic branches (*Fig. 114* A).

Portal hypertension arises as a result of obstruction either within the liver or extrahepatic in the portal or splenic veins. In such cases anastomotic channels form with filling of some of the branches of the portal vein (*Fig. 114* B). Commonly reflux occurs into the superior and inferior mesenteric veins as well as the left gastric vein. The latter anastomoses with the azygos system of veins in the lower end of the oesophagus with the production of oesophageal and gastric varices.

In competent hands there are few complications of the examination, but the patient should be observed carefully for a few hours afterwards in case bleeding occurs.

Alternative methods are necessary to demonstrate the portal venous system in patients who have had a splenectomy performed. Injection of contrast medium directly into a tributary of the portal vein can be done at laparotomy. Alternatively, selective arteriography of the superior mesenteric artery may on late films demonstrate the portal vein.

Liver Scanning with Radio-isotopes

It is possible to visualize the liver by using labelled colloids such as ^{99m}Tc sulphur colloid which is removed by the reticulo-endothelial system. It can also be shown by substances such as ^{131}I-labelled Rose Bengal which is taken up by the parenchymal cells. Using the former technique space-occupying lesions within the liver show up as areas of low activity as they do not contain reticulo-endothelial cells. It is not usually possible to see lesions within the liver smaller than 2 cm. in diameter.

This technique is particularly valuable for outlining the configuration of the liver, detection of space-occupying lesions, and in the differential diagnosis of upper abdominal masses. It is of particular value in the demonstration of liver metastases or possible liver abscesses.

^{131}I-labelled Rose Bengal is being increasingly used in the diagnosis of extrahepatic obstruction as normally this isotope is excreted into the intestine within 1 hour after injection. Failure to do so suggests a diagnosis of extrahepatic obstruction.

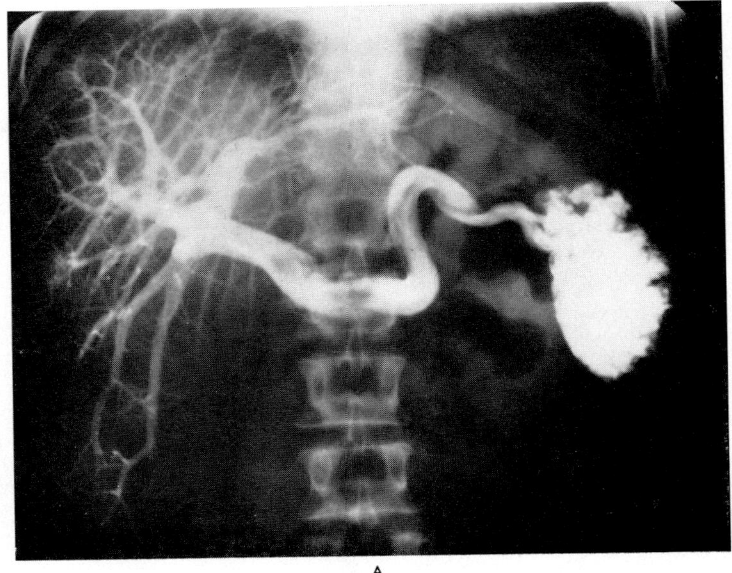

A

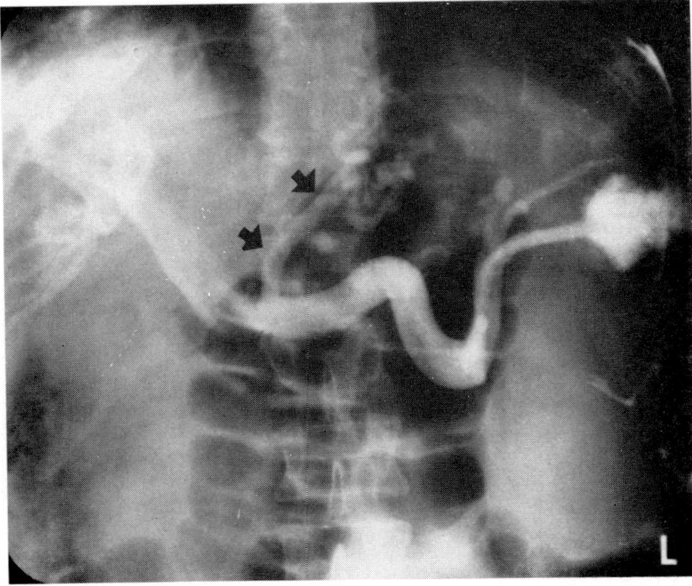

B

Fig. 114. **A**, Normal splenoportal venogram. **B**, Splenoportal venogram in a patient with portal hypertension due to cirrhosis of the liver. Note filling of the left gastric vein producing gastric and oesophageal varices.

Pancreatic Scanning with Radio-isotopes

Satisfactory demonstration of the pancreas has proved extremely difficult. Some good results have been obtained using ^{75}Se-labelled methionine analogue. The technique has the disadvantage that it is difficult to be certain whether the absence of uptake is a pathological or physiological phenomenon. Unfortunately the uptake of selenomethionine within the liver may obscure the pancreas. It is now possible by electronic processing to erase the activity due to selenium within the liver and similar techniques may well give more valuable results in the future.

Chapter 26

Special Investigations in Gastro-enterology

I. BIOPSY PROCEDURES

NEEDLE BIOPSY OF THE LIVER

THIS IS now established as a valuable diagnostic aid in such varied disorders as the following:

1. In cirrhosis to establish the diagnosis.

2. Liver cell jaundice—in establishing the diagnosis of virus hepatitis where this is uncertain and particularly where the clinical picture is atypical or prolonged.

3. Obstructive jaundice—to help to make adiagnosis of intrahepatic or extrahepatic biliary obstruction.

4. In the investigation of hepatomegaly of uncertain cause.

5. To confirm the diagnosis of general diseases such as sarcoidosis, amyloidosis, etc.

6. In differentiating patients with homozygous Wilson's disease from heterozygous sibs (*see* p. 185).

7. In the investigation of glycogen-storage disorders (*see* p. 158).

Special staining techniques for amyloid, iron, copper, and glycogen may be indicated in certain cases, otherwise routine reticulin and haematoxylin and eosin preparations suffice.

Biopsy Needles

The two types of needle which have largely superseded earlier apparatus are: (1) The Vim-Silverman. (2) The Menghini. Both are 'cutting' needles. The latter is the simpler to use and will be described in detail (*Fig. 115*). A disposable Vim-Silverman needle is now available and ensures sharp-cutting blades.

Preliminary Precautions

1. The prothrombin time should be between 80 and 100 per cent of normal. Vitamin K should be given if it is low.

2. There should be no significant anaemia and no thrombocytopaenia.

3. Severe jaundice—particularly liver cell jaundice—is a contra-indication.

4. Diminished hepatic dullness to percussion, suggesting a small liver or interposition of the gut between the ribs and the liver, is also a contra-indication. Ascites must be removed before biopsy is attempted.

Method

The procedure should be explained to the patient and if he is nervous premedication can be given. Young children may require heavy sedation. The proper 'respiratory drill' must be practised by the patient so that the biopsy can be performed in the apnoeic phase after expiration. The site for biopsy is the midaxillary line where liver dullness is maximal—usually the right eighth or ninth intercostal space. If the liver is enlarged the sub-costal route can be used.

The patient should lie supine with his right side close to the side of the bed on which there is only one pillow and a firm mattress. Another pillow under the opposite loin slopes the abdomen a little towards the operator. The patient's hands are best held above the head grasping the bars of the bed.

Steps in Biopsy Procedure

1. A skin disinfectant is applied to the right lower chest and upper abdomen.

2. Sterile towels are applied to demarcate the area of hepatic dullness. At the site of biopsy a mark is made and intradermal local anaesthetic introduced. Plenty of local anaesthetic (10 ml. of xylocaine 1 per cent) must be given to ensure anaesthesia of the subcutaneous tissues and the pleura.

3. A small nick is made in the skin. The biopsy needle is assembled and a syringe containing a few millilitres of sterile saline solution is attached to it. The proposed needle track can be 'opened up' with the reamer supplied with the needle or the process may be made easier by using a Menghini needle with a removable sharp trocar.

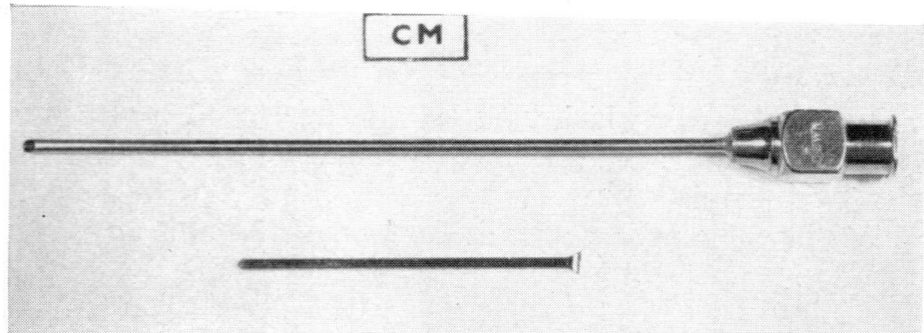

Fig. 115. The Menghini needle.

4. Otherwise the needle is pushed and rotated through the skin incision into the subcutaneous tissues and intercostal muscles down to and through the pleura. Expressing a few millilitres of saline ensures that none of these tissues enters the needle.

5. After a normal expiration, the patient is told to stop breathing and then the needle is rapidly advanced into the liver and withdrawn—suction being maintained on the plunger of the syringe.

6. The patient is instructed to breathe normally after the needle is withdrawn, and the specimen which remains in the needle is gently blown out into a saline solution prior to transfer to fixing fluid—usually 15 per cent formol–saline.

If the operation is unsuccessful, which is unusual, it may be repeated once more providing the patient is not distressed.

The biopsy specimen, usually 2 cm. or longer, may show macroscopic abnormality. It is dark green in obstructive jaundice, black in Dubin-Johnson syndrome, fragmented in cirrhosis, mottled in neoplasia, and yellowish when from a fatty liver.

Complications

Not serious—Pleural and right shoulder pain; a small amount of pleural fluid and basal collapse occasionally occur.

Serious—Haemorrhage. Pneumothorax. Biliary peritonitis (in patients with obstructive jaundice or following perforation of gall-bladder). Rupture of hydatid cyst (very rare).

Mortality—1 in 1000 biopsies (probably less if Menghini instrument is used and precautions fully observed).

After care

Keep in bed for 12 hours. Take 1-hourly blood-pressures and chart pulse.

In patients with cirrhosis fragmentation and the toughness of the liver may prevent a successful biopsy with this needle, in which case the Vim-Silverman needle may be preferable.

BIOPSY OF SMALL BOWEL MUCOSA

There are several varieties of apparatus: (1) The Shiner flexible biopsy tube. (2) The Rubin biopsy tube. (3) The Crosby capsule (*Fig. 116*).

Newer types of multiple biopsy machines, where the multiple specimens are washed to the surface, have also been described. The Crosby capsule is the most suitable apparatus for everyday use, so it will be described in some detail. It suffers from the disadvantage of only supplying one biopsy—and if the procedure fails there is no way of obtaining tissue short of reintubation.

The Crosby capsule is a small hollow capsule (approximately 2 cm. × 0·7 cm.) with a side-hole and detachable cap. Inside there is a spring-loaded knife, which in the loaded position leaves the side-hole clear, and is itself kept in position by the engagement of a notch in the upper surface of the circular blade with a small side-bar in the wall of the capsule. A knuckle of mucosa enters the side-hole when suction is applied to the apparatus through the attached polythene tube and the knife is then disengaged to sever it. Suction pulls the piece of rubber which fits between the capsule and its cap into the body of the capsule and so depresses the knife from its side mounting. The spiral spring provides the power to revolve the blade in the capsule. A child-size capsule is available and advisable for infants and small children, particularly if coeliac disease is suspected.

Method

The apparatus must be fully checked and the rubber diaphragm cut to size before use. Patients fast overnight, and most do not require a local anaesthetic 'gargle'.

The capsule is placed on the back of the tongue and if the patient sits upright it can be swallowed without difficulty. The length of tubing required to allow the capsule to enter the gastric antrum has been estimated and

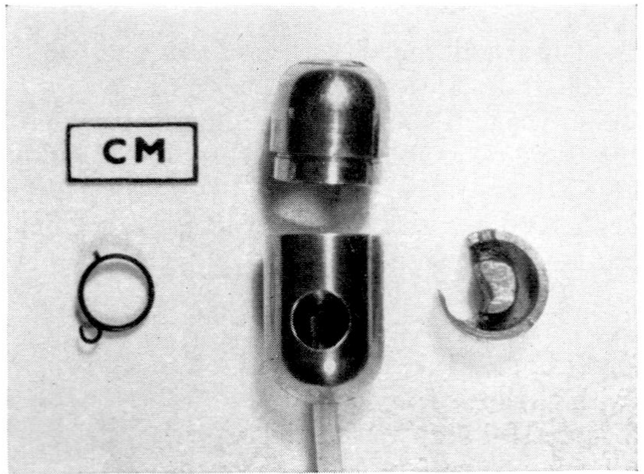

Fig. 116. The Crosby capsule.

this point marked with a piece of adhesive tape. When this is reached gastric peristalsis is encouraged by gently injecting air down the apparatus while the patient lies in the right lateral position for two hours. The efflux of bile-stained duodenal juice into the polythene tube indicates entry of the capsule into the duodenum. At this point the patient is turned into the supine position and is instructed to swallow another foot of tubing again marked with adhesive tape.

The end of the tube can be kept wrapped in two or three gauze swabs to soak up duodenal juice and strict instructions are given that on no account must suction be applied to the apparatus. At the end of three hours the position of the capsule must be confirmed radiologically. If the tube is not radio-opaque, sodium iodide or hypaque may be injected down the tube. When the capsule has reached the jejunum it can then be fired by applying forceful suction from a 20-ml. syringe several times to make sure the knife is released. A much quicker technique uses a semirigid radio-opaque catheter threaded over the polythene tubing. Under the image intensifier the capsule can be guided to and pushed through the pylorus into the duodenum. A biopsy may then be obtained within a few minutes of swallowing the capsule.

The capsule is withdrawn and opened. The specimen is gently removed and spread out on a piece of smooth paper. It is then fixed in formol–saline and sent for microscopical examination. Preliminary low-power examination is useful and often diagnostic in malabsorption due to sprue syndrome.

Dangers

1. Perforation of small bowel.
2. Intestinal haemorrhage (rare).
3. Abdominal pain and pyrexia presumably due to a local inflammatory reaction at the biopsy site.
4. Loss of the cap of the capsule—best prevented by using a screw-on type of cap.

BIOPSY OF OTHER REGIONS OF THE ALIMENTARY TRACT

Biopsy of the *gastric mucosa*—of value in diagnosing gastric mucosal atrophy and gastritis—is best done with a Wood's gastric biopsy tube. This is a thin flexible tube—a circular knife operated by a central wire being used to cut specimens of mucosa which are sucked into the distal capsule by a syringe attached to the tube. Several mucosal specimens can be taken, and a local anaesthetic gargle is all that is required. Biopsy may be obtained under direct vision via a fibre-optic duodenoscope.

A Crosby capsule can also be used to obtain a single specimen of gastric mucosa. *Rectal and colonic mucosa* may be required for histological examination in ulcerative colitis or schistosomiasis and specimens can be obtained with biopsy forceps inserted through a sigmoidoscope, or alternatively a suction type of apparatus similar to the Wood's tube can be used. The introduction of fibre-optic colonoscopes means that polyps and other pathological changes can now be visualized, photographed, and biopsied in virtually any part of the colon.

CYTOLOGICAL EXAMINATION

Though not widely practised in this country this method can be employed in the detection of neoplasms in the upper alimentary tract and the large bowel and also those causing ascites. Most reports concern its application in the diagnosis of gastric neoplasia, where its value is greatest in the detection of early lesions.

After an overnight fast a fine Levine tube is passed into the stomach; 50–100 ml. of normal saline used to wash out the stomach are then aspirated. It is important not to lubricate the Levine tube, as fat droplets make microscopy difficult. The aspirate is fixed with an equal volume of ethyl alcohol, centrifuged, and smears made of the deposit. After staining with Papanicolaou stain, particular attention is paid to the detection of cells with large hyperchromatic nuclei with an abnormal chromatin pattern.

The use of tetracycline to produce fluorescence in malignant cells showed earlier promise, but recently because of indifferent discriminatory results between normal patients and those with gastric cancer the administration of tetracycline prior to exfoliative studies has been abandoned. Brush cytology practised at endoscopy is less laborious and gives better results from both stomach and colon.

II. BIOCHEMICAL AND ISOTOPE PROCEDURES

1. THE ESTIMATION OF GASTRIC SECRETORY FUNCTIONS
(see p. 70)

2. INSULIN TEST MEAL

The completeness of a vagotomy may be tested for by insulin hypo-glycaemia (20 units sol. Insulin i.m.) or with 2-deoxy-D-glucose which also causes hypoglycaemia (blood-glucose level should be 40 mg. per cent or less). Basal acid and volume are compared with the same parameters after hypoglycaemic gastric stimulation. A complete vagotomy is *not* associated with an increase of acid secretion > 1 mEq. compared with the basal hour in the 2 hours after the stimulus. An early (within 45 minutes) and a late response are recognized. The first is of more significance.

3. STUDIES OF GASTRIC pH

A 24-hour analysis of gastric secretion by measurement of the pH of hourly samples of gastric juice has been used as a screening test of gastric secretory function. In normal subjects mean pH values throughout the day are from 2·0 to 3·5 and there is a rise in pH (fall in acidity) after food and at night. In ulcer subjects the pH pattern varies with the site of the ulcer.

In gastric ulcer the pH is normal or above normal and shows the usual postprandial and nocturnal rise.

In duodenal ulcer the mean pH tends to be low (high acidity), there is little postprandial rise, and a low nocturnal figure.

This type of gastric secretory analysis has been shown to be of value:

1. *In the Diagnosis of the Cause of Upper Alimentary Bleeding*

Patients bleeding from chronic duodenal ulceration maintain their pattern of acid hypersecretion with a low nocturnal pH. Patients bleeding from chronic gastric ulcers tend to neutralize their acid secretion at night and acute peptic ulceration is often associated with achlorhydria.

2. *In the Diagnosis of Duodenal Ulceration, Gastric Ulcer, and Carcinoma*

Diagnosis will obviously not depend on pH studies alone and radiological support will be essential. In the patient with ulcer-type dyspepsia who has no radiological evidence of peptic ulceration low pH values would certainly support the diagnosis of duodenal ulcer. Likewise achlorhydria would intensify the hunt for a neoplasm.

3. *In the Diagnosis of the Zollinger-Ellison Syndrome*

High volumes and low pH values are characteristic.

Table 28. CHANGES IN GASTRIC pH

	RESTING pH	CHANGE IN pH AFTER MAXIMAL STIMULATION
Pernicious anaemia	7·0	± 1
Achlorhydria	3·5	-1
Hypochlorhydria	3·5	> -1
Normal	2·0–3·5	> -1 unless very low resting pH

Changes in gastric pH before and after maximal histamine secretion are given in *Table 28* (Callender, Retief, and Witts, 1960). Similar figures hold for pentagastrin.

4. PEPSIN SECRETION

The most convenient way of measuring gastric pepsin secretion is by the estimation of uropepsinogen in the urine. The activity of this substance is derived from the proteolytic activity of acidified urine on a suitable protein substrate such as pooled dried plasma. By using a Folin and Ciocalteau reagent and comparing the colour obtained with that of a standard solution of tyrosine a measure of urinary peptic activity is obtained. Values are in agreement with pepsin measured in gastric juice.

The following table indicates the disorders in which estimations of uropepsin may be of value:

VALUE	LESION
Normal	Gastric ulcer (provided no duodenal ulcer is present)
Raised	Duodenal ulcer Zollinger-Ellison syndrome
Low	Pernicious anaemia Total gastrectomy Most patients with partial gastrectomy Iron-deficiency anaemia Carcinoma of stomach

5. TUBELESS GASTRIC ANALYSIS

The advantage of this method is that the patient's ability to secrete acid can be measured without the discomfort or inconvenience of obtaining a specimen of gastric juice. Various substances have been used including those resins tabulated below.

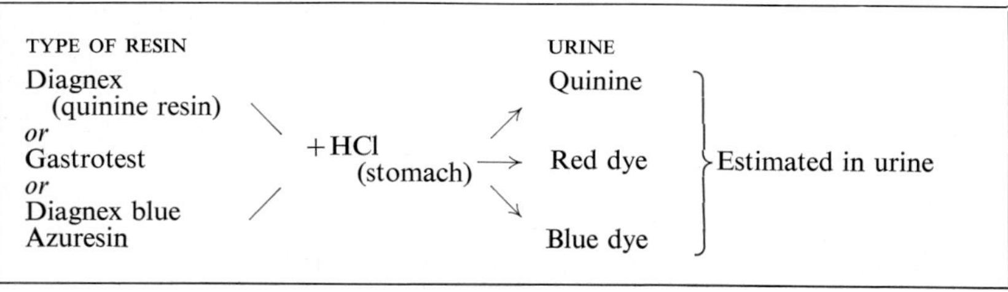

Pentagastrin 6 μg. per kg. body-weight may be given to stimulate acid production. A control specimen of urine collected over one hour is obtained after the bladder has been emptied and before the resin is given. Two hours after the test substance has been given urine is voided and the quinine or dye content determined.

These tests are useful for screening large numbers of patients for achlorhydria or for its detection in patients who cannot tolerate intubation.

LIVER FUNCTION TESTS

In many instances the so-called 'liver function tests' do not necessarily measure abnormalities related to liver disease. For example, the flocculation tests may be abnormal in any disease where there is excess production of globulins. The tests are best subdivided into the following groups:

1. *Estimation of Serum Bilirubin*

Normal value is 0·2–0·8 mg. per cent. Nearly all the normal pigment is unconjugated and gives a negative Van den Bergh reaction. Even if the serum bilirubin is within normal limits a positive direct Van den Bergh (due to the presence of conjugated bilirubin) indicates an abnormality.

2. *Detection of Urinary Bilirubin*

In obstructive and liver cell jaundice bilirubin is found in the urine. As well as altering the colour of the urine its presence can be confirmed by *Fouchet's test*. Urine is filtered after treatment with barium chloride. The precipitate which absorbs the bile-pigment turns blue when Fouchet's reagent (containing a diazo dye) is added. A tablet test based on the same type of reaction and colour change is also available (Ictotest, Ames Co.).

3. *Detection of Increased Urinary Urobilinogen*

Increased urinary urobilinogen is found in two conditions, haemolytic anaemia and liver cell dysfunction. In complete biliary obstruction urobilinogen disappears from the urine.

Urobilinogen is converted to urobilin after the urine has been exposed to air for some time. The easiest test to perform is that for urobilinogen in fresh urine, in which 8 drops of *Ehrlich's aldehyde* reagent are added to 5 ml. of freshly voided urine. A slight pink colour developing within a minute indicates a normal urobilinogen excretion and a cherry-red colour excess of this substance.

A rough quantitative estimate may be derived by tests on serial dilutions of urine. A pink colour obtained with a 1 : 20 or more dilution of urine indicates excess excretion. The pink colour can also be concentrated in chloroform, thus differentiating urobilinogen from porphobilinogen. In patients with bile-pigment in the urine, the test for urobilinogen is best performed after precipitation of bile-pigment with calcium chloride.

Van den Bergh Test

Students are often confused by this test. The application of Ehrlich's diazo-reagent (diazobenzene sulphonate) to icteric sera may give a red colour with sera from patients with obstructive or liver cell jaundice which contain conjugated bilirubin. This is a positive *direct* reaction. If alcohol is added to the reagents a positive reaction is also obtained in haemolytic jaundice. This is a positive *indirect* reaction.

The qualitative test may be of value in the diagnosis of jaundice because it allows a rough estimate to be made of the amount of conjugated and free bilirubin. In obstructive jaundice there may be a higher proportion of conjugated bilirubin than in patients with liver cell jaundice. In haemolytic jaundice and in normal subjects bilirubin is in the free form only. There is overlap, however, in the concentration of conjugated pigment in obstructive and liver cell disease.

The Serum Proteins

The normal total is 6·0–8·0 g. per 100 ml., albumin, 3·5–5·0 g per 100 ml., globulin (total), 2·0–3·3 g. per 100 ml. The albumin : globulin ratio is 1·2–2·4.

On electrophoresis, serum proteins can be divided into their components, namely, albumin and alpha-, beta-, and gamma-globulins. From the point of view of liver disease the protein fractions most susceptible to quantitative changes are the albumin, beta- and gamma-globulins.

Albumin levels fall if there is progressive liver cell disease because albumin is manufactured only by liver cells and because there may be an alteration of volume distribution. In acute liver cell disease albumin levels may remain within the normal range because of the comparatively slow turnover of this protein.

Increased levels of beta- and more particularly of gamma-globulin develop in response to liver cell injury, perhaps because of reticulo-endothelial proliferation. This increase is also responsible for another type of reaction—the altered flocculation tests. The common tests of this type depend on the fact that precipitation of beta- and gamma-globulin occurs when these proteins adhere to electronegative colloids such as colloidal gold, and to metallic salts such as zinc sulphate, or to organic compounds such as thymol. The colloidal gold turbidity, zinc sulphate turbidity, and thymol turbidity are positive because of hyperglobulinaemia and thus they are not specific for liver disease. Results of these tests are as follows:

NAME OF TEST	NORMAL RESULT	RESULT IN LIVER CELL DISEASE
Zinc sulphate turbidity	2–14 Kunkel units	May be raised > 14 Kunkel units
Thymol turbidity	0–4 units	May be raised > 5 units

Alteration of serum protein components in hepatocellular disease and in biliary obstruction where there is often a raised alpha-2 and beta-globulin level may be revealed by the electrophoretic strip, examples of which are shown in *Fig. 117*.

In many hospitals serum electrophoresis has completely replaced the flocculation tests. Separate analysis of immunoglobulins (gamma-globulins) is of little extra help in the diagnosis of liver disease though high IgM levels are of some diagnostic importance in patients with primary biliary cirrhosis.

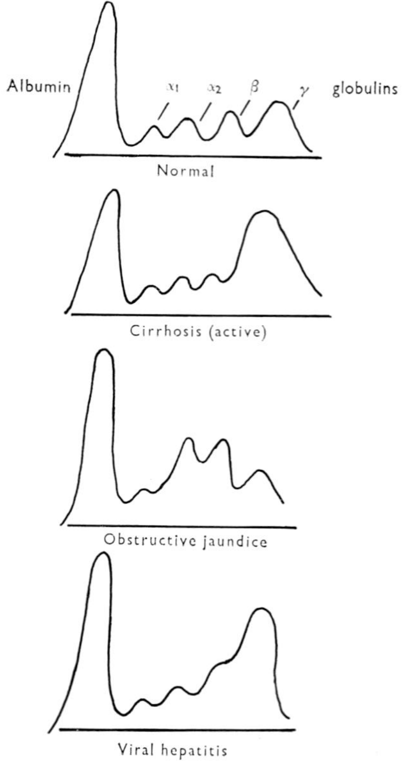

Fig. 117. Serum electrophoretic patterns in liver disease.

Alkaline Phosphatase

Normal serum value is 3–13 KA units. This enzyme is produced in bone as well as by liver cells. There are also contributions from the intestinal mucosa and in pregnancy from the placenta. The former is determined by the subject's blood group and secretor status, but in some disease states such as malabsorption this intestinal component may be raised. Excretion occurs through the biliary tract, so that patients with obstructive lesions at any site in the biliary tree have raised serum alkaline phosphatase values. In patients with obstructive jaundice the alkaline phosphatase is usually greater than 30 KA units, but it must not be forgotten that values in excess of this figure may be seen with liver cell disease and in other diseases such as Paget's and metabolic bone disease. Some help here in the distinction of bone from liver disease may be obtained by measuring the 5′-nucleotidase in the serum (normal serum level 2–17 i.u. per l). This enzyme is only elevated in liver disease and therefore distinguishes between a hepatic and an osseous cause for elevated alkaline phosphatase values in the serum—provided that both conditions are not present together. It is also now possible to separate chemically and electrophoretically the various isoenzymes of alkaline phosphatase and thus to determine their origin.

In the absence of jaundice the alkaline phosphatase can be elevated by partial biliary obstruction secondary to single or multiple hepatic lesions, e.g., cyst or neoplasm, or multiple granulomatous deposits of sarcoid. Tumours of various tissues are known to produce alkaline phosphatase and to cause elevation of serum values.

OTHER SERUM ENZYMES

Serum Transaminases

These enzymes are responsible for transfer of amino groups from donor alpha amino-acids to acceptor alpha keto-acids without the intermediate formation of ammonia. In tissues the only transaminases recognized are those utilizing a glutamic pyruvic system for amino transfer (serum glutamic pyruvic transaminase, or SGPT) and that using a glutamic oxaloacetic system (serum glutamic oxaloacetic transaminase, or SGOT). These enzymes have alternative names. SGOT is aspartate transaminase, whilst SGPT is alanine transaminase. Transamination plays a key role in intermediary metabolism as it provides a means for the synthesis and breakdown of amino-acids. The content of these two enzymes varies in different human tissues. A gramme of heart or liver tissue contains the same amount of GOT, but the liver contains six times more GPT than does the heart. When SGOT is elevated it usually exceeds SGPT, whatever the site of tissue destruction. When liver cells are damaged, SGOT and SGPT levels rise, but when destruction is severe, as in viral hepatitis or drug hepatitis, very high levels are found. Moderate elevations of serum transaminase activity in the serum occur in cirrhosis and in 50 per cent of patients with metastases or other space-occupying liver lesions. Serum transaminases are detected colorimetrically or spectrophotometrically.

RESULTS

	SGOT (*Int. units per ml.*)
Normal	Average 3–15
Hepatitis, etc.	Average 500–1000
Acute hepatic necrosis	Average 1000–2000
Cirrhosis	Average 40–200
Biliary obstruction	Average 40–300

Serum transaminase values are raised in non-hepatic disorders, e.g., in myocardial infarction, massive muscle and brain necrosis, etc., and are thus not specific for hepatobiliary disease.

Lactic Dehydrogenase (LDH)

This enzyme normally converts lactate into pyruvate. It is widely distributed in tissues, so that elevated levels appear in the serum whenever there is cell damage in the heart, liver, and muscles or there is disseminated malignant disease. It is comparatively easy to estimate. Substantial elevations are found in hepatitis, drug jaundice, certain anaemias, and infective mononucleosis, but in biliary obstruction, unless due to a neoplasm, normal values are usual. There are five iso-enzymes of LDH of which two—LD_4 and LD_5—are of hepatic origin. Estimation of the two fractions is therefore of value in the diagnosis of liver disease even when the serum total LDH is normal.

OTHER ENZYMES

Isocitric Dehydrogenase (ICD)

Two forms of this enzyme catalyse the oxidation of isocitrate to ketoglutarate. Though raised serum levels are occasionally found in non-hepatic disease, notably placental infarction, elevation is almost specific for liver cell lesions, such as virus and drug hepatitis, infective mononucleosis, and cirrhosis, and in some cases of intrahepatic malignancy. The specificity is helpful though sensitivity is low.

All these three enzymes can be estimated in the routine detection of liver disease, but the transaminases are estimated most often. ICD may be more helpful in the elucidation of hepatic problems.

Pseudocholinesterase

This enzyme, widely distributed in body tissues and plasma, acts on acetylcholine to produce choline. The liver is a good source of pseudocholinesterase and, in general, activity of this enzyme in the serum falls in chronic liver cell disease. A rise is of favourable prognostic import in cirrhosis. In obstructive jaundice normal levels are found.

OTHER LIVER FUNCTION TESTS

Serum Cholesterol and Lipoprotein X

Normal, 130–250 mg. per 100 ml. Esters, 60–75 per cent of total. The liver is an important source of cholesterol and damage to its cells causes the serum level to fall, whilst in biliary obstruction it rises. The proportion of cholesterol as an ester decreases in liver cell disease. The bile-salt-chelating agent cholestyramine causes a fall in serum cholesterol because of intensification of bile-salt synthesis from cholesterol. Lipoprotein X can also be detected immunologically in the serum of patients with obstructive jaundice.

Dye Extraction Tests

BROMSULPHTHALEIN (BSP)

This dye is removed from the circulation by the liver cell. Measurements to show the disappearance of the dye from the serum are therefore a delicate test, both of liver cell function and of the circulation to the liver. The test is invalidated by the presence of jaundice, but it is sensitive enough to detect slight impairments of function due to fatty infiltration or heart failure.

Method: Bromsulphthalein, 5 mg. per kg., is injected into a forearm vein. This should be done slowly because of the possibility of anaphylactoid reactions. Exactly 30 minutes later a specimen of 5 ml. of blood is taken from the opposite forearm and the hepatic BSP uptake is deduced from the amount retained in the serum. In normal persons the retention is up to 6 per cent and a figure greater than 10 per cent is abnormal. At 45 minutes retention of BSP greater than 5 per cent is also abnormal.

The metabolism of BSP depends on its uptake by the liver (and some other organs) and its excretion by the biliary apparatus after conjugation. The excretion rate into the bile (T_m) and the storage (S) of the dye in the liver can be calculated. Both of these parameters are reduced in liver disease though there is a differential effect depending on the type of pathology. Roughly speaking a diminution in S reflects a structural or functional decrease in liver tissue and a reduction in T_m mirrors an abnormality of biliary excretion. Together their estimation produces a highly sensitive test of liver function but the procedure demands two infusions of BSP at known concentration into the patient and multiple blood estimations as well as plasma-volume determination. Calculation is made by substitution in two equations obtained with different BSP concentrations, where $I = T_m + \Delta P(PV - S)$. I = infusion rate. T_m = transport maximum for BSP. ΔP = change in serum concentration. PV = plasma volume. S = storage of BSP. Normal values: T_m = 6–10 mg. per min, S = 50–90 mg. per mg. per cent.

Use of BSP to measure hepatic blood-flow: Bromsulphthalein has been used to measure hepatic blood-flow by utilizing the Fick principle. This necessitates infusing BSP into the patient until a constant blood-level is reached and then estimating its concentration in arterial and hepatic vein blood. As the blood-level remains constant, infusion is equal to hepatic extraction of dye, therefore the volume of blood flowing through the liver can be calculated from the difference between peripheral arterial and hepatic venous blood-dye levels.

Example

$$\frac{\text{Hepatic blood-flow}}{\text{(estimated)}} = \frac{\text{Rate of dye removal}}{\text{A} - \text{V dye difference}} \times \text{Haematocrit.}$$

If concentration in hepatic artery is kept constant:

$$\frac{\text{Hepatic blood-flow}}{\text{(ml. per min.)}} = \frac{\text{Rate of infusion}}{\text{A} - \text{V dye difference}} \times 100.$$

Liver blood-flow may also be measured from the plasma disappearance curve of a single injection of a radioactive colloid or indocyanine green. This method assumes complete extraction by one passage through the liver and is inaccurate where there is hepatic disease. Liver blood-flow studies are not of great clinical importance though there is no doubt that they would merit more attention if the separate contributions of the portal veins and hepatic artery could be easily and separately measured. This would be important particularly before portacaval anastomosis as post-operative complications may depend on the extent of the remaining hepatic artery flow.

CONGO RED TEST

Congo red, 15 ml. of 1·5 per cent, is injected intravenously and 5 minutes and 1 hour later 10 ml. of blood are withdrawn from the opposite forearm. Normally, less than 40 per cent of the amount of dye in the control (5-minutes) specimen disappears in the hour. In extensive amyloid disease the dye is taken up so rapidly from the blood that over 60 per cent may disappear. To make matters difficult, however, in cases of heavy proteinuria from whatever cause, excretion of the dye in the urine may lead to a rapid fall of serum levels.

ACTH Test

To distinguish between intrahepatic cholestasis due to virus hepatitis and other varieties of obstructive jaundice an ACTH or other corticosteroid test is often useful. After two or three daily determinations of serum bilirubin have shown a steady state, ACTH, 80 units intramuscularly, or prednisone 40 mg. (which is more convenient because it can be given orally) is given for five consecutive days and serum bilirubin estimations made. A steep fall in the serum bilirubin of more than 8 per cent daily suggests hepatitis. This 'test' can be misleading; we have personally seen jaundice caused by pancreatic carcinoma and gall-stones show a positive response.

SMALL-BOWEL FUNCTION

Proximal Small-bowel Function

a. GLUCOSE TOLERANCE TEST

A glucose tolerance curve is the result of many biochemical mechanisms; 50 g. of glucose in 200 ml. of fluid are administered by mouth to the fasting patient who should have received a full carbohydrate intake in the days before the test. Capillary or venous specimens are taken before and at half-hourly intervals after the glucose load and glucose levels are measured. Urine passed during the test is also analysed.

Examples of normal and abnormal glucose tolerance curves in gastro-intestinal disease are shown in the accompanying figure (*Fig. 118*). In patients with proximal gut lesions, e.g., due to the coeliac syndrome, 'flat' curves are usually obtained. In a flat glucose tolerance curve the rise in the blood-level is 40 mg. per cent or less.

It is often possible to detect whether malabsorption is due to a proximal mucosal defect or pancreatic disease by the shape of the curve, which is flat in the coeliac syndrome, or of diabetic type if pancreatic disease has interfered with the secretion of insulin. Patients with partial or total gastrectomy absorb glucose so quickly from the food which has passed rapidly into the jejunum that the first part of the curve is peaked. Increased insulin output may cause an equally rapid fall so that the rest of the curve is normal.

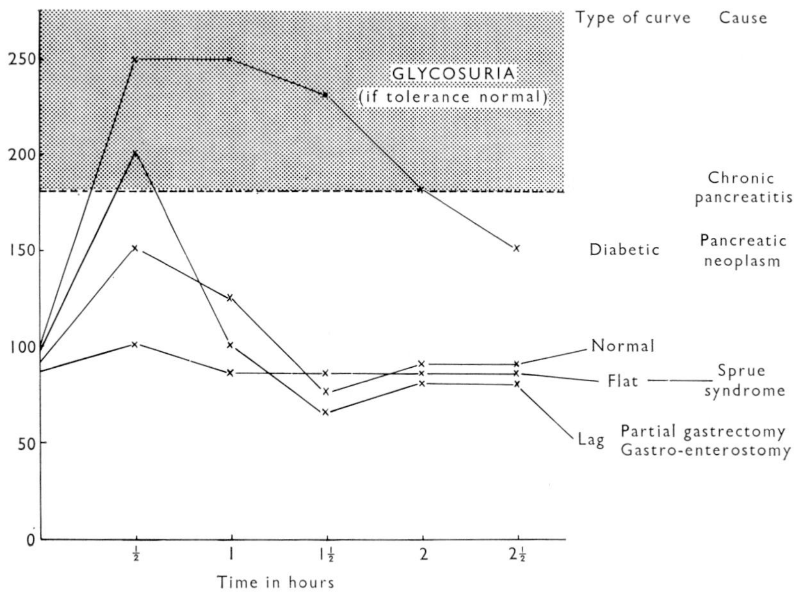

Fig. 118. Glucose tolerance in alimentary disease.

b. D-XYLOSE ABSORPTION

This pentose sugar has been used as an indicator of proximal small-bowel absorptive function. Although some have questioned the metabolic inertness of D-xylose it forms the basis of a clinically useful test. The patient fasts overnight and after emptying the bladder in the morning, 25 g. of xylose in 500 ml. of water are given by mouth. The urine is collected for the next 5 hours and its xylose content measured colorimetrically. Normal patients excrete more than 5 g. and those with a sprue syndrome less than this in the time allowed. Other diseases which affect the proximal small bowel can give a similar result. The D-xylose test is more usefully performed by using a 5-g. dose and by collecting specimens so that 2-hour and 5-hour urinary collections are made. The 5-g. dose avoids the possibility of diarrhoea and intestinal hurry seen with a 25-g. load and the 2- and 5-hour levels allow some estimate to be made of upper and lower small-bowel function. Normally the 2- and 5-hour excretion figures are 23 per cent and 35 per cent. A low 2-hour and normal 5-hour excretion suggests upper small-gut disease. Renal disease may limit its usefulness and allowance must be made for this in the elderly.

c. LACTOSE TOLERANCE TEST—LACTASE DEFICIENCY

Following 50 g. lactose orally the blood glucose should rise by more than 20 mg. per 100 ml. in a previously fasting subject. If there is no such rise 25 g. of glucose and 25 g. of galactose—the constituent monosaccharides —should produce a similar elevation of the respective blood levels. If these tests are negative this suggests a lactase deficiency which can be proved by estimating the enzyme in small intestinal mucosal specimens. Sucrase and maltase may also be estimated, though in primary lactase deficiency they are normal whereas when the syndrome is secondary to intestinal disease all three enzymes may be deficient.

'Mid' Small-bowel Function

THE INVESTIGATION OF FAT ABSORPTION

a. A 24-hour faecal collection.

In patients with gross steatorrhoea adequate chemical confirmation may be obtained by estimation of fat in a single day's collection.

b. The simplest, but probably least accurate, way of determining faulty fat absorption is to leave the patient on his normal diet, if this is not out of the ordinary, and to measure the daily fat excretion for three successive days. An excretion of over 18 g. in three days is diagnostic of steatorrhoea, but borderline cases or those with a wide scatter of daily values should have a 5-day fat balance.

c. Fat Balance. More satisfactory confirmation of steatorrhoea depends on balance studies. The principle is that the patient takes a constant fat intake and the faecal output is determined over five or more days. Some simple sources of error include the possibility that the patient does not consume all the dietary fat, which should be as near as possible to 100 g. daily, that faecal collections are incomplete, or that rest is a hospital bed so often causes constipation that the balance period is unrepresentative.

A preliminary period of three days on the diet is allowed so that equilibration takes place. A carmine marker can be administered at the beginning of the test and another at the end so that the period of collection is defined. Faeces are conveniently collected from a bed-pan with a detachable cellophane lining and transferred to disposable waxed cartons. The total collection is weighed, homogenized, and an aliquot for fat estimation dried and reweighed. The dried aliquot is extracted with ether and the lipids measured.

There has been a recent tendency to measure fat excretion in the faeces in relation to the concentration of non-absorbable marker, such as chromic oxide, which is administered by mouth and mixes with the intestinal contents. The necessity for long and tedious balance studies may be lessened by determining the fat and marker content of an aliquot of the faeces and calculating the daily fat excretion from knowledge of intake of the marker.

Results: Normal faecal fat, 15–22 per cent of dry weight (more than 25 per cent suggests steatorrhoea). Normal fat balance (on 100 g. fat diet) excretion of more than 6 g. per 24 hours suggests steatorrhoea.

Relatively little importance is now attached to split (15 per cent): unsplit (10 per cent) fat ratio. Normal faecal nitrogen, 1–2 g. per 24 hours.

d. Radioactive Fat Studies. Because of the length of time required for fat balance studies, and because of the unpleasant processes in the biochemical estimation, studies using radioactive fat have been well tried in certain centres. There are, however, grave sources of error, due particularly to the liberation of the labelled radioactive iodine (^{131}I) from the administered fat by the intestinal secretions before absorption. Further, stool collections are very likely to become contaminated by urine which will contain free ^{131}I.

In general the techniques are similar. After administering 600 mg. of potassium iodide thrice daily for three days before and throughout the study, neutral fat (triolein—^{131}I labelled) is administered to the fasting patient in a fatty vehicle such as milk or olive oil flavoured with fruit juice. The container is carefully washed out with the vehicle and a standard breakfast is eaten.

Serial specimens of blood for determination of radioactivity measure the absorption of fat into the blood-stream, and faeces, which are collected for three days, measure the fat excreted. If possible, urine should be collected separately and its radioactivity measured.

Steatorrhoea is characterized by the presence of a low plasma and high faecal radioactivity. Urine, if collected, will show a low activity in keeping with the serum.

Unfortunately, the snags prevent this method from displacing chemical estimations in the diagnosis of steatorrhoea. By using neutral (triolein) fat and fatty acid (oleic acid) tagged with ^{131}I some idea of pancreatic exocrine function can be obtained, for in pancreatic steatorrhoea fatty acid is more readily absorbed than neutral fat.

Microscopical Examination of Faeces

If performed properly this simple method can be used as a preliminary screening test for steatorrhoea.

Preparations of faeces are emulsified on a glass slide with ethyl alcohol and stained with alcoholic Sudan III. Neutral fat shows as yellow orange globules. Split fat in the form of soaps and glycerides is converted to free fatty acid by treatment with 36 per cent acetic acid followed by three periods of gentle heating to boiling point. Staining with Sudan III reveals free fatty acid as spherical droplets.

If there is gross faecal fat-loss, as in the sprue syndrome, a large number of fatty acid crystals are seen under the microscope. In pancreatic steatorrhoea neutral fat globules may be seen, but a large number of these may simply mean that the patient has taken liquid paraffin.

Distal Small-bowel Function

VITAMIN B_{12} STUDIES

Normal serum level, 140–900 μg. per ml. Vitamin B_{12} levels in the serum are determined by microbiological or immunoassay and in the various types of alimentary lesions a low level may be found. The organisms used in the microbiological assay are either *Lactobacillus leishmannii* or *Euglena gracilis*.

ABSORPTION STUDIES

Providing there is adequate gastric secretion of intrinsic factor the absorption of vitamin B_{12} is a measure of small-bowel function. By labelling with radioactive cobalt (usually [58]Co) this absorptive process can be followed. Various procedures are used:

1. After administration of an oral dose of [58]Co vitamin B_{12}, faeces are collected and the amount excreted subtracted from that administered, to give the amount absorbed.

2. *The Schilling Test.* A small dose (1 μg.) of radioactive vitamin B_{12} is administered by mouth to the fasting patient together with a large 'flushing' dose (1000 μg.) of vitamin B_{12} intramuscularly. The patient's urine is collected for twenty-four hours and the amount of the radioactive dose excreted in the urine expressed as a percentage of the administered dose. Normal patients excrete more than 15 per cent, patients with pernicious anaemia or after gastrectomy less than 5 per cent. The test can be repeated after antibiotics or with the addition of intrinsic factor in order to elucidate the cause of malabsorption. One slight objection to this test is the fact that the flushing dose adequately treats vitamin B_{12} deficiency and partially treats folic acid deficiency, so rendering further diagnostic tests difficult. A further modification is the use of a dose of vitamin B_{12} and another of vitamin B_{12} with intrinsic factor each being differentially labelled with separate isotopes ('Dicopac'). This allows the effect of the presence of intrinsic factor to be rapidly established in the same urine specimen.

3. By counting over the liver following an oral dose of [58]Co vitamin B_{12}. This method avoids the inaccuracy and unpleasantness of collecting faeces and will be described in detail.

A dose of 1 μg. of [58]Co vitamin B_{12} is given in 20 ml. of fluid to the fasting subject. Seven days later surface radioactivity over the liver is measured with a scintillation at two sites, usually in the midaxillary and midclavicular lines. If purgatives are used to clear unabsorbed radioactivity from the intestinal tract the count can be made three days after the oral dose. If radioactivity over the lower abdomen is high this suggests intestinal stasis, in which case hepatic counting should be deferred.

If you wish to know the percentage of the dose which is absorbed the procedure is repeated after an *intramuscular* injection of the same dose of [58]Co vitamin B_{12}. The hepatic radioactivity after the oral dose is then expressed as a percentage of that after the intramuscular dose.

Normally about one-third of the oral dose (more than 0·28 μg. of 1 μg.) is absorbed. The effects of antibiotics and intrinsic factor on vitamin B_{12} absorption can also be determined by this method.

OTHER TESTS RELEVANT TO MALABSORPTION

Tests of Folic Acid Metabolism

a. SERUM FOLATE LEVELS

Normal, 6–20 ng. per ml. (as *L. casei* activity). Deficiency of folic acid can be detected by estimation of its serum level by microbiological assay with the organism *Lactobacillus casei*. If there is deficiency the level is below 6 ng., and if this deficiency is responsible for megaloblastic anaemia levels below 4 ng. are usually found. Total *red-cell* folate is probably a more accurate test for folate deficiency and is performed on whole blood. Normal levels for red-cell folate are 160–700 ng. per ml. (assuming haematocrit is 45 per cent).

b. EXCRETION OF FORMIMINOGLUTAMIC ACID (FIGLU)

This substance is excreted in the urine in increased amounts in folic acid deficiency. FIGLU is a normal breakdown product of the essential amino-acid, histidine. Tetrahydrofolic acid is required for the conversion of FIGLU to glutamic acid.

This test is performed after histidine loading. The patient fasts overnight and on waking empties his bladder and then takes 15 g. of histidine dissolved in fruit juice. The patient then resumes a normal fluid intake and empties the bladder three hours after taking the histidine. The urine passed from 3 to 8 hours after the loading dose of histidine is collected in a sterile Winchester containing a few crystals of thymol and its volume recorded. The urine is examined electrophoretically.

A rough quantitative measure of the amount of FIGLU can be obtained by comparing the intensity of the 'spot' with that of controls of known FIGLU concentration, or more simply graded $+$ to $+ + +$. It can also be quantitated.

c. FOLIC ACID ABSORPTION

A folic acid absorption test has been developed to detect abnormal absorption resulting from small-bowel disease. The test is performed after previous saturation of the patient with intramuscular folic acid, 15 mg. daily for 3 days. The rise of serum folic acid is estimated by a bio-assay method after an oral dose of 40 μg. per kg. given 36 hours after the last of the loading doses. In normal subjects a rise of greater than 40 mμg. per ml. is obtained, but if absorption is impaired in patients with a widespread mucosal defect, as in the sprue syndrome, this level is not reached.

d. SERUM AMYLASE OR DIASTASE

Some of the amylase produced by the pancreas is absorbed into the bloodstream. The concentration of this enzyme expressed as Somogyi units is

18

estimated by determining the liberation of glucose per 100 ml. of plasma from excess starch at 37° C. and *p*H 7·2. In acute pancreatitis or complete obstruction of the pancreatic duct very high amylase concentrations occur in the plasma. In pancreatitis peak concentrations are usually reached 12 to 48 hours after the onset. Moderately elevated amylase levels can also occur in peritonitis, perforation, and obstruction of the alimentary tract, and inflammatory diseases of the salivary glands, e.g., mumps, etc. Other causes include a dilated afferent loop following Polya gastrectomy, and recently binding of amylase to globulin as macromolecular complexes has been noted as a further cause. In acute or chronic renal failure the serum level may be elevated from impaired excretion and this factor may also operate in acute pancreatitis. The measurement of urinary amylase levels may also be useful in the diagnosis of acute pancreatitis and the comparatively slow excretion may make it of value at a late stage when serum levels are near normal. In chronic pancreatitis the serum amylase is normal unless there are acute exacerbations.

Normal range is 60–180 Somogyi units; in acute pancreatitis, 300–2000 Somogyi units (usually more than 1000 units).

e. SERUM LIPASE

Though more difficult to estimate than amylase, serum lipase levels are raised in acute pancreatitis and stay higher for longer.

f. 5-HYDROXYINDOLACETIC ACID (5-HIAA)

The simplest procedure available for the diagnosis of serotonin excess in the carcinoid syndrome is the estimation in the urine of its breakdown product, 5-hydroxyindolacetic acid (5 HIAA). The easiest method is a colorimetric one using a nitrosonaphthol indicator after the extraction by chloroform of hydroxyindoles. In most cases the 5 HIAA is 10–100 times the normal value and is best estimated on an aliquot of a 24-hour specimen. This should be collected in a Winchester containing toluene and 20–25 ml. of glacial acetic acid.

Normal is 2·0–14 mg. per 24 hours; carcinoid (average), 100–800 mg. per 24 hours.

Various drugs such as reserpine and chlorpromazine interfere with the estimation of this substance. The patient must also avoid bananas.

g. URINARY INDOXYL SULPHATE

This is a valuable indicator of the presence of small intestinal bacteria and is easily estimated in an aliquot of a 24-hour urine specimen collected into a bottle containing a little chloroform or ether. The amount of indoxyl sulphate present is estimated colorimetrically following treatment with *p*-dimethylaminobenzaldehyde. Values of greater than 80 mg. per 24 hours are abnormal and values over 150 mg. per 24 hours suggest severe bacterial contamination.

INTUBATION OF THE SMALL BOWEL FOR BACTERIOLOGICAL STUDIES

A simple sterile polyvinyl tube is usually adequate and can be screened into the desired position. Specimens can be aspirated at intervals and should be obtained fasting and after food. Specimens are sent for aerobic and anaerobic culture and counts of $> 10^5$ organisms per ml. indicate significant bacterial contamination. *Esch. coli* and *Bacteroides* are the important organisms as regards the pathogenesis of the blind-loop syndrome.

PANCREATIC FUNCTION TESTS (*see* (*d*) *and* (*e*) *above*)

1. Exocrine Function

SECRETIN–PANCREOZYMIN TEST

A double-lumen tube is passed under fluoroscopic control so that its tip is in the third part of the duodenum and one lumen opens in the stomach. Continuous suction of the latter prevents the entry of gastric juice into the duodenum. A duodenal secretion consisting largely of pancreatic secretion can thus be obtained after twenty minutes, during which acid-contaminated duodenal juice is aspirated and discarded.

Secretin (1·0 unit per kg.), either alone or with pancreozymin (1·7 units per kg.) (Boots), is injected intravenously after two 10-minute periods of control in which secretions have been aspirated. A marked increase in the volume of the duodenal aspirate should follow the injection, and specimens aspirated in six 10-minute periods are collected in glass tubes standing in an ice-bath. After the volume of the aspirates has been measured specimens are diluted with an equal volume of glycerol and stored on ice until estimations of bicarbonate and amylase (and sometimes trypsin and lipase) can be made. Serial specimens of blood may also be taken for estimation of amylase at intervals up to 6 hours after the injection and again at 24 hours.

Results are shown in *Tables 29* and *30*. A simple version of this test measures the bicarbonate response (normal greater than 100 mEq. per l.) to secretin alone. This obviously avoids the collection for, and the estimation of enzyme levels.

SINGLE DUODENAL INTUBATION

A simple screening test for impaired pancreatic exocrine function consists in the aspiration of duodenal juice to test for tryptic activity. Tests of faecal tryptic activity may also be of value, providing that a sensitive method relatively specific for trypsin is used. This can be done by using a sulphonilic acid azocasein substrate and allowing digestion with faeces or duodenal juice to proceed at pH 8·3. The products of tryptic digestion are estimated colorimetrically.

Normal values are: duodenal trypsin, 10–60 units per ml.; faecal trypsin, 10–100 units per ml.

Table 29. RESULTS OF SECRETIN–PANCREOZYMIN TEST—
DUODENAL JUICE

	DUODENAL JUICE (*vol.*)	BICARBONATE	AMYLASE	TRYPSIN	LIPASE
				(*usually not estimated*)	
Normal	130–250 ml./hr.	90–130 mEq./l.	300–1200 units/hr.	20–40 units/hr.	7000– 14,000 units/hr.
Abnormal					
a. Carcinoma of pancreas (blocked pancreatic duct)	↓	↓	↓	↓	↓
b. Chronic pancreatitis	↓	↓	↓	↓	↓
c. Carcinoma of biliary tract	Slight ↓	Normal	Normal	Normal	Normal
d. Non-pancreatic steatorrhoea	Normal	Normal	Normal	Normal	Normal

Table 30. SERUM LEVELS AFTER SECRETIN–PANCREOZYMIN

	AMYLASE	LIPASE
Normal fasting	70–130 units/ml.	0·5–1·15 units/ml.
After secretin–pancreozymin	No change	No change
Carcinoma of pancreas		
After secretin–pancreozymin	Raised (normal fasting value)	Raised (raised fasting value)
Chronic pancreatitis		
After secretin–pancreozymin	Raised (raised fasting value)	Raised (raised fasting value)
Cancer of biliary tract		
After secretin–pancreozymin	Raised (normal fasting value)	Raised (normal fasting value)

THE LUNDH TEST MEAL

A weighted and perforated radio-opaque tube is screened into the region of the duodenojejunal flexure and a test meal comprising 18 g. of corn or soya-bean oil, 40 g. of glucose, and 15 g. of casilan is administered in 300 ml. of warm water. The duodenum is drained over 2 hours in half-hourly collections of which the *p*H, volume, and tryptic activity are measured. In normal subjects tryptic activity lies between 11 and 20 i.u. per 2 hours. Low values are seen in pancreatitis, pancreatic cancer, and steatorrhoea of various causes. Unlike other pancreatic function tests it is easy to perform and though probably less reliable than the secretin–pancreozymin test it is a useful screening test for chronic pancreatic disease.

2. Endocrine Function

There are three tests for endocrine function, the glucose tolerance test (*see* p. 420) the tolbutamide tolerance test, and serum insulin levels.

The *tolbutamide* tolerance test, in that it measures the ability of the pancreas to secrete insulin and does not, as does the *glucose* tolerance test, measure several parameters of carbohydrate metabolism including absorption, is a useful test of pancreatic function. The test measures impairment of pancreatic function as in chronic pancreatitis or pancreatic tumours.

Following a diet containing 300 g. of carbohydrate daily for three days the patient is fasted overnight. One gramme of sodium tolbutamide in 10 ml. of saline is administered intravenously after a fasting specimen of blood for glucose determination has been taken. Further specimens of blood are taken at 20, 30, and 60 minutes after the injection and then hourly for 3 hours. In normal subjects there is a fall of the 30-minute blood-glucose amounting to 75 per cent of the initial value. The fall is greater and more prolonged if an insulinoma is present.

SERUM INSULIN LEVELS

In conjunction with a glucose tolerance test serum insulin levels may confirm endocrine pancreatic deficiency in patients with suspected exocrine failure and may be useful in the diagnosis of insulinoma (*see* p. 240).

EXAMINATION OF THE FAECES FOR OCCULT BLOOD

If there is frank blood in the faeces tests are obviously not required for its detection, though it is surprising how often such specimens are sent to the laboratory. Tests for occult blood, however, are amongst the most valuable diagnostic aids available to the clinician.

The detection of occult blood in the faeces depends on the fact that certain substances such as benzidine and orthotoluidine are oxidized in the presence of blood to produce blue compounds. Orthotoluidine was the standard reagent used and was most conveniently used in the form of a tablet (Haematest, Ames Co.).

Recent legislation has restricted the use of these substances because of possible carcinogenic properties so that both benzidine and orthotoluidine have disappeared from the laboratory and clinic room. This is an unfortunate state of affairs as one is now without a sensitive and easily handled tablet test. Only guaiac, most conveniently used as a guaiac-impregnated filter paper with hydrogen peroxide developer, is left. Guaiac tests are sensitive to intestinal blood-loss of the order of 10 ml. per day. Reagents may deteriorate and must be checked at regular intervals.

Radioactive Methods

The patient's red blood-cells may be labelled with chromium (^{51}Cr) and stools collected for estimation of radioactivity. The technique can be made to detect blood-loss of less than 10 ml. of blood up to six weeks after labelling of the cells. As homogenization of faecal samples is necessary

18*

the technique is unpleasant unless complex counting equipment is available. The technique has the advantage that it only detects blood from non-dietary sources, but it is time-consuming and thus more suited to studies of faecal blood-loss over a period of several weeks in a small number of patients. It does allow a quantitative expression of faecal blood-loss.

Samples of small intestinal contents obtained through a tube which is progressively passed downwards may be assayed for radioactivity and thus information obtained as to the site of alimentary bleeding.

The String Test

This test may also help to decide from which point in the upper alimentary tract recurrent bleeding is occurring. The 'string' used in the test is a cotton tape about 0·5 cm. wide and 2 m. long with suitable radio-opaque markers at 30 cm. intervals along it. A small volume of mercury in a finger-cot enables the apparatus, when swallowed, to navigate the pylorus. The patient, who should be fasting, swallows the string after it has been immersed in water. Within two to three hours the end of the string should reach the duodenojejunal flexure if the patient has been lying on his right side. A plain film of the abdomen is taken. An intravenous injection of 20 ml. of 5 per cent fluorescein is given and after 5 minutes the apparatus is withdrawn. The string is examined in ultra-violet light. Intestinal bleeding is identified by fluorescence, but when bleeding is rapid there may be blood-staining as well.

The area of fluorescence is related to the appropriate radio-opaque markers on the plain film and the site of alimentary bleeding thus identified. The string can be left in situ for a longer period than 2–3 hours in order to obtain information about possible bleeding sites in the rest of the small bowel. Unfortunately string tests cannot always be relied on for an accurate answer and false positives may ensue from trauma to the mucosa from the string. Intestinal angiography may be a more successful procedure in the face of definite alimentary bleeding.

Estimation of Alimentary Protein Loss

In recent years it has been recognized that alimentary loss of protein occurs in a variety of intestinal lesions, including giant hypertrophic gastritis, the sprue syndrome, Crohn's disease, and ulcerative colitis. Methods have been devised to detect and estimate the magnitude of this loss.

If intravenous ^{131}I radioactive human albumin is given and faeces collected some radioactivity may be found in the faeces. Unfortunately, albumin which 'leaks' into the gut is digested so that the label is split off, reabsorbed, and re-excreted into the gut, thus giving very little idea of the amount lost into the gut. If an inert substance of similar particle size, such as polyvinylpyrrolidine, is labelled (^{131}I PVP) no such digestion takes place, and loss of labelled material in the faeces is a pointer to protein loss from the same route. There are, however, difficulties even with PVP, which is not a physiological substance, is of variable particle size, and tends to be removed by the reticulo-endothelial system. Its introduction was, however, a significant step forward in the investigation of protein loss from the gut.

The material is injected i.v. after suppression of thyroid uptake with oral iodine. The faeces are collected for 4 days and must not be contaminated by urine which will contain large amounts of radioactivity. Less than 1·5 per cent of the injected dose is normally found in the 4-day collection, but in patients with intestinal protein loss figures may reach 30 per cent or more.

Chromium-labelled albumin seems to be an improvement upon ^{131}I PVP, but the latter has a place in clinical practice, whilst substances such as ^{51}Fe-labelled iron dextran, Niobium–^{95}Nb–albumin and ^{67}Cu–caeruloplasmin have some advantages both in the detection of gut protein loss and in protein turnover studies.

III. ENDOSCOPY AND INVESTIGATION OF ALIMENTARY MOTILITY

ENDOSCOPY

With the introduction of fibre-optic instruments the necessity for using rigid and semi-rigid instruments for the examination of the stomach has passed. Not only has this made examination more comfortable and safer for the patient but it has allowed this type of procedure to be used in those who were not fit enough for conventional gastroscopy and endoscopy. The present instruments are flexible—easy to pass and possess facilities for biopsy under direct vision as well as photography (*Fig. 119*) and cytology. Distension of the stomach with air and cleaning of the lens may also be made semi-automatic with a suitable power unit. The Olympus or the A.C.M.I. fibre-optic oesophago-gastroduodenoscope offers excellent

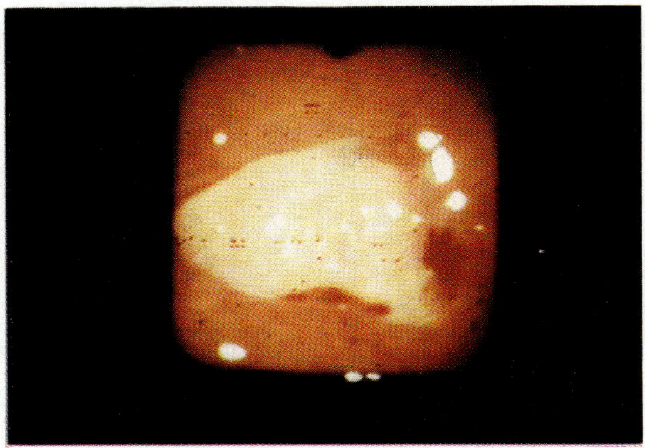

Fig. 119. A large duodenal ulcer seen at duodenoscopy.

visualization of the oesophagus, all areas of the stomach and proximal duodenal loop. Full visualization is obtained by means of the fully movable tip which can be directed through a range of 120°. Biopsy, photography, and exfoliative cytology of suspicious lesions are all possible. The examination of the colon with a flexible colonoscope offers similar facilities for examination of the whole colon, distal ileum, and caecum. The side-viewing duodenoscope allows visualization and cannulation of the ampulla of Vater so that the pancreatic and bile-duct systems can be opacified with radio-opaque contrast (*Fig. 120*).

There are no exact indications for fibre-endoscopy but its use is indicated in situations such as:

a. Dysphagia.

b. Upper alimentary bleeding.

c. The identification of acute and chronic gastric and duodenal ulcers. Chronic gastric ulcers may be photographed and biopsied and malignancy more confidently excluded.

d. The identification of gastric tumours both benign and malignant.

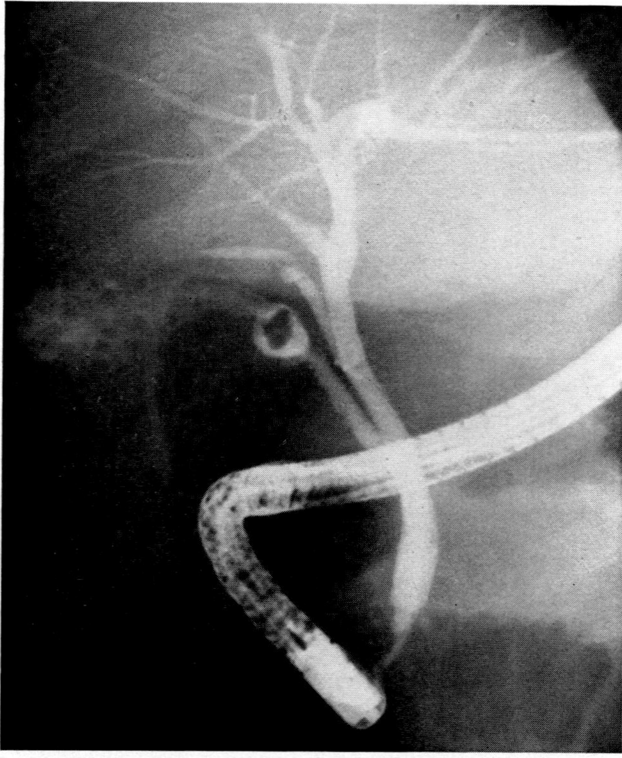

Fig. 120. Opacification of the biliary tract in a patient with attacks of right upper abdominal pain, using the technique of endoscopic retrograde cholangiopancreatography (ERCP). The cholecystogram was not helpful but ERCP shows multiple non-opaque gall-stones in the gall-bladder with a larger one in the cystic duct. The bile-ducts are normal.

e. The identification of duodenal ulcers particularly when barium X-rays are not helpful.

f. Examination of the duodenal bulb—second part of duodenum—and the identification and canalization of the pancreatic and biliary ducts have now considerably enlarged the diagnostic possibilities of endoscopy to include pancreatic and biliary disease.

Examination of the sigmoid and ascending colon by colonoscopy is of great value in the diagnosis of polyps, neoplastic and inflammatory disease of the colon, whilst the longer instruments enable visualization of the right side of the colon including the radiologically difficult caecal area. They have also been used to visualize the small bowel as far as the ileocaecal valve and removal of colonic polyps is now possible with the colonoscope and a snare.

Sigmoidoscopy

The onset of diarrhoea, lower intestinal bleeding, and other symptoms suggestive of colonic disease are indications for rectal examination followed by sigmoidoscopy. The latter can be performed under general anaesthesia, but using a small-calibre instrument such as the Lloyd Davis apparatus, the procedure is usually well tolerated without special preparation. Rectal wash-outs prior to examination hinder rather than help and providing that there is no gross constipation a simple bowel action, helped if necessary by a glycerin suppository, is all that is required. The examination can be performed in the left lateral or knee-elbow position. Patients prefer the former, in which case a sandbag under the left buttock and a firm mattress facilitate the procedure.

The apparatus is lubricated and thoroughly tested before use. With the obturator in position, and after preliminary digital examination of the rectum, the instrument is gently passed through the anal sphincter and directed towards the umbilicus into the rectal ampulla. The obturator is then withdrawn and the eyepiece, with its lighting and bellows attachment, fitted. The instrument is then advanced into the rectum using the bellows to separate the rectal walls. At about 15 cm. from the anal margin the instrument can usually be passed into the sigmoid colon. This may cause some discomfort to the patient as it is usually achieved by altering the line of direction of the instrument to navigate the angle between the rectum and sigmoid colon. Once round the flexure the instrument can be advanced to 25 cm.

If faeces bar the way, patient cleaning with swabs on the end of long-handled sigmoidoscopy forceps may allow progress. Careful attention is paid to the mucosa, its vascular pattern, surface, and friability. Biopsy of any ulcers or polyps can be done with biopsy forceps, and scrapings, rectal 'snips', or swabs sent for pathological examination. If sigmoidoscopy is unsuccessful the procedure is best repeated in hospital if necessary after bowel preparation and under general anaesthesia. Colonoscopy with a flexible fibre-optic instrument is an alternative approach and has the advantage of accessibility to the whole of the large bowel, but should follow sigmoidoscopy.

Peritoneoscopy

This is a valuable way in which to inspect certain abdominal viscera, particularly the liver, gall-bladder, spleen, and their peritoneal coverings. It had relatively few protagonists in this country until a year or two ago though it has been more popular in Europe.

After premedication and the marking of enlarged viscera on the abdominal wall a pneumoperitoneum is induced using a Maxwell pneumotherapy apparatus. Alternatively, carbon dioxide can be used and though still giving rise to discomfort in some patients it obviates the risk of air embolus. A small incision is made through the skin slightly away from the midline and midway between xiphisternum and umbilicus. Liberal injection of local anaesthetic agents, e.g., xylocaine 2 per cent, is important down to, and including, the peritoneum which is easily identified because of the pneumoperitoneum. The tissues are separated with sinus forceps and the trocar inserted. The apparatus, thoroughly tested and slightly warmed to prevent condensation on the eyepiece, is then introduced into the abdominal cavity. (*Note.*—In cases of considerable hepatomegaly the point of insertion of the trocar must be considerably lower.)

The liver and spleen are usually well seen and the examination is facilitated by the use of a tipping table and by making sure that the pneumoperitoneum is maintained by occasional refills. Biopsy of the liver can be carried out under direct vision.

This procedure is valuable in the detection of hepatic cirrhosis and hepatic metastases and saves the patient a formal laparotomy. It may be of value in the diagnosis of cirrhosis when liver biopsy is contra-indicated because of coagulation difficulties.

Motility and Pressure Changes in the Alimentary Tract

Recent workers have used pressure-sensitive radio-pills which are swallowed by the patient to detect changes in alimentary pressures and motility. These radiotelemetering capsules emit a radio-signal which can be detected and recorded by a suitable external recording system. Pressure variations in the gut are transferred to a rubber or perspex diaphragm in the capsule which, by its movement of a ferrite core, modifies inductance in the capsule circuit, thus emitting a signal. The apparatus is calibrated before use, and can be used with little inconvenience to the patient to record both pressure and mobility changes in the gut. Localization of the capsule is achieved by radiological screening with an image intensifier.

Gastro-intestinal motility has also been studied in man by recording the pressure changes within intraluminal balloons. There are, however, certain limitations of this method because, unless the balloons are small, they may well induce abnormal movements and pressure changes. Open-ended polythene tubes containing either air or water do not have this disadvantage and the pressure changes are recorded either electrically or with the aid of an optic manometer. Studies with open-ended tubes have given valuable information about pressure changes in the lower oesophagus and the motility of the colon. The changes in the colon are particularly important as hypermotility seems to be the basis for the syndrome of spastic or irritable colon and of its possible successor, diverticular disease.

PARACENTESIS ABDOMINIS

The indications for this procedure in patients with cirrhosis are given in Chapter 14.

The patient lies on a firm mattress, and a many-tailed bandage and macintosh sheet are placed under him. He empties his bladder at the start of this procedure. A site for puncture is chosen in the flank well below the point at which the central gut resonance to percussion is replaced by dullness due to fluid. A small amount of local anaesthetic is introduced into the skin and subcutaneous tissues, and with a longer needle a further amount is used to infiltrate the deeper structures and peritoneum. The trocar and cannula are inserted through a small skin incision and fluid is collected through attached tubing into a Winchester bottle. There seems to be little difference concerning the severity of side-effects when decompression is rapid or slow. Tightening the binder allows drainage to proceed more evenly and supports the abdomen.

Specimens of fluid may be sent for bacteriological, biochemical, and cytological examination. If diagnostic tapping only is required specimens may easily be obtained with an ordinary needle and a 10-ml. syringe.

Side-effects are few, but special hazards may exist in the cirrhotic patient.

FURTHER READING

Liver Needle Biopsy
MENGHINI, G. (1958), 'One-second Needle Biopsy of the Liver', *Gastroenterology*, **35**, 190.
READ, A. E. (1971), 'Needle Biopsy of the Liver', *Br. J. Hosp. Med.*, **5**, 84.
SHERLOCK, S. (1962), 'Needle Biopsy of the Liver. A Review', *J. clin. Path.*, **15**, 291.

Small-bowel Biopsy
BRANDBORG, L. L., RUBIN, C. E., and QUINTON, W. E. (1959), 'A Multipurpose Instrument for Suction Biopsy of the Oesophagus, Stomach, Small Bowel, and Colon', *Gastro-enterology*, **37**, 1.
CROSBY, W. H., and KUGLER, H. W. (1957), 'Intraluminal Biopsy of the Small Intestine', *Am. J. dig. Dis.*, **2**, 236.

Exfoliative Cytology
BURN, J. I., and SELLWOOD, R. A. (1962), 'The Results of Exfoliative Cytology Studies in 50 Patients with Symptoms of Large Bowel Disorder', *Gut*, **3**, 32.
GEPHART, T., and GRAHAM, R. M. (1959), 'The Cellular Detection of Carcinoma of the Esophagus', *Surgery Gynec. Obstet.*, **108**, 75.

Gastric Secretion
BARON, J. H. (1970), 'The Clinical Use of Gastric Function Tests', *Proc. 4th World Cong. of Gastroenterology, 1970, Scand. J. Gastroent.*, **5**, Suppl. 6, 9.
BOCK, O. A., and WITTS, L. J. (1961), 'Tubeless Gastric Analysis', *Br. med. J.*, **2**, 665.
CALLENDER, S. T., RETIEF, F. P., and WITTS, L. J. (1960), 'The Augmented Histamine Test with Special Reference to Achlorhydria', *Gut*, **1**, 326.
CHANDLER, G. N., and WATKINSON, G. (1959), 'The Early Diagnosis of the Causes of Haematemesis', *Q. Jl Med.*, **52**, 371.
HOLLANDER, F. (1946), 'The Insulin Test for the Presence of Intact Nerve Fibres after Vagal Operations for Peptic Ulcer', *Gastroenterology*, **7**, 607.
KAY, A. W. (1953), 'Effect of Large Doses of Histamine on Gastric Secretion of HCl', *Br. med. J.*, **2**, 77.
SIRCUS, W. (1954), 'Studies of Uropepsinogen Excretion in Gastrointestinal Disorders', *Q. Jl Med.*, **47**, 291.

Liver Function Tests

Bilirubin
BILLING, B. H. (1963), 'Bilirubin Metabolism', *Post-grad. med. J.*, **39**, 176.

Serum Proteins
HILL, P. G., and SAMMONS, H. G. (1967), 'An Assessment of 5'-nucleotidase as a Liver Function Test', *Q. Jl Med.*, **36**, 457.
MARTIN, N. H., and NEUBERGER, A. (1957), 'Protein Metabolism and the Liver', *Br. med. Bull.*, **13**, 113.
ZIMMERMAN, H. (1964), 'Serum Enzymes in Diagnosis of Hepatic Disease', *Gastroenterology*, **46**, 613.

Scintiscanning of the Liver
JONES, E. A., and JIRSA, M. (1967), 'Liver Scintillography', in *The Liver* (ed. READ, A. E.), vol. 4, p. 139, *The Colston Papers*. London: Butterworths.

Bromsulphthalein Metabolism
ZAMCHECK, N., CHALMERS, T. C., WHITE, F. W., and DAVIDSON, C. S. (1950), 'The BSP Test in the Early Diagnosis of Liver Disease in Gross Gastrointestinal Haemorrhage', *Gastroenterology*, **14**, 343.

Enzymes
HARGREAVES, T., JANOTA, I., and SMITH, M. J. (1961), 'Multiple Plasma Enzyme Activities in Liver Disease', *J. clin. Path.*, **14**, 283.

Transaminases
SOMMERVILLE, R., FLEISHER, G. A., DEARING, W. H., HALLENBECK, G. A., and DOCKERTY, M. B. (1960), 'Transaminases in Hepatic Tissue and Serum in Hepatic Disease', *Gastroenterology*, **38**, 926.

Isocitric Dehydrogenase
BELL, J. L., SHALDON, S., and BARON, D. N. (1962), 'Serum Isocitrate Dehydrogenase in Liver Disease and Other Conditions', *Clin. Sci.*, **23**, 57.

Hepatic Blood-flow
BRADLEY, S. E., INGELFINGER, F. J., and BRADLEY, G. P. (1952), 'Hepatic Circulation in Cirrhosis of the Liver', *Circulation*, **5**, 419.
DOBSON, E. L., and JONES, H. B. (1952), 'Behaviour of Intravenously Injected Particulate Material and its Rate of Disappearance from the Blood Stream as a Measure of Liver Blood Flow', *Acta med. scand.*, **144**, suppl. 273, 1.

Corticosteroid Test
SUMMERSKILL, W. H. J., and JONES, F. A. (1958), 'Corticotrophin and Steroids in the Diagnosis and Management of "Obstructive" Jaundice', *Br. med. J.*, **2**, 1499.

Small-bowel Function

Xylose Absorption
SAMMONS, H. G., MORGAN, D. B., FRAZER, A. C., MONTGOMERY, R. D., PHILIP, W. M., and PHILLIPS, M. J. (1967), 'Modification in the Xylose Absorption Test as an Index of Intestinal Function', *Gut*, **8**, 348.
SHINER, M., VAKIL, B. J., and WILCOX, P. B. (1962), 'Urinary Xylose Excretion in Steatorrhoea', *Ibid.*, **3**, 240.

Lactose Intolerance
MCMICHAEL, H. B., WEBB, J., and DAWSON, A. M. (1965), 'Lactose Deficiency in Adults', *Lancet*, **1**, 717.

Fat Metabolism
DRUMMEY, G. D., BENSON, J. A., and JONES, C. M. (1961), 'Microscopical Examination of the Stool for Steatorrhoea', *New Engl. J. Med.*, **264**, 85.
WALKER, W. F., STEWART, W. K., MORGAN, H. G., and MCKIE, J. (1960), 'Clinical Assessment of Intestinal Fat Absorption using Radioactive Fat', *Br. med. J.*, **1**, 1403.
WHITBY, L. G., and LANG, D. (1960), 'Experience with the Chromic Oxide Method of Faecal Marking in Metabolic Balance Investigations on Humans', *J. clin. Invest.*, **39**, 854.

Vitamin B_{12} Absorption
GLASS, G. B., BOYD, L. J., GELLIN, G. A., and STEPHANSON, L. (1954), 'Uptake of Radioactive Vitamin B_{12} by the Liver in Humans: Test for Measurement of Intestinal Absorption of Vitamin B_{12} and Intrinsic Factor Activity', *Archs Biochem. Biophys.*, **51**, 251.
SCHILLING, R. F. (1953), 'Intrinsic Factor Studies', *J. lab. clin. Med.*, **42**, 860.

Serum Vitamin B₁₂ Level
MATTHEWS, D. M. (1962), 'Observations on the Estimation of Serum Vitamin B_{12} using *Lacsobacillus Leishmannii*', *Clin. Sci.*, **22**, 101.

Serum Folate (Folic acid)
WATERS, A. H., and MOLLIN, D. L. (1961), 'Studies on the Folic Acid Activity of Human Serum', *J. clin. Path.*, **14**, 335.

Formiminoglutamic Acid (FIGLU) Excretion
KOHN, J., MOLLIN, D. L., and ROSENBACH, L. M. (1961), 'Conventional Voltage Electrophoresis for Formiminoglutamic Acid Determination in Folic Acid Deficiency', *Ibid.*, **14**, 345.

Pancreatic Function

Lundh Test
LUNDH, G. (1962), 'Pancreatic Function in Neoplastic and Inflammatory Diseases: A Simple and Reliable New Test', *Gastroenterology*, **42**, 275.

Secretin–Pancreozymin Test
BURTON, P., EVANS, D. G., HARPER, A. A., HOWAT, H. T., OLEESKY, S., SCOTT, J. E., and VARLEY, H. (1960), 'A Test of Pancreatic Function in Man based on the Analysis of Duodenal Contents after Administration of Secretin and Pancreozymin', *Gut*, **1**, 111.
— — HAMMOND, E. M., HARPER, A. A., HOWAT, H. T., SCOTT, J. E., and VARLEY, H. (1960), 'Serum Amylase and Serum Lipase Levels in Man after Administration of Secretin and Pancreozymin', *Ibid.*, **1**, 125.

Secretin Test
DREILING, D. A. (1971), 'Investigation of Pancreatic Function', in *The Exocrine Pancreas* (ed. BECK, I. T., and SINCLAIR, D. G.), p. 154. London: Churchill Livingstone.

Faecal Trypsin
MCGOWAN, G. K., and WILLS, M. R. (1962), 'The Diagnostic Value of Faecal Trypsin Estimation in Chronic Pancreatic Disease', *J. clin. Path.*, **15**, 62.

Intestinal Bleeding
CAMERON, A. D. (1960), 'Gastrointestinal Blood Loss measured by Radioactive Chromium', *Gut*, **1**, 177.
HAYNES, W. F., PITTMAN, F. E., and CHRISTAKIS, G. (1960), 'Location of Site of Upper Gastrointestinal Tract Haemorrhage by the Fluorescein String Test', *Surgery*, **48**, 821.
STEINGOLD, L., and ROBERTS, A. A. (1961), 'Laboratory Diagnosis of Gastro-intestinal Bleeding', *Gut*, **2**, 75.

Alimentary Protein Loss
JEEJEEBHOY, K. N., and COGHILL, N. F. (1961), 'The Measurement of Gastrointestinal Protein Loss by a New Method', *Ibid.*, **2**, 123.
GORDON, R. S. (1959), 'Gastrointestinal Protein Loss in Idiopathic (Hypercatabolic) Hypoproteinemia', *Lancet*, **1**, 327.

Mobility of the Alimentary Tract
CHAUDHARY, N. A., and TRUELOVE, S. C. (1961), 'Human Colonic Motility. A Comparative Study of Normal Subjects, Patients with Ulcerative Colitis, and Patients with Irritable Colon Syndrome', *Gastroenterology*, **40**, 1.
CONNELL, A. M. (1961), 'The Motility of the Pelvic Colon', *Gut*, **2**, 175.

Fibre-optic Endoscopy
CLASSEN, M. (1971), 'Fibre-endoscopy of the Intestines', *Ibid*, **12**, 330.

Index